ADVANCES IN

Pediatrics

Editor-in-Chief
Michael S. Kappy, MD, PhD

Professor, Department of Pediatrics,
University of Colorado Health Sciences Center,
The Children's Hospital, Denver, Colorado

ELSEVIER

PHILADELPHIA   LONDON   TORONTO   MONTREAL   SYDNEY   TOKYO

ADVANCES IN

Pediatrics

Editor-in-Chief
Michael S. Kappy, MD, PhD

MOSBY

ADVANCES IN
Pediatrics

VOLUMES 1 THROUGH 53 (OUT OF PRINT)

Vice President, Continuity Publishing: John A. Schrefer
Editor: Carla Holloway

Printed and bound in the United Kingdom
Transferred to Digital Print 2011

Editorial Office:
Elsevier
1600 John F. Kennedy Blvd,
Suite 1800
Philadelphia, PA 19103-2899

International Standard Serial Number: 0065-3101
International Standard Book Number: 13: 978-1-4160-5753-6
International Standard Book Number: 10: 1-4160-5753-6

ADVANCES IN
Pediatrics

Editor-in-Chief

MICHAEL S. KAPPY, MD, PhD, Professor, Department of Pediatrics, University
of Colorado Health Sciences Center, The Children's Hospital, Denver, Colorado

Associate Editors

LEWIS A. BARNESS, MD, DSci(hc), DPH(hc), Distinguished University Professor
Emeritus, Department of Pediatrics, University of South Florida College
of Medicine, Tampa, Florida

LESLIE L. BARTON, MD, Professor, Department of Pediatrics, Steele Memorial
Children's Research Center, University of Arizona, Tucson, Arizona

ENID GILBERT-BARNESS, AO, MD, MBBS, FRCPA, FRCPath, DSci(hc), MD(hc),
Professor, Departments of Pathology and Cell Biology, Pediatrics,
and Obstetrics and Gynecology, University of South Florida College
of Medicine, Tampa General Hospital, Tampa, Florida

MORITZ ZIEGLER, MD, Chief, Pediatric Surgery, The Children's Hospital, Denver,
Colorado

Editor-in-Chief

Associate Editors

ADVANCES IN
Pediatrics

CONTRIBUTORS

LISA ADCOCK, MD, Assistant Professor of Pediatrics, Neonatology Section, Pediatrics, Baylor College of Medicine, Houston, Texas

MARNI E. AXELRAD, PhD, Assistant Professor, Section of Psychology, Pediatrics, Baylor College of Medicine; and Psychology Service, Texas Children's Hospital, Houston, Texas

LESLIE AYENSU COKER, MD, Clinical Fellow, Pediatric and Adolescent Gynecology, Department of Obstetrics and Gynecology, Baylor College of Medicine, Texas Children's Hospital, Houston, Texas

CYNTHIA J. BARTOK, PhD, Assistant Professor of Kinesiology, Penn State College of Health and Human Development, University Park, Pennsylvania

JONATHAN S. BERG, MD, Assistant Professor, Department of Molecular and Human Genetics, Baylor College of Medicine, Texas Children's Hospital, Houston, Texas

CAROL D. BERKOWITZ, MD, Executive Vice-Chair and Professor of Clinical Pediatrics, Department of Pediatrics, Harbor-UCLA Medical Center, David Geffen School of Medicine at the University of California Los Angeles, Torrance, California

LEANN L. BIRCH, PhD, Distinguished Professor of Human Development, Penn State College of Health and Human Development, University Park, Pennsylvania

DANIEL J. BONTHIUS, MD, PhD, Professor of Pediatrics and Neurology, Department of Pediatrics, University of Iowa Hospital, Iowa City, Iowa

DONALD C. BROSS, JD, PhD, Professor in Pediatrics (Family Law); Director of Education; and Legal Counsel, Kempe Center for the Prevention and Treatment of Child Abuse and Neglect, University of Colorado School of Medicine, Aurora, Colorado

WEERASAK CHONCHAIYA, MD, Medical Investigation of Neurodevelopmental Disorders Institute, University of California-Davis Medical Center, Sacramento, California; Department of Pediatrics, Chulalongkorn University, Bangkok, Thailand

JULIE COY, MS, RN, CPNP, Instructor-APN, Department of Anesthesia, University of Colorado Denver; and The Children's Hospital, Acute Pain Service, Aurora, Colorado

HEATHER R. DAVIDS, MD, University of Colorado Denver, Aurora, Colorado

JENNIFER DIETRICH, MD, MSc, FACOG, Assistant Professor, Obstetrics and
Gynecology, Pediatric and Adolescent Gynecology, Department of Obstetrics and
Gynecology, Baylor College of Medicine, Texas Children's Hospital, Houston,
Texas

DANIELLE S. DOWNS, PhD, Associate Professor of Kinesiology, Penn State College of
Health and Human Development, University Park, Pennsylvania

BENARD P. DREYER, MD, Professor of Pediatrics, Department of Pediatrics, New York
University School of Medicine and Bellevue Hospital Center, New York, New
York

BURRIS DUNCAN, MD, Professor of Pediatrics and Public Health, Department of
Pediatrics and Public Health, Arizona Health Sciences Center, Mel and Enid
Zuckerman College of Public Health, Tucson, Arizona

RENATA FABIA, MD, PhD, Clinical Assistant Professor of Surgery, The Ohio State
University Collge of Medicine; and Associate Burn Director, Nationwide
Children's Hospital, Columbus, Ohio

GUIDO FILLER, MD, PhD, FRCPC, Professor and Chair, Department of Paediatrics,
Children's Hospital at London Health Sciences Centre, University of Western
Ontario, London, Ontario, Canada

SHANNON L. FRENCH, MD, Assistant Professor, Pediatrics-Endocrinology and
Metabolism, Baylor College of Medicine, Houston, Texas

NEIL FRIEDMAN, MBChB, Staff Physician, Center for Pediatric Neurology,
Neurological Institute, Cleveland Clinic, Cleveland, Ohio

ANITA DUHL GLICKEN, MSW, Professor and Section Head, Pediatrics; and Program
Director, Child Health Associate/Physician Assistant Program, University of
Colorado, Aurora, Colorado

EDWARD GOLDSON, MD, Professor, Department of Pediatrics, University of
Colorado Health Sciences Center, Denver, Colorado

RONALD GOTLIN, MD, Professor Emeritus, University of Colorado School of
Medicine, Aurora, Colorado

RONALD T. GRONDIN, MD, FRCSC, Assistant Professor, Department of
Neurosurgery, Nationwide Children's Hospital, The Ohio State University,
Columbus, Ohio

JONATHAN I. GRONER, MD, Professor of Clinical Surgery, Pediatric Surgery, The
Ohio State University College of Medicine; and Nationwide Children's Hospital,
Columbus, Ohio

SHEILA GUNN, MD, Assistant Professor, Pediatrics-Endocrinology and Metabolism, Baylor College of Medicine, Houston, Texas

RANDI J. HAGERMAN, MD, Medical Director and Endowed Chair in Fragile X Research, Medical Investigation of Neurodevelopmental Disorders Institute, University of California-Davis Medical Center; and Department of Pediatrics, University of California-Davis Health System, Sacramento, California

KAM-LUN HON, MD(CUHK), FAAP, FCCM, Professor of Paediatrics, Department of Paediatrics, Prince of Wales Hospital, The Chinese University of Hong Kong, Shatin, Hong Kong

LEFKOTHEA P. KARAVITI, MD, PhD, Professor, Pediatrics-Endocrinology and Metabolism, Baylor College of Medicine, Houston, Texas

RUTH KEMPE, MD, Professor Emerita, Departments of Pediatrics and Psychiatry, University of Colorado School of Medicine, Aurora, Colorado

PERRI KLASS, MD, Professor of Pediatrics, Department of Pediatrics, New York University School of Medicine and Bellevue Hospital Center, New York, New York

RICHARD D. KRUGMAN, MD, Vice Chancellor for Health Affairs and Dean, School of Medicine, University of Colorado, Aurora, Colorado

NATHALIE LEPAGE, PhD, Associate Professor, Department of Pathology and Laboratory Medicine, Children's Hospital of Eastern Ontario, Ottawa, Ontario, Canada

ALEXANDER K.C. LEUNG, MBBS, FRCPC, FRCP(UK&Irel), FRCPCH, FAAP, Department of Pediatrics, The Alberta Children's Hospital, University of Calgary, Calgary, Alberta, Canada

B. LEE LIGON, PhD, Instructor, Department of Pediatrics, Baylor College of Medicine, Houston, Texas

MARIA J. MANDT, MD, Assistant Professor, University of Colorado School of Medicine, The Children's Hospital, Aurora, Colorado

LAWRENCE B. McCULLOUGH, PhD, Dalton Tomlin Chair in Medical Ethics; Health Policy Professor of Medicine; and Medical Ethics Associate Director, Education Center for Medical Ethics and Health Policy, Baylor College of Medicine, Houston, Texas

ANNE MARIE McKENNA, MD, BSc, Schulich School of Medicine and Dentistry, University of Western Ontario, London, Ontario, Canada

ALAN L. MENDELSOHN, MD, Associate Professor of Pediatrics, Department of Pediatrics, New York University School of Medicine and Bellevue Hospital Center, New York, New York

AYESHA MIRZA, MD, Department of Pediatrics, University of Florida, Pediatric Infectious Diseases and Immunology, Jacksonville, Florida

ED NIEUWENHUYS, BSc, Sanquin-Research Academic Medical Center, Landsteiner Laboratory, Amesterdam, The Netherlands

IAN M. PAUL, MD, MSc, Associate Professor of Pediatrics and Public Health Sciences, Penn State College of Medicine, Department of Pediatrics, Hershey, Pennsylvania

LARA D. RAPPAPORT, MD, MPH, Assistant Professor, University of Colorado School of Medicine, The Children's Hospital, Aurora, Colorado

MOBEEN H. RATHORE, MD, CPE, FAAP, FIDSA, FACPE, Department of Pediatrics, University of Florida, Pediatric Infectious Diseases and Immunology; and Wolfson Children's Hospital, Jacksonville, Florida

ANDREA SCHNEIDER, PhD, Medical Investigation of Neurodevelopmental Disorders Institute, University of California-Davis Medical Center; and Department of Psychiatry and Behavioral Sciences, University of California-Davis Health System, Sacramento, California

R. MICHAEL SCOTT, MD, Professor, Department of Neurosurgery, Children's Hospital Boston, Harvard Medical School, Boston, Massachusetts

AJAY P. SHARMA, MD, Associate Professor, Department of Paediatrics, Children's Hospital at London Health Sciences Centre, University of Western Ontario, London, Ontario, Canada

ANDY SILVER, MD, Denver, Colorado

EDWARD R. SMITH, MD, Assistant Professor, Department of Neurosurgery, Children's Hospital Boston, Harvard Medical School, Boston, Massachusetts

ROBIN SLOVER, MD, Director, The Children's Hospital Chronic Pain Clinic; and Associate Professor, University of Colorado Denver, Interventional Pain Management Pain Medicine Clinic, Aurora, Colorado

DIANE M. STRAUB, MD, MPH, Associate Professor of Pediatrics and Chief, Division of Adolescent Medicine, University of South Florida, Tampa, Florida

CYNTHIA A. STIFTER, PhD, Professor of Human Development and Psychology, Penn State College of Health and Human Development, University Park, Pennsylvania

V. REID SUTTON, MD, Associate Professor, Department of Molecular and Human Genetics, Baylor College of Medicine, Houston, Texas

ALISON K. VENTURA, PhD, Postdoctoral Fellow, Monell Chemical Sciences Center, Philadelphia, Pennsylvania

ADVANCES IN
Pediatrics

CONTENTS   VOLUME 56 • 2009

Immunization Update II
By Ayesha Mirza and Mobeen H. Rathore

Severe Childhood Respiratory Viral Infections
By Kam-Lun Hon and Alexander K.C. Leung

Lymphocytic Choriomeningitis Virus: A Prenatal and Postnatal Threat
By Daniel J. Bonthius

Sexually Transmitted Diseases in Adolescents
By Diane M. Straub

Opportunities for the Primary Prevention of Obesity during Infancy
By Ian M. Paul, Cynthia J. Bartok, Danielle S. Downs, Cynthia A. Stifter, Alison K. Ventura, and Leann L. Birch

Relationships Among Serum Iron, Inflammation, and Body Mass Index in Children
By Ajay P. Sharma, Ann Marie McKenna, Nathalie Lepage, Ed Nieuwenhuys, and Guido Filler

The Gender Medicine Team: "It Takes a Village"
By Marni E. Axelrad, Jonathan S. Berg, Leslie Ayensu Coker, Jennifer Dietrich, Lisa Adcock, Shannon L. French, Sheila Gunn, B. Lee Ligon, Laurence B. McCullough, V. Reid Sutton, and Lefkothea P. Karaviti

Fragile X: A Family of Disorders
By Weerasak Chonchaiya, Andrea Schneider, and Randi J. Hagerman

Pediatric Brain Tumors

By Ronald T. Grondin, R. Michael Scott, and Edward R. Smith

Pediatric Stroke: Past, Present and Future

By Neil Friedman

Global Child Health: Promises Made to Children—Not Yet Kept

By Burris Duncan

Advances in the Management of Pain in Children: Acute Pain

By Robin Slover, Julie Coy, and Heather R. Davids

Update in Pediatric Resuscitation
By Maria J. Mandt and Lara D. Rappaport

Advances in Pediatrics 56 (2009) xxi–xxii

ADVANCES IN PEDIATRICS

Introduction

Michael S. Kappy, MD, PhD, FAAP

We are pleased to present Volume 56 to you. We continue with the honoring of individuals who have made significant contributions to pediatrics with our "Foundations of Pediatrics" section. In this volume, we honor Dr. Henry K. Silver, an individual who made far-reaching contributions in several areas. Thus, there is the need for several authors, each with a unique view of Henry's life, starting with his son, Andrew Silver, MD.

We are instituting a new feature, "International Health" issues, with this volume (see the article by Duncan) and will include articles in this area in future volumes. We believe this to be particularly relevant in view of the global health care problems faced by children, and also the risk of the spread of a variety of infectious diseases due to the increased mobility of populations in general.

The Reach Out and Read program (see the article by Klass and colleagues) has made significant improvements in children's literacy, and is focused in primary care settings, making it an ideal program for the pediatrician's office. Contact information is given at the end of the "milestone" chart for those pediatricians who would like to add this program to their office activities.

Our biannual update on immunizations is presented by Rathore and Mizra, and specific conclusions regarding the lack of association of autism with immunizations are given in the article "Autism: An Update" by Goldson. Three additional articles in the infectious disease field are by Hon and Leung ("Severe Childhood Respiratory Viral Infections", which includes information in H1N1), Bonthius ("Lymphocytic Choriomeningitis Virus"), and Straub ("Sexually Transmitted Diseases in Adolescents").

The critical issue of early prevention of obesity is addressed by Paul, and is particularly relevant in our current obesity "epidemic" or "endemic" climate, with the metabolic syndrome and type 2 diabetes as potential resultant morbidities, also addressed by Sharma and colleagues. A novel team approach to the diagnosis and care of children with disorders of sexual development is presented by Axelrad and colleagues at Texas Children's Hospital, and Hagerman provides a recent update on Fragile X.

Dr. Berkowitz provides guidelines to the primary care physician for the support of children who have been subject to "pornographic abuse."

Surgical topics are presented by Fabia and Groner ("Advances in the Care of Children with Burns"), and Grondin and Scott give an update on the

0065-3101/09/$ – see front matter
doi:10.1016/j.yapd.2009.08.018

evaluation of brain tumors in children. Other articles include "Pediatric Stroke: Past, Present and Future" by Friedman, "Update in Pediatric Resuscitation" by Mandt and Rappaport, and part one of a two-part presentation by Slover and colleagues, "Advances in the Management of Pain in Children: Acute Pain." Part two (chronic pain) will be included in our next volume (57).

As always, the editors welcome suggestions for future topics to be included in *Advances in Pediatrics*.

Michael S. Kappy, MD, PhD, FAAP
University of Colorado Health Sciences Center
The Children's Hospital
13123 East 16th Avenue, B-265
Aurora, CO 80045, USA
E-mail address: kappy.michael@tchden.org

Advances in Pediatrics 56 (2009) 1–9

ADVANCES IN PEDIATRICS

Foundations of Pediatrics:
Henry K. Silver, MD (1918–1991)

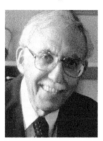

Henry K. Silver, MD

Andy Silver, MD, Ronald Gotlin, MD, Ruth Kempe, MD[†],
Donald C. Bross, JD, PhD, Richard D. Krugman, MD,
Anita Duhl Glicken, MSW*

[†] *Ruth Svibergson Kempe, M.D., Emerita Professor of Psychiatry and Pediatrics at the University of Colorado School of Medicine passed away Friday, July 24, 2009 at the age of 87. Her professional life was devoted to practice in child psychiatry and, in partnership with her husband, C. Henry Kempe, MD, to the prevention and treatment of child abuse. Ruth was one of only two women in her class at the Yale School of Medicine in the 1940's. Her publications included Child Abuse, part of Brunner's Developing Child Series and a best-seller in the United Kingdom, and the last two editions of The Battered Child, for which she was a lead Editor as well as a chapter contributor. She was a wonderful mother and grandmother and is survived by her five daughters, Karin, Annie, Miriam, Allison and Jenny, and sixteen grandchildren.*

Vision, passion, loyalty, and wisdom are all words often used to describe Henry K. Silver. The following stories and anecdotes, collected from some of Henry's colleagues, friends, and family, paint a picture of a man steadfastly committed to improving the lives of children and families; a man whose vision and tenacity gave birth to an enduring legacy. His many contributions to pediatric endocrinology, the diagnosis and treatment of child abuse and neglect, as well as his efforts to change

*Corresponding author. E-mail address: anita.glicken@ucdenver.edu (A. Duhl Glicken).

0065-3101/09/$ – see front matter
doi:10.1016/j.yapd.2009.08.004

the culture of medical education would have been sufficient to rank him among the world's most influential pediatricians. However, these pale in comparison to his significant contributions to the health care workforce through the creation of innovative education programs for nonphysician providers at the University of Colorado School of Medicine. These programs, specifically designed to address provider shortages, would change the face of the medical workforce both in the United States and abroad. Henry, a true futurist, would likely not have been surprised to learn that 40 years later, over 200,000 nurse practitioners and physician assistants have entered the workforce, primary contributors to a health care system that continues to struggle in the face of unmet needs.

HENRY SILVER—THE MAN
BY ANDY SILVER, MD

My father, Henry K. Silver, MD, was born in Philadelphia on April 22, 1918. Several years later his family moved to Los Angeles, where his parents ran a small, open-air grocery store, and where he later graduated from Fairfax High School. He went to the University of California, Los Angeles for undergraduate work and received his MD in 1942 from the University of California, San Francisco (UCSF). Dr. Silver did his internship at the University Hospital in San Francisco and then went to the Children's Hospital of Philadelphia for residency. He returned to UCSF from 1944 to 1952 as a research assistant, Instructor, and Assistant Professor in Pediatrics. It was during this time he met C. Henry Kempe, MD, and for the next 40 years, formed a mutual bond of friendship, respect, admiration, and understanding. They would later be known at the University of Colorado as the "two Henrys." Many of Henry Silver's first papers were co-authored by Dr. Kempe. From 1952 to 1957, Dr Silver was an Associate Professor of Pediatrics at Yale University School of Medicine. In 1953, he published his first significant paper in pediatrics [1], describing congenital asymmetry, short stature, and variations in sexual development, known as the "Silver-Russell Syndrome."

In 1957 Henry Kempe, now Chairman of the Department of Pediatrics at the University of Colorado School of Medicine, asked Henry Silver to join him in Denver. My father did and remained there until his death in 1991. During this time he was Professor of Pediatrics, Vice-Chairman of the Department of Pediatrics, Director of the Child Health Associate Program (CHAP) (1969–1991), and Associate Dean of Admissions for the School of Medicine (1977–1991). Henry Silver was devoted to the University of Colorado, loved the climate of Denver, and greatly enjoyed the yearly pediatric summer symposiums held in the Rocky Mountains, initially in Estes Park and later in Aspen. He had a deep respect for the people of Colorado, whose progressive thinking would enable him to forge ahead with many of his innovative projects.

The early years in Colorado focused on child abuse and pediatric endocrinology. The first paper on abuse was "Problem of parental criminal neglect and severe physical abuse of children," published in 1959 [2]. This was followed by the landmark article "The battered child syndrome" in the *Journal of the American Medical Association* in 1962 [3], recently reviewed as a JAMA Classic in 2008. Also during this time, Henry Silver established the first academic department of pediatric endocrinology, with emphasis on growth and pubertal problems in children.

The second phase of Henry Silver's career would mark his legacy. In the early 1960s he realized that many children were not receiving adequate medical care. He developed 3 programs to help address this need: in 1967, the Pediatric Nurse Practitioner Program [4], in 1968, the CHAP [5], and in 1970, the School Nurse Practitioner Program [6]. Dr. Silver and the University of Colorado soon became recognized nationally and internationally as leaders in the allied health care field. In 1966, my father was invited to attend the signing of the Allied Health Professions Personnel Training Act by President Johnson at the White House. In 1990, he received the Gustav Lienhard Medal for the Advancement of Health Care from the Institute of Medicine of the National Academy of Sciences.

My father's final major focus was as Associate Dean of Admissions for the medical school in Denver. Under his leadership, there was a shift toward more women and minority applicant admissions; more applicants majoring in nonbiology fields were being considered; and the previously "rarely discussed" problem of medical student abuse was brought to light [7].

Henry K. Silver was a remarkable and brilliant innovator, advocate, teacher, mentor, and friend. In addition to his professional "creations" previously described, in his private life he created his own brand of art, combining fabrics and wood pieces in framed pictures. There was the perpetual scribbling of notes during the middle of the night. Was it that he was always thinking of ways to improve things and never slept, or was he trying to turn his dreams into reality? Personally, I think it was the latter.

My father was the ultimate advocate for those most in need. He always strove to help improve the lives of children, be they undergrown, maltreated, or undertreated. He was a champion for the "underqualified," be they "less than perfect" nurse practitioner/child health associate/medical school applicants, or "just not quite there" junior faculty. Many of the programs or individuals my father advocated for were often controversial, but I must admit, as he would, that he loved a good intellectual fight. An example of this was during the period that the child health associates were being considered for acceptance/licensure in the state of Colorado. The major challenges did not come from the legislatures, but from fellow pediatricians and some in the nursing profession. Physicians did not want "assistants," and nurses did not want "extenders." With tenacity, and some luck, Henry Silver won over these early skeptics.

One of Dr. Silver's favorite passions was teaching. His sessions with the house staff at the old Fitzsimons Medical Center were known as "Silver Pearls." Early CHAP classes were small and held in his office, where no one escaped from participating. He was always challenging the students, as he did all of us, to expand our way of thinking. Finally, along with Dr. Kempe, Dr. Silver was the editor of *Handbook of Pediatrics* and *Current Pediatric Diagnosis and Treatment* for many years.

My father was a mentor to many fellow peers and junior faculty, particularly when it came time to writing papers for publication in various medical and nursing journals. The rewrite after rewrite drove many individuals crazy, but in the end their paper would inevitably be accepted. In his latter years, he spent many hours with applicants who had failed to get into medical school, the "life coach" of today.

Finally, Henry K. Silver, MD was a friend to countless physician and nursing colleagues, and to nurse practitioners, CHAP, and medical students. He spearheaded the nomination of Henry Kempe for the Nobel Peace Prize in 1984, and described his deeply cherished friend as "the best of what a human being ought to be." Always supportive and nonjudgmental, I am proud that Henry Silver was not only my father, but my best friend as well.

HENRY SILVER—THE ENDOCRINOLOGIST
BY RONALD GOTLIN, MD

My first memory of Dr. Henry Silver is from 1962. I was a third-year medical student early in my first clinical year. He was the featured lecturer in a required afternoon lecture series. I still remember that the subject was coagulation in a problem-solving format. Dr. Silver was a pediatrician and pediatric endocrinologist, but was also well versed in hematology and infectious diseases. His contributions to academic pediatrics and health care were many, and he published over 120 articles in various pediatric fields. His clinical work in endocrinology produced many publications, but perhaps 3 were most memorable. His initial description in 1953 of a syndrome characterized by hemihypertrophy, short stature, and gonadal insufficiency (elevated urinary gonadotropins) [1] is now well recognized as Silver or Silver-Russell syndrome. Later, in 1958, he was one of the first to associate long-standing primary hypothyroidism with precocious puberty [8], and during his activism in child abuse recognition in the 1960s, he identified a specific syndrome of growth retardation and behavioral abnormalities in emotionally deprived children, "deprivational dwarfism" or psychosocial short stature [9].

More memorable was Dr. Silver himself. He was tall, slim, well groomed, and he wore the traditional long white coat. Beneath the coat he wore a white shirt, dark thin tie, black trousers, and black military oxford shoes (more about the oxfords later). His stethoscope was neatly contained in a waist pocket. There was no need for the symbolic round-the-neck ornament. He was easily identified as a doctor and a professor.

Dr. Silver's delivery was calm and his manner very engaging. He always seemed to have a reassuring, ever so slight smile. This composure remained a constant whether he was lecturing, seeing patients, or stressing a viewpoint in a large faculty discourse. His countenance gave the impression that he was ready to accept contrasting viewpoints, but this was not necessarily the case.

His conclusions were reached after considerable thought and once he had reached a conclusion or viewpoint, he was prepared to defend it.

One of the most memorable training highlights was Dr. Silver's "Silver Nuggets." These were small group problem-solving sessions in which he would present general pediatric cases and the trainees would attempt to solve the problem. To this day, former pediatric trainees remember these cases, particularly the infant who had not passed a stool for 1, 2, 3 or more days.

With the exception of 2 years when I was on active duty in the navy, Dr. Silver and I saw patients with endocrine disorders together from 1965 through the 1970s. Beginning in the early 1970s, he became more involved in the development of training programs for pediatric caregivers in nonresidency traditional programs. The Nurse Practitioner Program was first, but was soon followed by the CHAP. Both programs continue to this day (see later discussion).

I also learned early in my experience with Dr. Silver that he was troubled by moderate (at times severe) problems with his back, which required a specific chair in clinics and was aided by the military oxfords mentioned earlier. He indicated that these were the only shoes that afforded him some comfort with his back, and indicated that he lived in some degree of continuous pain. He did so always without complaint or significant change in his composure or interaction with others. Moreover, pain did not dampen his sense of humor or change his love of wit. For example, Dr. Silver always attended medical school graduation in cap and gown. His cap and gown were rented, and when asked at a faculty lunch why he had not already purchased the regalia, he replied that he already had too much invested in rentals. These light moments came through daily, and I found him to be a delight to know and with whom to work.

While there are other memories, I believe those mentioned here provide a clear picture of one of our pediatric masters. Those of us who had the opportunity to know him were indeed fortunate. I have purposely avoided excessive use of superlatives or mawkish embellishments. However, it should be clear that in Dr. Silver we saw an exceptional human being. He hoped for and worked for a better mankind, society, and planet his entire life. Were it not for his untimely death, his work in seeking better models of teaching, patient care for children, and the human race in general would have continued indefinitely and continues through the efforts of others today.

HENRY SILVER—THE ADVOCATE AGAINST CHILD ABUSE
BY RUTH KEMPE, MD, AND DONALD C. BROSS, JD, PhD

Henry Silver and C. Henry Kempe probably met when Henry Kempe was a medical student on the pediatric service and Henry Silver was a pediatric resident at UCSF.

Their personal friendship and collaboration was important to both men because it was totally supportive and noncompetitive. Despite their different personalities and somewhat different professional interests, they shared many cultural and ethical values. Both also kept a deep interest in medical education. They shared not only ideas but helped one another in practical ways, such as the work required to communicate to legislators and to lobby for much-needed legislation, whether it be for child protection or provision of medical manpower.

Concerned about the large number of injured children they were seeing on the 4 pediatric wards in Denver, they were distressed by unwillingness on the part of doctors to believe abuse could happen. The Two Henrys wrote a paper that was printed in 1959 in abstract only, entitled "The problem of parental criminal neglect and severe physical abuse of children" [2]. The article presented a "review of several incidents of criminal neglect and severe physical assault on more than one sibling in a family," and discussed the need for pediatricians to become aware of the problem so they could make a firm diagnosis and provide protection for children.

From the Department of Psychiatry, Dr. Brandt Steele was persuaded to see one of the parents of an abused infant, and became very much interested in her history. That marked the beginning of his major contributions to the understanding of the difficulties in caregiving which led to abuse and neglect—and added another member to the "team" that proved so necessary. In 1962, the "Battered child syndrome" [3], authored by Kempe, Silverman, Steele, Droegmueller, and Silver, was published in JAMA. This was a true multidisciplinary discussion of the problem of child abuse, with descriptions of the clinical findings, the convincing radiographic evidence to document the injuries, and the history of psychiatric evaluations of the parents. It also described the development of the diagnosis, and of a treatment and management plan for this condition.

As time went on, Dr. Silver went on to focus on other problems in pediatrics, and mainly to develop his interest in alternative medical care providers. This did not mean that his concern about child abuse and neglect had ended, and as an example, he published an early paper on deprivation dwarfism in 1967 [9].

Dr. Silver's long involvement with the recruitment and training of young physicians led him to question whether some aspects of medical education might be abusive and detrimental to the development of future physicians, and in 1984 he and Dr. Donna Rosenberg published their classic paper entitled "Medical student abuse: an unnecessary and preventable cause of stress" [7].

Whereas the development of pediatric physician assistants and nurse practitioners in pediatric care is addressed elsewhere, Henry Silver's 1967 article [4] on these developments coincided with C. Henry Kempe's early efforts to use health visitors to prevent child abuse.

In a 1984 letter to his old friend, Henry Silver, thanking him for his part in nominating him for the Nobel Peace Prize, Dr. Kempe said:

> You did accomplish, and are still doing so much, that only now the full implications of what you have begun in health care is being felt—and it has revolutionized child care at all levels, by many professionals.

HENRY SILVER—INNOVATOR IN ALLIED HEALTH AND MEDICAL SCHOOL EDUCATION
BY RICHARD D. KRUGMAN, MD,
AND ANITA DUHL GLICKEN, MSW

Following his outstanding career in pediatric endocrinology, Henry's primary interest in pediatrics turned to health care delivery and the delivery of primary care services to children. He was interested in medical education, which he thought was unfocused, not competency based, wasted a lot of time, and was not geared to preparing physicians for what they were eventually going to do in practice. During the period 1964 to 1981 he pursued approaches to changing both how health professional education and the provision of primary care services to children and adults would be organized and delivered.

During this time, Henry and his colleagues searched for additional solutions to address health care disparities and a predicted shortfall in the pediatric workforce. In 1965, a revolution, generally unrecognized at the time, occurred in the Unites States health care system when Henry and Loretta Ford launched an experiment to see whether it was possible to give pediatric nurses enough additional training and skills to be able to assist in the provision of primary care for children. Henry assumed that if he took someone who had basic nursing training and 5 years of experience as a pediatric nurse in an ambulatory setting, and then provided 4 months of additional training in history taking and physical diagnosis, that the nurse could provide much of the ambulatory primary care services that children needed. These "pediatric nurse practitioners (PNPs)" were educated to answer 3 questions:

1. Is this child sick or well?
2. If the child is sick, is it a mild or self-limited illness?
3. Does a physician need to see this child now or later?

The program was a success [10]. PNPs were able to care for 90% of children who came to pediatric offices for health maintenance and minor acute illnesses, demonstrating that nonphysicians could provide many of the health care services previously assigned only to phsyicians. The nurses worked collaboratively with physicians, who reported that they had at least one-third more time than they formerly had for patient care and other activities. Although the program began in the Department of Pediatrics in the School of Medicine, the School of Nursing later took over the program, lengthened the training, and provided a Master's degree.

There are now about 120,000 practicing NPs in the United States, with 6000 new NPs prepared each year in over 325 educational programs. NPs continue to have education beyond their registered nurse preparation; but most now have Master's degrees and many have doctorates. In addition to the limited role that Silver envisioned, NPs now provide an expanded range of services including diagnosis and treatment of acute and chronic conditions, and cover almost 600 million patient visits each year. A subgroup of the profession still specialize in pediatric/child health, whereas others now specialize in acute care, adult health, family health, gerontology, neonatology, oncology, psychiatry, women's health, and many other variations on this original theme.

At the time, Henry also wondered what curriculum would be necessary to provide someone with no previous health care experience the competencies necessary to do much of the primary care in ambulatory settings as well as low-risk nursery. Thus in 1968, Henry created a second program designed to meet the workforce shortage, Henry's own version of a physician assistant. Unlike their NP colleagues, the child health associate (CHA) entered the program without prior training in medicine. The 3-year program represented a significant shift from traditional medical education in preparing nonphysicians to provide extensive primary care, including diagnosis and treatment of patients. Henry's intent was to train graduates in problem-solving and decision-making that would approach that of physicians and allow them to provide extensive health care to most patients. Within clearly defined limits they would make independent decisions, and assume responsibility and accountability for decisions and performance. The first class enrolled in 1969, the same year the Colorado general assembly, in partnership with the Colorado Board of Medical Examiners (BME), passed the Child Health Associate Act, which was the first in the United States to establish a framework for certification of an allied health profession, a nonphysician, to practice pediatrics [11]. Henry was instrumental in moving this act through the legislature; this groundbreaking legislative process became the precursor to many subsequent state practice acts. Overall, the training program prepared the graduate to care for 80% to 90% of patients seen in pediatric practice. Extensive evaluations of early graduates demonstrated that they provided high-quality, comprehensive primary care to infants, children, and adolescents including diagnostic, preventive, and therapeutic services. The graduates also provided extensive parent and patient education, counseling, and support. In 1973, under Henry's leadership, the program achieved another milestone; it was the first in the country to offer a Master of Science degree.

In 1981, Henry became Associate Dean for Admissions at the University of Colorado School of Medicine, and he held this post for 12 years until his death. He completely changed the face of the School's graduates by admitting large numbers of women, minorities, and middle-aged students who came to medical school after having had previous careers. He had no doubt about the motivation of individuals to be physicians if they left a well-paid job to come to medical school, whereas it was often not clear how to gauge the motivation of a 22-year-old student who was on the "pre-med track" from preschool on.

Henry also made an important observation while Associate Dean. He noticed that when the class sat at graduation 4 years later, they had changed. I (Glicken) remember him telling me one day: "I wonder what causes so many of our medical students to go from such happy, excited, altruistic young people in their first week to such cynical, flat, almost depressed men and women at their graduation? It reminds me of the children Henry Kempe and I saw in the early sixties. Do you think they are abused?" This led to his study published with Donna Rosenberg in 1984 [7] and then to his further studies published in 1990 [12]. Medical student abuse is now recognized as so prevalent that the Liaison Committee on Medical Education has issued standards to assure that Schools of Medicine recognize and address the issue.

Three months before Henry died in 1991, I (A.G.) sat in his office and reflected on the work ahead. There was still so much to be done. We planned to share an office and, in our "free time," envision new models of health care delivery and better ways to educate students. As in the case of countless others, I had already learned invaluable lessons from Henry about passion, tenacity, commitment, and hope, but I was particularly excited about the concept of using multidisciplinary/interprofessional teams to reintegrate an increasingly fragmented health care system, and to expand safety and access to patient care.

As we face another projected workforce shortage, Henry's spirit and wisdom continue to inspire and lead us to better solutions. I can think of few individuals in health care that have had the breadth and depth of influence of Henry K. Silver. The full implications of Henry's work have yet to be realized. As a mentor, colleague, friend, and father he is clearly missed, but his legacy continues through the programs he inspired and the work of countless generations of new health care providers.

References

[1] Silver HK, Kiyusu W, George J, et al. Syndrome of congenital hemihypertrophy, shortness of stature and elevated urinary gonadotropins (Silver syndrome). Pediatrics 1953;12: 368–76.

[2] Silver HK, Kempe CH. Problem of parental criminal neglect and severe physical abuse of children. Am J Dis Child 1959;95:528.

[3] Kempe CH, Silverman FN, Steele BF, et al. The battered child. J Am Med Assoc 1962;181: 19–24.

[4] Silver HK, Ford LC, Stearly SG. A program to increase health care for children: the pediatric nurse practitioner. Pediatrics 1967;39:756–60.

[5] Silver HK, Hecker JA. The pediatric nurse practitioner and the child health associate: new types of health professionals. J Med Educ 1970;45(3):171–6.

[6] Silver HK, Nelson N. The school nurse practitioner program: a new concept in providing health care. Medical Tribune 1970.

[7] Rosenberg DA, Silver HK. Medical student abuse: an unnecessary and preventable cause of stress. JAMA 1984;251:739–42.

[8] Silver HK. Juvenile hypothyroidism with precocious sexual development. J Clin Endocrinol Metab 1958;18:886–91.

[9] Silver HK, Finkelstein M. Deprivational dwarfism. J Pediatr 1967;70:317–24.

[10] Silver HK. Use of new types of allied health professionals in providing care for children. Am J Dis Child 1968;116:486–90.

[11] Jones AA, Krugman RD. The Child Health Associate Act: licensure of an allied health profession. Ethics Sci Med 1976;3:65–9.

[12] Silver HK, Glicken AD. Medical student abuse: incidence, severity and significance. J Amer Med Assoc 1990;263:527–32.

Advances in Pediatrics 56 (2009) 11–27

ELSEVIER
MOSBY

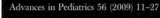

ADVANCES IN PEDIATRICS

Reach Out and Read: Literacy Promotion in Pediatric Primary Care

Perri Klass, MD*, Benard P. Dreyer, MD,
Alan L. Mendelsohn, MD

Department of Pediatrics, New York University School of Medicine and Bellevue Hospital Center,
550 First Avenue, New York, NY 10016, USA

Anyone who works with children, and especially with child development, balances the quantifiable and the ineffable. When one looks at social–emotional development, and specifically at infant attachment and parent–child interactions, one must take into account the carefully argued theories of mental and social development that define the history of developmental psychology, a vast literature of observation and experimentation, the variations described by cultural anthropologists, and the clashes of the nature–nurture debate. But it would be naïve to think that any of these intellectual endeavors fully captures what goes on between a parent and a child. To round out the picture, or gallery, one must include fiction, poetry, memoir, art, music, and all the complexities of emotion they evoke. Even if it does not have any clear place in scientific inquiry or evidence-based medicine, when one considers child development, one must make room for elements of spirit, serendipity, and occasionally magic.

This is also true when one thinks about how children learn, how children read, and how children learn to read. On one hand, the mechanics of teaching and learning the technical skills of reading can be studied and quantified and can engender passionate debate among different schools of educational thought. Yet, on the other hand, the relationships between children and books, both before and after literacy acquisition, can go far beyond quantification. What books can mean in a child's life—what a specific book can mean to a specific child—is not something that can be broken down into components easily, or understood by formula. The explanation of why that specific book means so much to that specific child defies analysis and quantification, as does the phenomenon of mass appeal. Just watch the publishing companies flail as they search for another Harry Potter.

Reach Out and Read (ROR) is an evidence-based national pediatric literacy program through which medical providers, as part of routine primary care for young children, are trained to offer parents anticipatory guidance about the

*Corresponding author. E-mail address: perri.klass@nyu.edu (P. Klass).

0065-3101/09/$ – see front matter
doi:10.1016/j.yapd.2009.08.009

importance of reading aloud. The program model focuses on children from 6 months to 5 years of age, and at each health supervision visit during that period, each child receives a new book to take home and keep. The book is chosen carefully to be developmentally appropriate. The family leaves the health supervision visit with the parents understanding the importance of reading aloud and primed with age-appropriate techniques to make it work (Fig. 1). This article reviews the history and development of the ROR program, the ROR model, and the recommended strategies for literacy promotion in the examination room, along with the evidence that the model is effective and the current structure that exists to support clinics that incorporate the model into daily practice. The article considers what books can mean in the lives of children, in both quantifiable and unquantifiable ways.

ROR is designed to promote books and reading aloud in the preschool years. The program's mission is to help children grow up with books and a love of reading. Although that mission does not mention the process of learning to read explicitly, one major goal of preschool literacy activities is to provide children with some of the cognitive skills they need for successfully learning to read once they get to school. Early exposure to books and reading aloud contributes to a child's readiness to read and learn at school entry, as does more general language exposure [1,2]. Successfully learning to read on time and on grade level is an essential key to overall school success [3]. Children who require remedial reading help in the first grade are statistically at increased risk to remain in remedial reading groups [4]. Children who go through school reading below grade level are at risk in their other subjects, especially once they get beyond the third grade, because school assignments and tests rely increasingly on printed texts and the fluency, efficiency, and accuracy with which the child can interpret, manipulate, and respond to text. To go from printed words to meaning is an essential part of the intellectual journey of

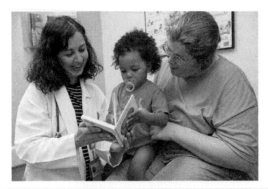

Fig. 1. The Reach Out and Read program is incorporated into routine primary care visits for young children. (*Courtesy of* the Reach Out and Read National Center.)

education, including early education. The child who struggles with the mechanics of decoding print is a child who may struggle with a whole range of aspects of school achievement and school function.

For children too young to read, picture books offer an attractive introduction to the mechanics of book handling and story structure (Fig. 2). They offer occasions for language exposure and language practice, both expressive and receptive, for naming and for dialogue and discussion as the child's verbal ability grows. "Dialogic reading" techniques, as elaborated by Whitehurst and the Stony Brook Reading Project [5], enhance the back-and-forth between adult reader and read-to child, which promotes pleasure and learning as the child becomes the teller of the story. Books and the routine of reading aloud also form links between child and parent/caretaker, because reading aloud to young children provides them with opportunities for close contact and concentrated parental attention. The stories and pictures that constitute the content of children's books can enrich and enlarge a young child's world with everything from animals (real, extinct, imaginary) to silly rhymes [6]. Books should serve young children as both mirrors and windows, reflecting back aspects of their own family's life and also offering a vision of the great wide world and all of its possibilities [7]. Given the current dominance of television and electronic media, reading aloud may be more important than ever. A growing body of evidence has documented the degree to which television exposure is associated with reduced reading, teaching and verbal interactions, reduced early learning, and reduced later achievement in school [8–11].

The authors will state their prejudice at the outset, that storybooks and picture books for young children teach their many, varied, valuable, and somewhat unpredictable lessons best when they are not explicitly educational. Children have an excellent eye for a message and a moral, and they seem to know immediately when a book has been concocted to improve them, rather than confected to engross and excite them. Real books, whether classics that have been calling out to children successfully for decades, or new flashes of mysterious picture book genius, cannot be replaced by carefully weighed and measured doses of approved vocabulary and character-building message. Anyone who has lived with a young child also knows that sometimes all the time-tested childhood classics, along with this year's expensively produced and stunning award-winning works of art, fade for an individual child compared with some particular inexplicable (and often highly tedious) work that becomes that particular child's particular obsession for some period of time. Parents of a 2-year old boy, for example, found it tedious to read *Bernie Drives a Truck* night after night, for some number of weeks (actually, it felt like months, if not years), but the boy was satisfied with nothing else. This must be considered a triumphant demonstration of the individuality and personality of the developing brain and the tenacity and determination of the 2-year-old will.

Books and stories and pictures enlarge a child's world and a child's vocabulary. Reading aloud to a young child fosters attachment to books and also

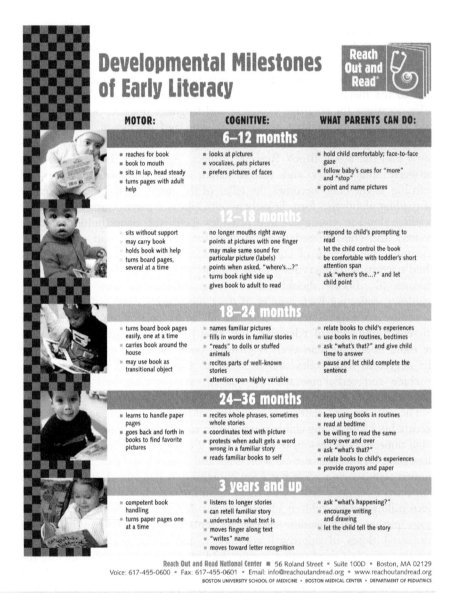

Developmental Milestones of Early Literacy

Reach Out and Read®

MOTOR:	COGNITIVE:	WHAT PARENTS CAN DO:
6–12 months		
▪ reaches for book ▪ book to mouth ▪ sits in lap, head steady ▪ turns pages with adult help	▪ looks at pictures ▪ vocalizes, pats pictures ▪ prefers pictures of faces	▪ hold child comfortably; face-to-face gaze ▪ follow baby's cues for "more" and "stop" ▪ point and name pictures
12–18 months		
▪ sits without support ▪ may carry book ▪ holds book with help ▪ turns board pages, several at a time	▪ no longer mouths right away ▪ points at pictures with one finger ▪ may make same sound for particular picture (labels) ▪ points when asked, "where's...?" ▪ turns book right side up ▪ gives book to adult to read	▪ respond to child's prompting to read ▪ let the child control the book ▪ be comfortable with toddler's short attention span ▪ ask "where's the...?" and let child point
18–24 months		
▪ turns board book pages easily, one at a time ▪ carries book around the house ▪ may use book as transitional object	▪ names familiar pictures ▪ fills in words in familiar stories ▪ "reads" to dolls or stuffed animals ▪ recites parts of well-known stories ▪ attention span highly variable	▪ relate books to child's experiences ▪ use books in routines, bedtimes ▪ ask "what's that?" and give child time to answer ▪ pause and let child complete the sentence
24–36 months		
▪ learns to handle paper pages ▪ goes back and forth in books to find favorite pictures	▪ recites whole phrases, sometimes whole stories ▪ coordinates text with picture ▪ protests when adult gets a word wrong in a familiar story ▪ reads familiar books to self	▪ keep using books in routines ▪ read at bedtime ▪ be willing to read the same story over and over ▪ ask "what's that?" ▪ relate books to child's experiences ▪ provide crayons and paper
3 years and up		
▪ competent book handling ▪ turns paper pages one at a time	▪ listens to longer stories ▪ can retell familiar story ▪ understands what text is ▪ moves finger along text ▪ "writes" name ▪ moves toward letter recognition	▪ ask "what's happening?" ▪ encourage writing and drawing ▪ let the child tell the story

Reach Out and Read National Center ▪ 56 Roland Street ▪ Suite 100D ▪ Boston, MA 02129
Voice: 617-455-0600 ▪ Fax: 617-455-0601 ▪ Email: info@reachoutandread.org ▪ www.reachoutandread.org
BOSTON UNIVERSITY SCHOOL OF MEDICINE ▪ BOSTON MEDICAL CENTER ▪ DEPARTMENT OF PEDIATRICS

Fig. 2. Developmental milestones of early literacy. (*Courtesy of* the Reach Out and Read National Center.)

promotes the language-rich attachment between parent and child. Part of the curriculum of ROR, included in the section describing techniques for literacy promotion in primary care, involves using books in the examination room to reinforce other important behavioral and developmental messages, including dialogic language with young children and building routines and rituals into toddlers' days. Books and literacy promotion in the examination room can offer providers avenues for anticipatory guidance and intervention that support families with young children on a level that is practical, pleasurable, and rewarding for the provider, parent, and child.

TWENTY YEARS, TWENTY MILLION BOOKS

ROR was born 20 years ago in Boston. The program was an intervention in the primary care clinic at what was then Boston City Hospital. Other pediatric clinics, especially those serving children growing up at risk and in poverty heard about ROR, and the group in Boston developed materials and a training curriculum to replicate ROR. The Reach Out and Read Manual was published with support from the Association of American Publishers and with an initial grant from the Annie E. Casey Foundation. Several additional teaching hospitals were given seed money to start programs. Over the course of the 1990s, the Reach Out and Read National Center, still based in Boston and affiliated with what is now Boston Medical Center, became a national nonprofit organization, assisting clinics, health centers, hospitals, and practices around the United States to develop ROR programs, train their medical providers and staff, choose and order appropriate books, and raise the money needed to buy books on a continuing basis. As the program reaches its 20th anniversary, there are over 4500 ROR sites operating in all 50 states, the District of Columbia, Guam, Puerto Rico, and the US Virgin Islands. Currently, the program reaches about 25% of the children in the United States who live in or near poverty. Most US sites are organized into more than 30 state and regional coalitions, which provide resources ranging from training to fundraising and advocacy. In addition, ROR programs operate in several foreign countries. The National Center collects reports from ROR sites twice a year and compiles information based on those data. As of this writing, ROR has trained 50,000 doctors and nurse-practitioners, and in this 2009 anniversary year, will present an estimated 5.4 million books to 3.3 million children in the United States. Since its inception, the program has distributed more than 20 million books to children [12].

In the recent revision of Bright Futures by the American Academy of Pediatrics, ROR is discussed as an evidence-based intervention, and reading milestones are incorporated into developmental assessment at pediatric visits [13]. The National Center has targeted residency programs and teaching hospitals as important sites for the ROR intervention because of opportunities to provide primary care to children at social and economic risk and change the culture of pediatric and family medicine practice by training doctors to incorporate books and literacy promotion into the delivery of primary care.

THE REACH OUT AND READ MODEL

The model was developed by busy primary care providers in health centers or clinic environments who consider the reality of primary care sites where the work of ROR is done, visit by visit. ROR offers opportunities to enhance the powerful relationship between parent and the primary care provider, who balances the many imperatives of the visit with attention to the patient's development and home environment. An important goal of ROR is to influence early attitudes and behaviors related to shared reading beginning in infancy and continuing into the preschool period. This period is critical both to child development and school readiness and to development of long-term patterns of parent–child interaction related to reading aloud [14].

The basic Reach Out and Read model has three components.

Literacy-rich waiting rooms

First, there is a waiting room intervention, which is scaled to the particular clinic, health center, or practice. The original ROR model took advantage of a big pediatric primary clinic waiting room full of children and deployed volunteer readers, who brought books to read to the waiting children. When this is possible, volunteer readers enhance the ROR intervention to a tremendous degree. They model techniques for reading aloud to parents who may perhaps not be familiar with the practice and show by example that the same books work with children of different ages, that the reader can put exaggerated expression into the reading voice, or use different voices for characters or animals. Volunteer readers make reading aloud a participatory adventure, with children calling out suggestions, answering questions, or jumping up to point to pictures on the page. And parents of very young children can experience the power of the reading aloud experience as they watch their child, wide-eyed and with rapt attention, listen to the reader and look at the pictures and words in the book. In addition, readers change the quality of the waiting room by changing the experience of waiting to be seen in the clinic. ROR sites report that children and parents, even after a "too-long" wait, do not want to leave the waiting room when they are called, because they want to hear the end of the story.

There are many ROR sites where consistent coverage by volunteer readers is not practical or realistic. Some sites do not have many children waiting regularly, while others do not have the facilities to recruit, screen, train, and supervise volunteers. Although sites are encouraged to consider volunteer readers, there are other waiting room interventions that support the message of ROR. The National Center has developed the concept of a literacy-rich waiting room that includes book displays and information on family literacy, libraries, and reading aloud. Some sites supply gently used books in the waiting room for children to read and take home. Others sites have success with videotapes of adults reading books aloud to cover times when there are no readers present. Some waiting rooms offer professional counselors who work with parents. Sites may invite a librarian into the waiting room to provide information on story hour and to issue library cards. These methods can be combined to meet the needs and the resources of each site. The literacy-rich waiting room introduces and reinforces the importance of reading and of having books in children's lives, making every clinic visit to some degree connected to books and reading.

Anticipatory guidance

The second major component is anticipatory guidance, which is at the heart of ROR's mission [15]. The primary care provider helps parents understand the importance of reading aloud to young children and offers parents age- and developmentally appropriate strategies for enjoying books with their children. Successful anticipatory guidance needs to be keyed to the child's developmental level, to the parent's skills and understanding, and to the family's situation. There are some general principles for ROR anticipatory guidance, however, that can help the intervention be maximally effective:

> Bring the book in early. Providers should come into the examination room with a book, or keep a selection available in the room. Children who are old enough should be offered at least a few books and invited to choose. By offering a book to the child early in the examination (before the otoscopy or immunization), providers can use the book, the child's reaction to the book, and the parent's reaction to the child's reaction as a way to assess development and discuss developmental stimulation [16]. The child's use of the book is an interactional and conversational tool that allows the provider to incorporate literacy into other aspects of anticipatory guidance offered during the visit.

> Give age-appropriate guidance about enjoying books with the child and about the child's ability to handle the book. Parents may need to be reassured that it is okay for 6-month-olds to put books in their mouths, or that it is normal for a 1-year-old to experiment with throwing a book on the floor.

> Emphasize that this should be fun. Reinforce the importance to babies and young children of having face time with their parents and hearing the sound of the parent's voice.

> Comment on the way the child handles the book in the examination room. Notice the 6-month-old who tries to grasp the book with her fist, the 12-month-old who points to a particular picture, the 12-month-old who uses a pincer grasp to turn one board page at a time. These responses represent developmental stages and progress that a parent can see.

> Make the connection for parents between the associations young children form by being on the parent's lap, listening to the parent's voice, and the later importance of literacy in school and enjoying books as a reader. This connection can be made more strongly as children get closer to school age and as their ability to understand and discuss books, stories, and illustrations becomes more sophisticated.

> Model dialogic reading and interactive behavior around books. For young children, point and name (Where's the baby? There's the baby! Where's the baby's nose? Where's your nose?). Ask the child specific questions. (What's that? Right, that's a dog! What does a dog say?) Allow the child to master new developmental tasks (Look, he turned the book right-side up, and now he's turning the pages one by one!) In the preschool years, a child might identify colors and name objects. Older children might tell a story and

describe story elements in illustrations [17]. Encourage the child's verbal language with interest, questions, and comments.

Use books as tools in anticipatory guidance that is not explicitly about literacy. Books can be an important part of bedtime and other transitions/routines. Books can help calm a child during a difficult wait or offer a parent strategies to spend one-on-one special time with an older child when a new baby arrives. In short, the book that is offered to the child to take home is in fact a small but real intervention to modify the child's home environment.

A book to take home

Through ROR, each child receives a new, developmentally appropriate book given by the primary care provider during the course of every health supervision visit, from the age of 6 months to 5 years. By kindergarten age, the child will have a ROR home library of 9 or 10 books provided by a consistent figure in the family's life and the child's growth and development.

Books are selected by each ROR site with specialized populations considered (books are available in English and Spanish, with more limited availability in many other languages). Sites access the National Center's research, reviews, and negotiated discounted prices. The books may include children's classics like *Goodnight Moon* and *Curious George*, as well as delightful and innovative newcomers.

Part of the ROR training curriculum involves reviews developmentally appropriate books. The program starts with simple board books for babies, which have the advantage of being chewable, and progresses to more complex board books for toddlers Such books can have more complex concepts or stories, but they are also simple and durable. By age 2, children are enjoying books with rhymes, humor, counting, and question-and-answer. Furthermore, sometime around age 2, they develop the fine motor skills needed to handle paper pages. As they grow into the preschool years, children enjoy alphabet books, counting books, and stories that increase in complexity and length [18].

PRACTICAL TIPS FOR THE EXAMINATION ROOM: MAKING IT WORK

Pediatric primary care providers who undertake the ROR intervention sometimes are concerned that literacy promotion may be just one more worthy item on an already too long laundry list of anticipatory guidance strategies and preventive interventions to perform, in the setting of waiting rooms at capacity and an already busy day of patient visits. ROR providers, however, often find that literacy guidance actually makes the visit more efficient and effective. The basic strategies for anticipatory guidance, as discussed previously, also can be used as practical strategies; by incorporating the book into our interaction with the child and parent, one can establish more effective connections, gather information, and deliver useful advice.

Early in the visit, hand the book directly to the child; make it clear that the book is coming from the primary care provider, and that it is intended for the child. The authors reiterate this advice, because it is probably the single most important strategy.

Allow older children to choose from a small selection of possible books.

Comment on the child's interest, or on developmentally appropriate book-handling behavior ("You expect a six-month-old to put the book directly into his mouth. That's normal, and that's why we give him a board book.").

Use the child's behavior with the book to assess the child's development and the parent's ability to respond to the child's cues.

Make the connection between growing up with books and being ready for school.

Be enthusiastic about the child's interest, pleasure, and potential as a reader and about the parent's ability to help the child achieve that potential.

In summary, effective use of the book in the examination room is most likely when the book is in the child's hands throughout the visit, when the child's book-handling behaviors and reactions to the book and pictures provide natural opportunities for the provider's comments and guidance about reading aloud and early literacy skills, and when the provider is able to incorporate books and reading into the other topics of anticipatory guidance including bedtime and daily routines and school readiness.

BEYOND THE BASICS: THE BOOK AS ASSESSMENT TOOL

In the authors' experience, practitioners comment on the power and the potential of the book as a developmental assessment tool. The book in the examination room elicits spontaneous language from many children. Providers observe gross and fine motor skills as the 6-month-old sits alone, reaches for the book, grasps it in his or her whole hand, and transfers it to his or her mouth. The 18-month-old holds the book and walks around; the 3-year-old turns paper pages with no difficulty. Practitioners see evidence of cognitive progress in the 18-month old who turns a book right-side up. The provider and parent enjoy listening to the 2-year-old who is beginning to name the animals. Practitioners hear pronoun use or complex sentences as the older child comments on illustrations.

Notice evidence of attentive parenting behavior in the way the parent follows the child's interest. Does the 6-month-old slap the page with her whole hand and the 1-year-old point to pictures? How does the parent respond to the 2-year-old who insistently demands to hear a story again and again? Observe the interaction as the child calls the parent's attention to pictures or to elements of the story.

A child's book-handling skills demonstrate both gross motor and fine motor progress, and the illustrations offer opportunities for the child to show language and communication skills, vocabulary range, and specific school readiness skills such as letter recognition and an understanding of print and its properties.

BEYOND THE BASICS: SPECIAL INITIATIVES

ROR has made efforts to provide better and more tailored literacy promotion to several specific populations.

Military families

An initiative supported by the Department of Defense will open 20 sites on military bases in 2009 and expand to more sites. The program is based on the idea that the best possible pediatric care includes early literacy promotion with the ROR model, and military families deserve that best possible care. Books about some of the issues that military families face, including separation and the deployment of a parent, will also be available to these programs.

Spanish-speaking families

Through the Leyendo Juntos initiative, the ROR National Center has assembled a team of bilingual and bicultural pediatric primary care providers who are assessing how best to provide anticipatory guidance to Spanish-speaking families. Through focus groups with Spanish-speaking parents, this initiative has identified several messages about reading to young children that are particularly welcome and effective with Latino families. The providers have assembled a Spanish phrase book and guide for discussing literacy and reading aloud with parents at the visit. The guide provides medical Spanish vocabulary and phrase book assistance for those who are not bilingual. The Leyendo Juntos initiative also includes more Spanish and Spanish–English books available to sites, and participation in research and advocacy groups concerned with health care for Spanish-speaking families [19].

American Indian/Alaska Native children

The ROR National Center has partnered with the American Academy of Pediatrics Committee on Native American Child Health, working with the Indian Health Service to reach more children who are American Indians and Alaska Natives. This initiative includes an effort to locate, make available, and sometimes help produce books in Native American languages, and books with stories and illustrations that reflect Native American families and traditions.

Children with special needs

There are several ROR programs in clinics for children with special needs and many children with special needs who receive their care at clinics where ROR is offered. Specialists in behavior and development have offered insights on how books can best be employed and enjoyed with children who have special needs including those who have hearing, visual, or neurodevelopmental challenges (M. Ultmann, personal communication, 2008).

READING TO YOUNG CHILDREN: LANGUAGE, SCHOOL READINESS, AND RISK

Reading aloud has been identified as an important precursor of successful literacy acquisition. Children who are read to in their preschool years are more likely to learn to read on schedule in school. Although reading aloud is also a marker for more educated parents and more generally literacy-rich environments, the amount of time children spend listening to books being read aloud is clearly associated with their language skills at school entry, and reading aloud in the preschool years is associated with childhood literacy acquisition [20,21]. After controlling for family education and socioeconomic status, the literacy qualities of a child's home are associated with language skills [22,23]. Other studies have shown that being read to from an earlier age is associated with better preschool language skills and with increased interest in reading [24]. Reading aloud to young children has been found to increase the richness of the vocabulary to which they are exposed and the complexity of syntax [25]. Books have been shown to stimulate increased interaction between adult and child [26,27].

Children with reading problems are at risk for school difficulties and school failure. By fourth grade in most school curricula, all school success is to some extent dependent on the child's ability to extract information and meaning efficiently from a printed text. Homework assignments, class assignments, and tests all favor the child who has achieved fluent reading, while the child who continues to struggle is likely to find every aspect of schoolwork more time-consuming and burdensome. Homework is more frustrating. Tests are more terrifying. Reading problems in the early grades are one very potent risk factor for later school problems, and there is a real danger that school will become a scene of struggle and failure [28]. The children who are most at risk may be the children whose parents are less able to advocate for them, to get them special help or additional tutoring, and to work with them outside of school to help them catch up.

The study by Hart and Risley pointed to dramatic socioeconomic differences in language exposure with children in families receiving economic assistance hearing on average only 620 words an hour, compared with an average of 2150 words per hour for children in professional families and 1250 words per hour for children in working class families. The study also examined the quality of the language to which these children were exposed, pointing up distinct gaps in the amount of feedback and interaction experienced by the children in poorer families. The vocabulary differences were impressive by age 3 and persisted into school age [29].

Children's literacy skills at school entry, kindergarten, and first grade predict their later reading success. In one study, 88% of children who had reading problems in kindergarten were still struggling with reading in the fourth grade [3]. Even reading skills in 11th or 12th grade can be predicted from reading skills in first grade [30].

Reading problems are significantly more common in children from low socioeconomic backgrounds. Children coming from these backgrounds are also significantly more likely to be retained in a grade and to be diagnosed with learning disabilities [31,32].

In national survey data from 2000, 37% of American fourth graders did not have basic grade level reading skills. By 12th grade, when many poor readers may have left school, 23% of the students still do not have basic reading skills. Poor reading skills in adults are associated with poor economic potential and with the perpetuation of cycles of poverty and dependency [33].

ROR is designed as an intervention to encourage parent–child interactions at home, which increase language and book-reading exposure, integral parts of literacy. Parents learn the importance of reading aloud and using developmentally appropriate strategies for enjoying books with young children.

LITERACY PROMOTION IN PRIMARY CARE: THE EVIDENCE

In more than 12 studies, the ROR model intervention was effective in several different populations and settings. Parents participating in ROR report a more positive attitude toward books and reading. For example, when asked to name favorite activities with their child or their child's favorite activities, parents are significantly more likely to mention looking at books and reading aloud than are parents in control groups who have not received the ROR intervention [34,35]. This significant increase in parents viewing reading with young children as a favorite activity has been found in English and Spanish-speaking parents, including recent immigrant populations [36]. One study looked at families who spoke languages in which no books were available. These families were given English books and still showed increased positive attitudes and practices [37].

Several studies have found differences in children's expressive and receptive language either by parent report or by direct testing of the children [38]. In one paper, there was a 6-month developmental increase in the receptive language skills of the children (average age was 4 years old) whose families were participating in ROR. Children with more contacts with ROR had larger increases in their language skills [39]. Follow-up of children receiving care at the control site of that study demonstrated similar increases in language skill after implementation of ROR [40]. ROR also has been found to contribute positively to a child's home literacy environment [41]. Additionally, a multicenter study of 19 sites before and after ROR showed increased parental support for reading aloud after the program was implemented in 19 pediatric primary care sites in 10 states [42].

In summary, research shows that in populations at risk, participation in the ROR intervention is associated with markedly more positive attitudes toward reading aloud, with more frequent reading aloud by parents, with improvements in the home literacy environment, and with significant increases in expressive and receptive language among children in the critical preschool age range [43].

FUTURE RESEARCH

Future studies could track children into adolescence and adulthood and explore the longitudinal effects of ROR components. Studies on comprehensive early childhood programs have demonstrated the importance of investing in programs that target the early childhood years. The Perry Preschool Project and the Abecedarian study are cited, for example, by Heckmann in his argument for the increased return on dollars invested in early childhood programs [44].

Even though ROR interventions are valuable, the program should not be compared with comprehensive preschool programs or with interventions that touch the lives of children and families for hours over time. At its best, the ROR intervention is performed in 10 primary care visits, each lasting perhaps 30 minutes. ROR directly forms some part of 5 hours plus waiting room time over the course of a child's first 5 years of life; the further effects of the program take place through the parent behaviors in the child's home.

Any longitudinal study of ROR interventions has to contend with a range of confounding variables, from family circumstances to learning disabilities as follow-up stretches into years, and the children enter school. Some researchers are now attempting to correlate the ROR exposures of school age children with reading success. Because it may be difficult to credit the ROR effect years after the intervention, researchers may construct shorter-term studies. There is already a much greater weight of evidence supporting ROR's effectiveness, however, than exists for many other primary care interventions that routinely are accepted as standard practice.

By counseling parents, early and often, about the importance of books and reading aloud, practitioners hope that parents seek out day care and preschool programs that support interactive literacy and look for other opportunities at library story hours and book fairs to increase their children's exposure to books.

PARENTAL LITERACY AND HEALTH LITERACY

What if the parent cannot read or cannot read very well? Many of the most at-risk children have parents who themselves struggled in school, who are not fluently literate themselves, who may feel uncomfortable reading aloud, who may not be inclined to look to the printed word for entertainment and edification. Some non-English speaking parents may be literate in their native language, while others may not be.

In many medical settings, patients or parents are not asked formally about their level of comfort with the written word, because practitioners feel the question would be intrusive or because they feel they can generally tell who is literate and who is not. In fact, inadequate literacy skills are extremely common among adults in the United States. In the 2003 National Assessment of Adult Literacy, 14% of US adults were found to have below basic prose literacy skills with another 29% at a basic level [33].

Poor parental literacy skills are a risk factor that can affect children's health and development in many ways [45]. How can there be what educators call "the intergenerational transfer of literacy," if there is limited literacy to transfer? Low parental literacy increases the likelihood that children will grow up in a print-poor environment, because a parent with limited skills is unlikely to use print to receive or to transmit information [46]. It may mean that the parent has had a difficult experience in school and is less likely to be comfortable in the school environment, which eventually may translate into the parent's unwillingness to connect with the child's teachers and participate in parent-teacher conferences, and to inability to understand materials sent home by the school. If the child struggles in school, a parent with poor literacy skills may be less likely or less able to advocate for the child and obtain help, interventions, or explanations. Significantly, the parent is not easily able to help the child with homework assignments, especially as those assignments get more complicated [47]. Finally, poor parental health literacy is a risk factor for children's health. Parents who cannot read print easily may struggle with prescriptions, asthma action plans, and with medical handouts [48].

What should primary care providers do to identify these parents whose children may be most at risk for reading problems and school issues? In one study [49], asking about the number of children's books in the home was a useful indicator for parent health literacy. A Chicago clinic has increased literacy referrals by asking a nonjudgmental question about whether the parent is interested in improving his or her reading ability (M. Glusman, personal communication, 2009). Asking all parents some basic screening question about literacy skills or about the home environment might help physicians identify more families where this risk factor is an issue, and might make it more possible to intervene. Parents need to know that help is available if they want to improve their own reading skills. ROR sites need to refer parents to adult or family literacy programs. Site coordinators are encouraged to form links with local literacy programs, networks, and coalitions.

When the provider knows or suspects that a parent is not necessarily comfortable with the written word, it is still possible to offer anticipatory guidance and a book for the child. Choose books with few words on the page or wordless books. Encourage the parent to look at books with the child and talk with the child about the pictures and the story the pictures tell. The parent can name objects and respond to the child's communications. The basic advice holds; the child will form positive associations with books and reading because of the connection with the parent's voice and the parent's attention.

REACH OUT AND READ: NATIONAL CENTER, COALITIONS, AND SITES

The Reach Out and Read National Center is a 501(c)3, a national nonprofit organization that supports and promotes the ROR model of early literacy promotion through primary care. The National Center maintains connections directly with individual sites and helps 34 state and city coalitions with training, fund-raising, book ordering, and other logistics. Every coalition has a coalition leader and a medical director, and each has resources for training, program support, and fundraising. Each ROR site has an on-site coordinator who is in charge of program logistics including book ordering and stocking, and reporting on the site's activities. All programs should have on-site medical directors, providers who take responsibility for medical leadership and provider training. The National Center and the coalitions foster dialogue through newsletters, on-line discussion forums, conference calls, continuing education, medical meetings, and conferences.

STARTING AN ROR PROGRAM

ROR targets its message and book funding to pediatric primary care practices that see children at social and economic risk. This article suggests some of the reasons why the provider's guidance to parents and the accompanying books given to the child may be particularly critical in the lives of children who are growing up with limited resources, often in print-poor environments [50]. ROR messages and strategies, however, are important for all families, regardless of income level and education. ROR recognizes the importance of reading to young children, and details developmentally appropriate techniques that help parents enjoy books with babies, toddlers, and preschoolers. ROR supports the vital and glorious role that books can play in the lives of children and families.

Practitioners who would like to incorporate ROR into clinical practice can contact a local ROR coalition or the National Center to discuss the possibility of starting a program. The National Center can help make connections to state or city-wide coalitions. ROR advocates for incorporating literacy promotion into standard pediatric primary care, and for understanding language and literacy development as an intrinsic part of the pediatrician's goal in helping children grow. When pediatricians and family physicians and nurse practitioners become literacy advocates, literacy becomes part of children's health, and books are part of every healthy childhood.

BOOKS IN CHILDREN'S LIVES

The ROR intervention relies on the primary care provider, the relationship between the provider and the family, and the power of the book. The advice that providers give parents is practical, modeled and rehearsed in the examination room. The child goes home with a book that can be incorporated into parent–child interactions and routines. Anecdotally, providers hear from parents who report that children ask to have the book read over and over or that children expect to hear the book read before going to sleep.

Giving early literacy guidance at the primary care visit, accompanied by an age-appropriate children's book, is a way to modify the home environment, stimulate and enrich the child's language, foster positive parent–child interactions, promote attachment, develop routines and strategies for daily life with a small child, and ultimately promote school readiness and literacy.

References
[1] Bus AG, Van Ijzendoorn MH, Pellegrini AD. Joint book reading makes for success in learning to read: a meta-analysis on intergenerational transmission of literacy. Rev Educ Res 1995;65:1–21.
[2] NICHD Early Child Care Research Network. Pathways to reading: the role of oral language in the transition to reading. Dev Psychol 2005;41:428–42.
[3] Juel C. Learning to read and write: a longitudinal study of 54 children from first through fourth grades. J Educ Psychol 1988;80:437–47.
[4] Foster WA, Miller M. Development of the literacy achievement gap: a longitudinal study of kindergarten through third grade. Lang Speech Hear Serv Sch 2007;38:173–81.

[5] Whitehurst CJ, Falco FL, Lonigan CJ, et al. Accelerating language development through picture book reading. Dev Psychol 1988;24:552–9.

[6] Senechal M, LeFevre JA. Parental involvement in the development of children's reading skill: a five-year longitudinal study. Child Dev 2002;72:445–60.

[7] Teale WH, Sulzby E, editors. Emergent literacy: writing and reading. Norwood (NJ): Ablex Publishing Corp.; 1986.

[8] Tomopoulos S, Valdez PT, Dreyer BP, et al. Is exposure to media intended for preschool children associated with less parent–child shared reading aloud and teaching activities? Ambul Pediatr 2007;7:18–24.

[9] Mendelsohn AL, Berkule SB, Tomopoulos S, et al. Infant television exposure associated with limited parent–child verbal interactions. Arch Pediatr Adolesc Med 2008;162(5):411–7.

[10] Zimmerman FJ, Christakis DA. Children's television viewing and cognitive outcomes: a longitudinal analysis of national data. Arch Pediatr Adolesc Med 2005;159(7):619–25.

[11] Kuhl PK, Tsao FM, Liu HM. Foreign language experience in infancy: effects of short-term exposure and social interaction on phonetic learning. Proc Natl Acad Sci U S A 2003;100(15):9096–101.

[12] Reach Out and Read: a national pediatric literacy program. Available at: http://reachoutandread.org.

[13] Hagan JF, Shaw JS, Duncan PM, editors. Bright futures: guidelines for health supervision of infants, children, and adolescents. 3rd edition. Elk Grove Village (IL): American Academy of Pediatrics; 2008.

[14] Berkule SB, Dreyer BP, Klass PE, et al. Mothers' expectations for shared reading following delivery: implications for reading activities at 6 months. Ambul Pediatr 2008;8(3):169–74.

[15] Klass P, Needlman R, Zuckerman B, et al. Reach out and read training manual. 2nd edition. Boston: Reach Out and Read National Center; 1999.

[16] ROR National Center. ROR on-line CME course in pediatric literacy promotion. Available at: http://www.bu.edu/cme/ror.

[17] Schickedanz JA. Much more than the ABCs: the early stages of reading and writing. Washington DC: NAEYC; 1999.

[18] Lipson ER. The New York Times parent's guide to the best books for children. Revised and updated. 3rd edition. New York: Three Rivers Press; 2000.

[19] ROR National Center. Available at: http://www.reachoutandread.org/about_special.html#rt.

[20] Duursma E, Augustyn M, Zuckerman B. Reading aloud to children: the evidence. Arch Dis Child 2008;93:554–7.

[21] Wells G. Language development in the preschool years. New York: Cambridge University Press; 1985.

[22] Raz IS, Bryant P. Social background, phonological awareness, and children's reading. Br J Dev Psychol 1990;8:209–25.

[23] Sticht TG. Adult literacy education. Rev Educ Res 1988;15:59–96.

[24] Payne AC, Whitehurst GJ, Angell AL. The role of literacy environment in the language development of children from low-income families. Early Child Res Q 1994;9:427–40.

[25] Hoff-Ginsberg E. Mother–child conversation in different social classes and communicative settings. Child Dev 1991;62:782–96.

[26] Neuman SB. Guiding young children's participation in early literacy development: a family literacy program for adolescent mothers. Early Child Dev Care 1997;127–128:119–29.

[27] Tomopoulos S, Dreyer BP, Flynn V, et al. Books, toys, parent–child interaction, and development in young Latino children. Ambul Pediatr 2006;6(2):72–8.

[28] Weitzman M, Siegel D. What we have not learned from, what we know about excessive school absence and school dropout. J Dev Behav Pediatr 1992;13:55–8.

[29] Hart B, Risley TR. Meaningful differences in the everyday experience of young American children. Baltimore (MD): Paul Brookes Publishing Company; 1995.

[30] Cunningham AE, Stanovich KE. Early reading acquisition and its relation to reading experience and ability 10 years later. Dev Psychol 1997;33:934–45.

[31] Byrd RS. Predictors of early grade retention among children in the United States. Pediatrics 1994;93:481–7.

[32] White KR. The relation between socioeconomic status ad academic achievement. Psychol Bull 1982;91:461–81.

[33] National Center for Education Statistics. A first look at the literacy of America's adults in the 21st century. Number: 2006470. Washington DC: NCES; 2005.

[34] Needlman R, Fried L, Morley D, et al. Clinic-based intervention to promote literacy. Am J Dis Child 1991;145:881–4.

[35] High P, Hopman M, LaGasse L, et al. Evaluation of a clinic-based program to promote book sharing and bedtime routines among low-income urban families with young children. Arch Pediatr Adolesc Med 1998;152:459–65.

[36] Sanders LM, Gershon TD, Huffman LC, et al. Prescribing books for immigrant children. Arch Pediatr Adolesc Med 2000;154:771–7.

[37] Silverstein M, Iverson L, Lozano P. An English-language clinic-based literacy program is effective for a multilingual population. Pediatrics 2002;109:E76.

[38] Golova N, Alario A, Vivier P, et al. Literacy promotion for Hispanic families in a primary care setting: a randomized, controlled trial. Pediatrics 1999;103:993–7.

[39] Mendelsohn A, Mogliner L, Dreyer B, et al. The impact of a clinic-based literacy intervention on language development in inner-city preschool children. Pediatrics 2001;107:130–4.

[40] Mendelsohn AL. Promoting language and literacy through reading aloud: the role of the pediatrician. Curr Probl Pediatr Adolesc Health Care 2002;32(6):183–210.

[41] Weitzman CC, Roy L, Walls T, et al. More evidence for reach out and read: a home-based study. Pediatrics 2004;113:1248–53.

[42] Needlman R, Toker KH, Dreyer BP, et al. Effectiveness of a primary care intervention to support reading aloud: a multicenter evaluation. Ambul Pediatr 2005;5:209–15.

[43] Needlman R, Silverstein M. Pediatric interventions to support reading aloud: how good is the evidence? J Devel Behav Pediatr 2004;25:352–63.

[44] Heckmann J. Catch 'em young: investing in disadvantaged young children is both fair and efficient. Wall St J January 10, 2006;A14.

[45] DeWalt DA, Berkman ND, Sheridan SL, et al. Literacy and health outcomes: a systematic review of the literature. J Gen Intern Med 2004;19:1228–39.

[46] Green CM, Berkule SB, Dreyer BP, et al. Does maternal literacy account for associations between education and parenting in low socioeconomic status families? Arch Pediatr Adolesc Med, in press.

[47] Hannon P. Literacy, home, and school: research and practice in teaching literacy with parents. London: The Falmer Press; 1995.

[48] Robinson LD, Calmes DP, Bazargan M. The impact of literacy enhancement on asthma-related outcomes among underserved children. J Natl Med Assoc 2008;100:892–6.

[49] Sanders LM, Zacur G, Haecker T, et al. Number of children's books in the home: an indicator of parent health literacy. Ambul Pediatr 2004;4:424–8.

[50] Bradley RH, Caldwell BM. The relation of infants' home environments to achievement test performance in first grade: a follow-up study. Child Dev 1984;55:803–9.

Advances in Pediatrics 56 (2009) 29–46

ADVANCES IN PEDIATRICS

Immunization Update II

Ayesha Mirza, MD[a],
Mobeen H. Rathore, MD, CPE, FAAP, FIDSA, FACPE[a,b,*]

[a]Department of Pediatrics, University of Florida, Pediatric Infectious Diseases & Immunology, 653-1 West 8th Street, LRC 3rd Floor, L-13 Jacksonville, FL 32209, USA
[b]Wolfson Children's Hospital, Jacksonville, FL 32209, USA

A dvances in the realm of immunizations continue to occur with amazing speed. In their previous article the authors discussed all the new vaccines and updated vaccination recommendations [1]. Information regarding the safety and efficacy of these vaccines continues to emerge as they become incorporated in the regular childhood and adolescent immunization schedules. The purpose of this article is to summarize all such information as well as provide readers with updates on any new vaccines that may be on the horizon.

ADOLESCENT VACCINES

Vaccinating adolescents continues to present numerous challenges because adolescents do not frequently seek preventive health services, some do not have health insurance, and some may visit multiple providers or nontraditional providers who vary in immunization practices. Even when adolescents visit their health care providers, missed opportunities are common [2]. Health care providers traditionally have been in the practice of simply trying to "catch up" with vaccines not given during childhood. With the licensure of several new vaccines for adolescents in 2005 to 2006, this approach changed. A *Healthy People 2010* objective is to achieve 90% or more vaccination coverage among adolescents 13 to 15 years old for certain vaccines [3]. For the first time in 2006, the National Immunization Survey (NIS) collected *provider-reported* vaccination information for adolescents aged 13 to 17 years for certain vaccines. Data collected for 2006, and now 2007, shows a steady increase in the percentage of adolescents obtaining certain recommended vaccines [4,5].

Tetanus, reduced diphtheria toxoids, and acellular pertussis vaccines
Pertussis remains one of the leading causes of morbidity and mortality from illness and death related to vaccine-preventable diseases. The overall burden

*Corresponding author. Department of Pediatrics, University of Florida, Pediatric Infectious Diseases & immunology, 653-1 West 8th Street, LRC 3rd Floor, L-13, Jacksonville, FL 32209. *E-mail address:* mobeen.rathore@jax.ufl.edu (M.H. Rathore).

0065-3101/09/$ – see front matter
doi:10.1016/j.yapd.2009.08.011

of disease from pertussis also remains steady, at around 600,000 estimated cases annually just among adults [6]. During 2006 a total of 15,632 cases of pertussis were reported, with 16 pertussis-related deaths. Fourteen (88%) deaths occurred among infants, who remain at greatest risk in terms of morbidity and mortality associated with the infection [7].

Mathematical modeling evaluating different vaccine strategies for the United States has suggested that pertussis vaccination of 90% of household contacts (children, adolescents, and adults) of newborns, in addition to pertussis vaccination of 75% of adolescents, would prevent approximately 75% of pertussis cases among infants aged 0 to 23 months [8]. Implementation of pertussis booster vaccination in adolescents also seems to be the simplest and most economical strategy to reduce societal costs as well as decrease morbidity and mortality associated with pertussis infections. Cost-benefit analysis shows that immunization of all adolescents 10 to 19 years old may prevent 0.4 to 1.8 million cases of pertussis and save the United States 0.3 to 1.6 billion dollars in a decade [9]. According to the NIS, coverage for tetanus, reduced diphtheria toxoids, and acellular pertussis vaccine (Tdap) among adolescents increased from 10.8% in 2006 to 30.4% in 2007 [4,5]. These numbers, though still far below the *Healthy People 2010* target of 90% for one or more doses of tetanus-diphtheria booster, are encouraging.

Another model estimated that vaccination of both parents of an infant before discharge from the hospital could prevent 38% of infant cases and deaths [10]. In fact it has been suggested that parents of hospitalized neonates in the intensive care unit be considered for immunization [11]. Consideration should also be given to pertussis vaccination of health care workers. These workers have been the source of pertussis outbreak in the newborn nursery [12]. Several other reports have described outbreaks of pertussis in the health care setting as well, in which the index patient has been a patient, health care worker, or visitor [13–15]. The Advisory Committee on Immunization Practices (ACIP) recommends vaccination for all health care workers [16].

Yet another option worth considering would be to initiate pertussis vaccine at an earlier age, that is, at 6 weeks rather than 2 months of age. This option has the potential to decrease the number of cases, hospitalizations, and deaths attributable to pertussis each year [17]. In fact the World Health Organization guidelines, which focus primarily on developing countries, recommend that pertussis-containing vaccine be given on a 6-, 10-, and 14-week schedule. These guidelines are already in place in several developing countries, and might be an option worth considering in the United States.

Whereas there is no question that Tdap vaccination for adolescents and adults is essential to decrease the spread of infection in the community and particularly amongst children younger than 1 year, there remains debate on the timing of Tdap in relation to the last dose of pediatric tetanus, diphtheria and tetanus toxoid and acellular pertussis vaccine (DTaP) as well as the need for future booster doses of Tdap. Tdap is currently licensed for one dose that may be given 5 years after the last dose of DTaP, although it could possibly also be given as early as 2 years after the last DTaP dose. This possibility arises due to the concern for severe injection site reactions, including Arthus type reactions, in anyone vaccinated too soon after the last DTaP vaccine is given. The results of a Canadian study on 7156 children and adolescents showed that the vaccine maybe given as early as 18 months after a previous dose of tetanus, diphtheria/tetanus, reduced diphtheria (TD/Td), with only a slight increase in injection site reactions [18].

Other studies looking at humoral immune responses measured by geometric mean titers 1 month and subsequently at 1, 3, and 5 years following immunization with Tdap showed persistent antibody levels exceeding the preimmunization levels, thus suggesting the persistence of immunity for extended periods of time [19]. This information will help further determine the need for acellular pertussis booster immunizations in the future. There are studies that support Tdap booster doses every 10 years following the current Td vaccination schedule; their results are based on mathematical modeling from 5-year serologic studies designed to predict antibody decay for pertussis antigens. No definite recommendations for Tdap boosters following initial vaccination have been made so far [20].

Tetravalent meningococcal conjugate vaccine

According to the 2007 NIS, tetravalent meningococcal A, C, Y, W135 conjugate vaccine (MCV4) (Menactra; SanofiPasteur, Swiftwater, PA) has been received by 32.4% of adolescents compared with 11.7% of adolescents aged 13 to 17 years in 2006. Receipt of the vaccine was fairly evenly distributed amongst the different ages in 2007 compared with 2006, when more adolescents aged 15 years (13%) had received the vaccine compared with those who were 17 years old (7.1%) [4,5].

In June 2007 the ACIP revised its recommendations to include routine vaccination of all persons aged 11 to 18 years with one dose of MCV4 at the earliest opportunity [21]. Previous recommendations called for immunization of children between the ages of 11 and 12 years with catch-up immunization at entry into high school or 15 years of age, whichever came first. These updated recommendations were based on MCV4 use and supply projections as well as the available data on safety and cost-effectiveness of the vaccine. This update should also simplify provider decisions to vaccinate.

Although MCV4 is now approved by the Food and Drug Administration (FDA) for children 2 years of age and older, the ACIP in its February 2008 meeting decided not to recommend routine vaccination of children 2 to 10 years old unless the child was at increased risk for the disease. This decision was based on immunogenicity, cost-effectiveness, and disease burden in this age group [22].

Since recommendations for immunization of adolescents with meningococcal conjugate vaccine were made by the ACIP, as of February 25, 2008, 26 confirmed cases of Guillain-Barré Syndrome (GBS) have been reported to the Centers for Disease Control and Prevention (CDC). All cases, which were temporally associated to MCV4 administration, occurred within 6 weeks of receiving the vaccine. To keep things in perspective, more than 15 million doses of MVC4 had been distributed by this time. That being said, the timing of the vaccine and onset of neurologic symptoms warranted further investigation. At the present time the CDC and FDA are investigating those cases of GBS that occurred after receiving the vaccine. Until the investigation is complete, the CDC is unable to determine if MCV4 increases the risk of GBS in people who received the vaccine, therefore the present recommendation is to continue with the immunization [23].

The incidence of typical GBS has been reported to be relatively uniform, between 0.6 and 4 cases per 100,000 per year throughout the world [24]. Compared with this incidence, there are between 1400 and 3000 cases of invasive meningococcal disease in the United States each year with an annual incidence of 0.5 to 1.1 per 100,000 population. Adolescents have the highest case fatality rate as well as increased incidence of complications compared with infants and children. It is estimated that 75% to 80% of adolescent meningococcal disease can be accounted for by serogroups A, C, Y, and W135, all of which are contained in MCV4 [1].

Other meningococcal vaccines

Currently there are 2 tetravalent A, C, Y, W 135 (polysaccharide and conjugate) meningococcal vaccines available in the United States. In the United Kingdom, a vaccine against serogroup C disease is also available for use. However, to date there is no vaccine that provides protection against serogroup B disease. Although serogroup B has a worldwide distribution, most cases are seen in the United States, South America, Europe, and Australia [25]. Most recently serogroup X has been reported as an emerging cause of invasive meningococcal disease in North America, Europe, and Africa [26].

Difficulty with developing a vaccine against serogroup B disease may be due to the structural similarity between the capsular polysaccharide and a glycoprotein found in human neural tissue, making it poorly immunogenic. Theoretical concerns also arise about the potential for the development of autoimmunity [27,28]. There are meningococcal serogroup B vaccines based on the outer membrane vesicle (OMV) that have been utilized in localized outbreaks of disease [29,30]. However, their usefulness for large-scale global immunization is limited due to the great antigenic variability of the meningococcal outer membrane structures [31]. These vaccines are also poorly immunogenic in children [30,32].

Using a technique called "reverse vaccinology," Novartis has developed a candidate serogroup B vaccine. This unique approach capitalizes on the availability of the bacterial genome sequences to identify potential protein antigens [33]. Using this method, the entire genetic makeup of the pathogenic meningococcal serogroup B strain was decoded and 600 novel proteins were discovered. Then a panel of 85 meningitis B strains was developed and used to engineer the vaccine with the antigens that showed the greatest ability to stimulate the immune system and kill bacteria [33,34]. The selected 85 strains were representative of global diversity.

Data from phase 2 studies of the recombinant meningococcal group B (MenB; Novartis) vaccine given to healthy term infants starting at 2 months of age produced a protective immune response. The vaccine was repeated at age 4, 6 and 12 months. Responses for those who also received the vaccine at age 12 months indicated not only a protective immune response but also a memory response [35]. The vaccine entered phase 3 clinical trials in early 2008. Other recent data released by Novartis show that this investigational vaccine may be the first to also protect infants age 6 months and older against multiple strains of serogroup B [36].

In addition, data from phase 3 studies of Men ACWY-CRM (Menveo; Novartis), another investigational conjugate vaccine, suggest that it has the potential to become the first meningococcal vaccine to protect all age groups from the 4 common vaccine preventable serogroups (A, C, Y, W135) [36,37].

Human papilloma virus vaccine

In the United States there is currently one licensed prophylactic, quadrivalent (types 6, 11, 16, and 18) human papilloma virus (HPV) vaccine, Gardasil (Merck, Whitehouse Station, NJ). Papers for another prophylactic, bivalent (types 16 and 18) HPV vaccine, Cervarix (GlaxoSmith Kline, Brentford, Middlesex, UK) have been submitted to the FDA for approval [38]. Cervarix has been approved for use in 67 countries around the world. Both vaccines provide greater than 90% protection against cervical infection for up to 5 years after vaccination. Since its approval in June 2006, the ACIP issued recommendations for routine vaccination of females 11 to 12 years old with 3 doses of the quadrivalent HPV vaccine along with catch-up vaccination for those between the ages of 9 to 26 years. There is as yet insufficient evidence to recommend vaccination for women older than 26 years.

In May 2007, the American Academy of Pediatrics (AAP) issued provisional recommendations for use of the HPV vaccine that were similar to the recommendations issued by the ACIP [39]. Although only 2% of women completed HPV vaccination 1 year after FDA approval, there are encouraging data from the NIS teen survey showing that 25% of adolescents have initiated the vaccination series, 44.2% had received 2 doses, and 23.5% had received 3 doses [5,40].

Nevertheless, despite recommendations from the ACIP and AAP, implementation and acceptance of HPV vaccine in the United States remains a source of ongoing debate. Various factors contributing to this debate include awareness and attitudes of parents and clinicians regarding the vaccine, cost-effectiveness of the vaccine, and issues related to vaccine financing.

Efforts to mandate the vaccine as a requirement for school have only been passed by the State of Virginia; however, at the time of writing a bill to delay that requirement, which would have become effective in 2009, is under consideration. The authors also wrote in their previous article that Texas had become the first state to mandate HPV vaccination. Since then, the Texas state legislature passed a law overriding the governor's order, thus prohibiting schools to require vaccination. In at least 41 states, and Washington DC legislation has been introduced to require, fund, or educate the public about the HPV vaccine [41].

Because Gardasil is the most expensive childhood vaccine ever marketed, currently priced at $375.00 retail [42] for the 3-dose series, cost-effectiveness and vaccine financing also play a significant role in vaccine delivery to the public. The vaccine is being provided free of charge under the Vaccines for Children Program (VFC) for women and young girls younger than 18 years who are uninsured. Recent studies using mathematical models show that the cost-effectiveness of HPV vaccination will depend on the duration of vaccine immunity and will be optimized by achieving high coverage in preadolescent girls, targeting initial catch-up efforts in women up to 18 or 21 years old, and revising screening policies [43]. Results of the cost-effectiveness analysis showed that extending routine vaccination from 12-year-olds to 26-year-olds had a cost per quality adjusted life-year gain of $150,000 compared with $43,600 for 12-year-olds when compared with screening alone [43].

Several objections have been raised by opponents of Gardasil, one of them being that the vaccine is aimed at personal rather than public health, and payment should therefore be an individual responsibility. In addition, there is also the concern that vaccination may lead to more promiscuity, making children and adolescents believe that they are less vulnerable to infections. Most authorities, however, doubt that this would be the case [44].

It is also important to mention that although the discussion thus far has concerned immunization in women, it would not be complete without mentioning immunization of boys and young men. Because the disease is sexually transmitted, it seems logical to consider immunization of men as well. In addition, male vaccination will become an important issue as female immunization rates increase. It is also hoped that vaccination would reduce the incidence of certain genital cancers in men. However, immunization in males will depend on efficacy of the vaccine and cost-effectiveness. Ongoing studies of efficacy in men are currently underway, although available data support gender-neutral immunization [45]. In certain countries, such as Mexico and Australia, HPV vaccines are licensed for use in males 9 to 15 years old [46].

Following the licensure of Gardasil, as of June 30, 2008, there have been reports of 20 deaths occurring in individuals after receiving the vaccine, as reported to the vaccine adverse event reporting system (VAERS). There have also been some reports of GBS and thromboembolic events. However, based on available data the FDA has determined that administration of Gardasil remains safe and effective, and the benefits far outweigh the risks. Reports of adverse events to VAERS should continue to be closely monitored, however [47].

VACCINES FOR CHILDREN
Rotavirus vaccines

A second oral rotavirus vaccine (Rotarix; GlaxoSmithKline) was licensed by the FDA on April 3, 2008 [48]. This vaccine is given as a 2-dose series at age 2 months and 4 months. The first dose can be given as early as 6 weeks of age and the second dose may be given 4 weeks later, but no later than 24 weeks of age. The vaccine may be used interchangeably with Rotateq (Merck & Co. Inc., Whitehouse Station, NJ), although whenever possible vaccination should be completed with the same product. To make it easier to schedule immunizations, the ACIP has recommended that both vaccines can be given up to age 32 weeks [49]. Although Rotarix contains only a single common strain of human rotavirus in the United States, G1P, it shares neutralizing epitopes with G1, G3, G4, and G9, but not G2 rotavirus serotypes. The 2 rotavirus vaccines are equally efficacious, conferring 85% to 98% protection against severe rotavirus disease and 72% to 87% protection against any rotavirus disease [50,51]. Rotarix was being used in several countries prior to licensure in the United States. Because the oral applicator of Rotarix contains latex (Rotateq does not), any infant with a severe anaphylactic reaction to latex should not receive Rotarix. Rotarix is also contraindicated in any infant with a history of an uncorrected congenital malformation of the gastrointestinal tract, or any infant who has exhibited severe hypersensitivity to any component of the vaccine or who has experienced a severe allergic reaction to a previous dose of rotavirus vaccine.

Post licensure monitoring of intussusception following Rotateq administration has not shown an increased risk following immunization. Using data obtained from VAERS, between February 1, 2006 and September 25, 2007 the observed versus expected rate ratios were 0.53 and 0.91 for the 1- to 21-day and 1- to 7-day interval after vaccination, respectively. In the Vaccine Safety Datalink, 3 cases of intussusception occurred within 30 days after 111,521 Rotateq vaccinations compared with 6 cases after 186,722 non-Rotateq vaccinations during the same period [52].

As to overall vaccine effectiveness, preliminary data show that from November 2007 to May 2008, there seems to be delayed onset and diminished magnitude of rotavirus activity in the United States [53]. These data were obtained by the CDC from the National Respiratory and Enteric Virus Surveillance Network (NREVSS) and the New Vaccine Surveillance Network (NVSN). NREVSS is a voluntary network of United States laboratories that provides CDC with weekly reports of the number of tests performed and positive results obtained for a variety of pathogens. Based on the NREVSS data, the onset of rotavirus activity during the 2007 to 2008 seasons appears to be delayed by 2 to 4 months when compared with the 15 prevaccine rotavirus seasons (July 1991 to June 2006). The data also show that the number of positive tests for rotavirus was lower by a median of 78.5% from January 1, 2008 to May 3, 2008 when compared with the same weeks in each of the preceding rotavirus seasons. Although the 2008 season is not yet over and the numbers reported are subject to certain other limitations as well (ie, incomplete reporting of results due to delays, different testing practices at different institutions, and lack of clinical patient data), the overall trend looks promising because these numbers coincide with the increasing use of rotavirus vaccine among infants.

The NVSN conducted prospective, population-based surveillance from January through May for rotavirus gastroenteritis among children younger than 3 years living in 3 United States counties (Monroe County, New York; Hamilton County, Ohio; Davidson County, Tennessee). The overall percentage of fecal specimens testing positive for rotavirus was 51% in 2006, 54% in 2007, and 6% in 2008. Smaller percentages of positive results were observed in all inpatient, emergency department, and outpatient clinic sites in 2008 compared with the previous 2 years.

In their own children's hospital in northeast Florida, the authors have observed similar trends (unpublished data; abstract currently submitted for review, PAS 2009). There was a 41% decrease in the average number of rotavirus tests ordered as well as a 72% decrease in the number of positive tests between April 2007 and thus far in 2008. Compared with rotavirus admissions in 2006, the admission rate in 2008 had decreased by 91%. Another interesting observation has been the delay in the onset of the rotavirus season from January to September, with the peak occurring in October/November as opposed to March/April in previous years. Whether these trends will continue to be observed remains to be determined.

Several additional reports also support the findings of the NREVSS and NVSN as well as the authors' own preliminary findings [54–57]. These numbers also suggest that the changes in rotavirus activity might be more pronounced than what might be attributable to the direct protective effects of vaccination alone. It could be surmised that vaccination may provide some indirect benefits to unvaccinated children (ie, herd immunity) by reducing transmission of rotavirus in the community. Surveillance is ongoing.

Influenza vaccines

With the 2008 influenza season, we continue to inch gradually toward the concept of universal influenza immunization. The ACIP has recommended influenza vaccination for all children aged 6 months to 18 years, in addition to all household members of high-risk patients and household contacts and caregivers of children younger than 5 years and adults 50 years or older, with particular emphasis on immunization of contacts of children younger than 6 months. This population is in addition to individuals aged 50 years or older, pregnant women, individuals with chronic medical conditions or immunosuppression, residents of nursing homes or chronic care facilities, and health care personnel [58]. Immunizing pregnant women is particularly important because this has been shown to provide protection to their newborn babies up to age 5 months [59].

Six influenza vaccines have been approved for use in the United States for the 2008 to 2009 influenza season (Table 1). The 3 strains used in the vaccine

Table 1
Influenza vaccines available in the United States

Vaccine Type	Vaccine Name	Age Indication	Doses Required	Preservative	Route
Trivalent inactivated	Fluzone (Sanofi Pasteur)	≥6 mo	1 or 2	Thimerosal	IM
		6–35 mo	1 or 2	None	
		≥36 mo	1 or 2	None	
	Fluvirin (Novartis)	≥4 y	1 or 2	Thimerosal in multidose vial None in prefilled syringe	IM
	Fluarix (GlaxoSmithKline)	≥18 y	1	None	IM
	Afluria (CSL Biotherapies)	≥18 y	1	Thimerosal in multidose vial None in prefilled syringe	IM
	Flulaval (GlaxoSmithKline)	≥18 y	1	Thimerosal	IM
Live activated	Flumist (MedImmune)	2–49 y[a]	1 or 2	None	Intranasal

IM, intramuscular.

[a]Healthy, nonpregnant adults and children younger than 5 years with no history of reactive airways disease or recurrent wheezing.

for the 2008 to 2009 vaccines are different from those in the previous vaccine used in the 2007 to 2008 season. Live attenuated influenza vaccine is not recommended for individuals who are immunocompromised, younger than 2 years or older than 49 years, as well as children younger than 5 years old with a history of reactive airways disease or recurrent wheezing. Older children with severe asthma should also not receive the live vaccine.

When immunizing children, it is important to follow the recommendations to give the influenza vaccine in 2 doses when given for the first time. Information obtained through the NVSN regarding influenza vaccine effectiveness for the 2003 to 2004 and 2004 to 2005 influenza seasons shows that receipt of all recommended doses in children 6 to 59 months old reduced by half the number of medical visits due to laboratory-confirmed influenza-related illnesses, whereas partial vaccination was not effective in either season [60].

Over the last several years there has been increasing emphasis on vaccinating children, which has arisen because of the increasing recognition of the burden of influenza in young children as well as school-aged children, who are responsible for much of influenza transmission [61,62]. Not only is illness in school-aged children related to significant absenteeism from school but also results in workdays missed by parents and subsequent illness amongst other family members [63]. School-based immunization programs have been shown to work, and perhaps this is the way to proceed to improve influenza immunization rates in the United States [64,65]. Ultimately the success of such programs would hinge on a multidisciplinary approach, with education and communication in the community as a whole being an integral component of successful school-based programs.

Current influenza immunization rates overall in children in the United States are unacceptably low [66]. The *Healthy People 2010* target of achieving 90% or greater coverage in adults aged 65 years and older and among nursing home residents, and 60% coverage in all other risk groups is still far from being close [67]. However, there is no question that over the last few years there has been great emphasis on improving influenza vaccination rates. Efforts have included increased media advertising and public education campaigns. Improvement in the vaccine supply and increased availability of the vaccine at common retail and grocery stores, airports, and even drive-through clinics has also allowed greater access to the public. These efforts need to be sustained and improved.

New combination vaccines

As the list of required vaccines continues to grow, as does the list of combination vaccines. The 2 most recently licensed combination vaccines include DTap-IPV (Kinrix; GlaxoSmithKline) and DTaP-PV/Hib (Pentacel; Sanofi Pasteur). Both these vaccines have been included in the VFC program. The VFC resolution states that DTaP-IPV and DTaP-IPV/Hib may be used if one of the component antigens is indicated and the others are not contraindicated. Both vaccines are thimerosal-free.

Diphtheria, tetanus toxoid, acellular pertussis, and inactivated poliovirus vaccine

This combination, DTaP and inactivated poliovirus vaccine (IPV), was licensed by the FDA on June 24, 2008 (Kinrix; GlaxoSmithKline) [68]. Kinrix is approved for use in the 4- to 6-year-old child as the fifth dose in the DTaP series, and as the fourth dose in the IPV series in infants who had previously received other combination vaccines, because the components of Kinrix are identical to those vaccines. The vaccine contains identical antigens and amounts of diphtheria toxoid, tetanus toxoid and inactivated pertussis toxin, filamentous hemagglutinin, and pertactin as those in Infanrix and Pediarix; and inactivated poliovirus types 1, 2, and 3 as in Pediarix. The vaccine demonstrated an immune response and safety profile that was comparable to separately administered DTaP and IPV vaccines, and if used would reduce the number of vaccines given at the 4- to 6-year visit by one shot. The rate of adverse reactions was similar to those following separate administration of DTaP and IPV. This combination vaccine was first licensed in France in 1996 and is now available in 33 countries worldwide.

Although the AAP and ACIP recommend that, when feasible, the same manufacturer's DTaP be used for each dose in the series, vaccination should not be deferred because the type of DTaP used previously is either not available or unknown. The same is not the case for IPV, however, which may be substituted for that from a different manufacturer in the same series. Therefore, if necessary Kinrix may be used as the fifth dose regardless of what the type of DTaP and IPV were previously used.

Diphtheria, tetanus toxoid, acellular pertussis, inactivated poliovirus, and *haemophilus influenzae* type b vaccine

The FDA licensed the combined DTaP, IPV, and *Haemophilus influenzae* type b (Hib) conjugate vaccine (Pentacel; Sanofi Pasteur Ltd., Swiftwater, PA) on June 20, 2008 [69]. The vaccine is licensed for use as a 4-dose series in infants and children at 2, 4, 6, and 15 through 18 months of age. Similar to other combination vaccines (Pediarix, Kinrix, Comvax, Proquad), Pentacel when used may reduce by 1 to 2 injections the number of shots a child may need. Pentacel is the first combination vaccine to overcome the immunogenicity challenges of a single product that can be given in a primary series to protect against both pertussis and Hib-invasive disease. In comparative studies, there was no difference in the frequency of local or systemic adverse events for the combination versus separately administered DTaP, IPV, and Hib control vaccines.

Immunologic responses following the third and fourth doses of DTaP-IPV/Hib vaccine were similar to those following respective, separately administered component vaccines. Antibody responses following the first and second doses of DTaP-IPV/Hib were not measured.

For certain American Indian/Alaskan native children at increased risk for Hib disease, particularly in the first 6 months of life, it is recommended that Hib vaccine containing the outer membrane protein (OMP) of meningococcus be used. This vaccine is associated with a more rapid seroconversion to protective antibody concentrations within the first 6 months of life with the use of 2 doses, and some protection even after the first dose of the vaccine. Use of Hib-OMP vaccines should be recommended in these populations preferentially unless there is unavailability or shortage of these vaccines, in which case DTaP-IPV/Hib may be used.

The current shortage of Hib vaccine due to manufacturing problems for Merck & Co. (West Point, PA), which produces 2 OMP-containing Hib vaccines, Pedvax HIB a monovalent conjugate vaccine, and Comvax, a conjugate vaccine that contains both Hib and hepatitis B, may necessitate the use of DTap-IPV/Hib in these high-risk populations depending on the duration of the Hib vaccine shortage, which is expected to last until mid 2009 at this point. The CDC currently recommends not giving the 12- to 15-month booster to healthy children while continuing to immunize all high-risk children [70].

For IPV, whereas 4 doses are recommended at 2, 4, 6 to 18 months, and 4 through 6 years of age, under ACIP recommendations of minimum intervals between doses, DTaP-IPV/Hib may be given at 2, 4, 6, and 15 to 18 months, providing 4 valid doses of IPV [71]. This dosage would obviate the need for IPV at 4 to 6 years of age except in states that mandate IPV at that age. DTaP-IPV/Hib may be given concurrently with other inactivated and live vaccines when they are indicated. The vaccines should be administered at separate injection sites.

OTHER CHANGES TO THE RECOMMENDATIONS FOR IMMUNIZATION

Mumps, measles, rubella, and varicella combination vaccine

A CDC postlicensure safety study found that the rate of febrile seizures 7 to 10 days after vaccination was about 2 times higher in children who received mumps, measles, rubella, and varicella combination vaccine (MMRV) compared with children who received mumps, measles, and rubella (MMR) and varicella vaccines at separate injection sites at the same visit. Therefore one additional seizure would be anticipated for every 2000 children immunized with MMRV. Interim analysis of the Merck postmarketing study have shown similar results [72].

Given the data on the increased risk of febrile seizures after vaccination with MMRV, the ACIP voted on February 27, 2008 to no longer express a preference for MMRV over separate MMR and Varicella vaccines in children 12 to 23 months old. It is not known whether the risk of febrile seizures is higher in the 4- to 6-year age group; however, febrile seizures in general are not common in this age group. MMRV is currently not available due to manufacturing issues that are unrelated to vaccine safety or efficacy.

Hepatitis a vaccine

Immunization with hepatitis A vaccine is recommended for all children in the United States beginning at 12 months of age. In addition, preexposure vaccination for high-risk individuals is recommended. This group includes travelers to endemic areas. Based on a study done in Kazakhstan, hepatitis A vaccine is also now recommended for postexposure prophylaxis in healthy individuals between the ages of 2 to 40 years with no evidence of underlying liver disease or immunocompromise. The vaccine should be given as soon as possible, within 2 weeks of exposure [73]. Individuals who are younger than 2 or older than 40 years, have underlying liver disease, or are immuno-compromised should still receive immune globulin simultaneously with the vaccine at a separate site. The second dose of hepatitis A vaccine should be given at the appropriate interval. Only monovalent hepatitis A vaccine should be used in these situations.

VACCINE UPDATES FROM AROUND THE WORLD

Unlike the United States and other industrialized nations, most of the world's underresourced countries continue to struggle with vaccine-preventable diseases. While those of us who live in the industrialized world are faced with different challenges such as vaccine financing, vaccine shortages, and the growing alliance against immunizations, outbreaks of diseases like measles bring with them the sobering reality of how much work still needs to be done globally. Certain new initiatives undertaken under the umbrella of the Global Alliance for Vaccine Initiative (GAVI) with the help of industrialized nations, and the Bill and Melinda Gates Foundation provide some encouraging news. Introduction of pneumococcal and rotavirus vaccines, accelerating access to Hib vaccines, as well as utilization of combination vaccines against diphtheria, pertussis, polio, tetanus, Hib, and hepatitis B are all part of a strategy to reduce by 66% child mortality rates in 33 countries by 2015. In addition, there are plans to increase support for vaccines against 6 other deadly diseases, namely cholera, Japanese encephalitis, rabies, rubella, typhoid, and cervical cancer [74]. In addition to this, global polio eradication efforts continue despite reports of increasing cases in Pakistan which, along with India, Nigeria, and Afghanistan, remains one of the 4 polio-endemic countries.

VACCINE FINANCING AND NEW IMMUNIZATION ALLIANCE

Finally, this review would be incomplete without at least mentioning some key issues that are directly and indirectly related to the delivery of immunizations to patients in the United States. The first issues that come to mind are those related to vaccine financing. With the licensure of new vaccines, physicians are continuously under pressure to find funding for increased office costs related to the purchase, storage, and costs of obtaining new vaccines, some of which the authors have mentioned here (eg, HPV vaccine). At the same time they must also offset dwindling revenues due to poor reimbursement from insurance companies for these very same vaccines. The problem lies in the private as well as the public sectors. The National Vaccine Advisory Committee's Vaccine Financing Working Group is working on proposals to try to address these issues [75].

In addition to the growing pressures associated with vaccine financing, pediatricians are being faced with yet another dilemma concerning the growing numbers of parents and families with questions about vaccine safety. This growing hostility toward vaccines is alarming. One just needs to look at the recent measles outbreak from an imported case that spread across 9 states to realize that we are far from immune from these deadly infectious diseases, which once took hundreds of lives and continue to do so in underresourced countries. The total number of cases of measles reported in the United States in 2008 shows that this number is the highest increase to date since 1996.This increase is not due to imported cases alone, but is also the result of higher viral transmission after importation to the United States among children who were unvaccinated [76]. To help answer some of these growing fears and dispel the rumors and untruths about vaccines, a new Immunization Alliance was formed early in 2008 [77]. The goals of this alliance are to facilitate a multipronged approach to recapture the public's trust in immunization, and develop compelling messages for parents over both the long and short term before one starts to see a decrease in immunization rates. Along with several other groups, which include but are not limited to the American Medical Association, the American College of Obstetrics and Gynecology, and the American Academy of Family Practitioners, the AAP is represented on the alliance. Research suggests that reasons why parents may refuse vaccines may be severalfold [78].

Despite all the challenges faced within the United States and globally, the work toward development of new vaccines and eradication of old vaccine-preventable diseases must continue. As the end of the first decade of this millennium nears, while there is good reason to celebrate, there is much work still to be done.

References

[1] Mirza A, Rathore MH. Immunization update. Adv Pediatr 2007;54:135–71.
[2] Lee GM, Suchita AL, Pfoh E, et al. Adolescent immunizations: missed opportunities for prevention. Pediatrics 2008;122:711–7.
[3] U.S. Department of Health and Human Services. Healthy people 2010. Available at: http://www.healthypeople.gov/document/HTML/Volume1/14Immunization.htm#_Toc494510242. Accessed October 30, 2008.
[4] CDC. National vaccination coverage among adolescents aged 13-17 years—United States, 2006. MMWR Morb Mortal Wkly Rep 2007;56:885–8.
[5] CDC. Vaccination coverage among adolescents aged 13-17 years—United States, 2007. MMWR Morb Mortal Wkly Rep 2008;57:1100–3.
[6] Cortese MM, Baughman AL, Brown K, et al. A "new age" in pertussis prevention. New opportunities through adult vaccination. Am J Prev Med 2007;32:177–85.
[7] CDC. Prevention of pertussis, tetanus and diphtheria among pregnant and post partum women and their infants. Recommendations of the Advisory Committee on Immunization Practices (ACIP). MMWR Morb Mortal Wkly Rep 2008;57:1–47.
[8] Van Rie A, Hethcote HW. Adolescent and adult pertussis vaccination: computer simulations of five new strategies. Vaccine 2004;22:3154–65.
[9] Hay JW, Ward JI. Economic considerations for pertussis booster vaccination in adolescents. Pediatr Infect Dis J 2005;24:S127–33.

[10] Scuffham PA, McIntyre PB. Pertussis vaccination strategies for neonates—an exploratory cost-effectiveness analysis. Vaccine 2004;22:2953–64.

[11] Shah S, Caprio M, Mally P, et al. Rationale for the administration of acellular pertussis vaccine to parents of infants in the neonatal intensive care unit. J Perinatol 2007;27:1–3.

[12] Hospital acquired pertussis among newborns—Texas 2004. Available at: http://www.cdc.gov/mmwr/preview/mmwrhtml/mm5722a2.htm. Accessed October 29, 2008.

[13] Matlow AG, Nelson S, Wray R, et al. Nosocomial acquisition of pertussis diagnosed by polymerase chain reaction. Infect Control Hosp Epidemiol 1997;18:715–6.

[14] Friedman DS, Curtis CR, Schauer SL, et al. Surveillance for transmission and antibiotic adverse events among neonates and adults exposed to a health care worker with pertussis. Infect Control Hosp Epidemiol 2004;25:967–73.

[15] Spearing NM, Horvath RL, McCormack JG. Pertussis: adults as a source in health care settings. Med J Aust 2002;177:568–9.

[16] Kretsinger K, Broder KR, Cortese MM, et al. Preventing tetanus, diphtheria, and pertussis among adults: use of tetanus toxoid, reduced diphtheria toxoid and acellular pertussis vaccine (Tdap). Recommendations of the Advisory Committee on Immunization Practices (ACIP) and supported by the Healthcare Infection Control Practices Advisory Committee (HICPAC), for use of Tdap among health-care personnel. MMWR Recomm Rep 2006;55:1–37.

[17] Shinall MC, Peters TR, Yuwei Z, et al. Potential impact of acceleration of the pertussis vaccine primary series for infants. Pediatrics 2008;122:1021–6.

[18] Halperin SA, Sweet L, Baxendale D, et al. How soon after a prior tetanus-diphtheria vaccination can one give adult formulation tetanus-diphtheria-acellular pertussis vaccine? Pediatr Infect Dis J 2006;25:195–200.

[19] Edelman K, He Q, Mäkinen J, et al. Immunity to pertussis 5 years after booster immunization during adolescence. Clin Infect Dis 2007;44:1271–7.

[20] Barilleux F, Coudeville L, Kolenc-Saban A, et al. Predicted long term persistence of pertussis antibodies in adolescents after an adolescent and adult formulation combined tetanus, diphtheria and 5 component acellular pertussis vaccine, based on mathematical modeling and 5 year observed data. Vaccine 2008;26:3903–8.

[21] CDC. Revised recommendations of the Advisory Committee on Immunization Practices (ACIP) to vaccinate all persons aged 11-18 years with meningococcal conjugate vaccine. MMWR Morb Mortal Wkly Rep 2007;56:794–5.

[22] CDC. Report from the Advisory Committee on Immunization Practices (ACIP): decision not to recommend routine vaccination of all children aged 2-10 years with quadrivalent meningococcal conjugate vaccine (MCV4). MMWR Morb Mortal Wkly Rep 2008;57:462–5.

[23] GBS and Menactra® meningococcal vaccine. Available at: http://www.cdc.gov/vaccinesafety/concerns/gbsfactsheet.htm. Accessed October 29, 2008.

[24] Hughes RA, Cornblath DR. Guillain-Barré syndrome. Lancet 2005;366:1653–66.

[25] Stephens DS, Greenwood B, Brandtzaeg P. Epidemic meningitis, meningococcemia and *Neisseria meningitidis*. Lancet 2007;369:2196–210.

[26] Materu S, Cox HS, Isaakidis P, et al. Serogroup X in meningococcal disease, Western Kenya. Emerg Infect Dis 2007;13:944–5.

[27] Harrison LH. Prospects for vaccine prevention of meningococcal infection. Clin Microbiol Rev 2006;19:142–64.

[28] Hayrinen J, Jennings H, Raff HV, et al. Antibodies to polysialic acid and its N-propyl derivative: binding properties and interaction with human embryonal brain glycopeptides. J Infect Dis 1995;171:1481–90.

[29] Granoff DM, Harrison LH, Borrow R. Meningococcal vaccines. In: Plotkin S, Orenstein WA, Offit PA, editors. Vaccines: expert consult. 5th edition. Philadelphia: WB Saunders; 2008. p. 399–434.

[30] Kelly C, Arnold R, Galloway Y, et al. A prospective study of the effectiveness of the New Zealand meningococcal B vaccine. Am J Epidemiol 2007;166:817–23.

[31] Pizza M, Scarlato V, Masignani V, et al. Identification of vaccine candidates against serogroup B meningococcus by whole genome sequencing. Science 2000;287:1816–20.

[32] Noronha CP, Struchiner CJ, Halloran ME. Assessment of the direct effectiveness of the BC meningococcal vaccine in Rio de Janeiro, Brazil: a case control study. Int J Epidemiol 1995;24:1050–7.

[33] Rappouli R. Reverse vaccinology, a genome based approach to vaccine development. Vaccine 2001;19:2688–91.

[34] Giulani MM, Adu-Bobie J, Comanducci M, et al. A universal vaccine for serogroup B meningococcus. Proc Natl Acad Sci U S A 2006;103:10834–9.

[35] Miller E, Pollard AJ, Borrow R, et al. Safety and immunogenicity of Novartis meningococcal serogroup B vaccine (MenB vaccine) after three doses administered in infancy. Presented at the 28th Annual Meeting of the European Society for Pediatric Infectious Diseases (abstract 133), May 13–17, 2008, Graz, Austria.

[36] Novartis website. New phase II data show Novartis investigational meningitis B vaccine may also protect infants six months and older. Available at: http://www.novartis.com/newsroom/media-releases/en/2008/1250239.shtml. Accessed November 14, 2008.

[37] Snape MD, Perrett KP, Ford KJ, et al. Immunogenicity of a tetravalent meningococcal glycoconjugate vaccine in infants: a randomized controlled trial. JAMA 2008;299:173–84.

[38] GlaxoSmith Kline website. Response to FDA on Cervarix®. Available at: http://www.gsk.com/media/pressreleases/2008/2008_pressrelease_10073.htm. Accessed November 14, 2008.

[39] American Academy of Pediatrics, policy statement. Prevention of human papillomavirus infection: provisional recommendations for immunization of females with quadrivalent human papillomavirus vaccine. Available at: www.cispimmunize.org/ill/pdf/HPVprovisional.pdf. Accessed November 14, 2008.

[40] Gorin SS. HPV vaccinations one year post FDA approval. Annual Meeting American Society of Clinical Oncology, abstract #1513. May 30-June 3, 2008, Chicago (IL).

[41] The National Conference of Sate Legislature. HPV vaccine. Available at: http://www.ncsl.org/programs/health/HPVvaccine.htm. Accessed November 14, 2008.

[42] CDC. HPV vaccine information for young women. Available at: http://www.cdc.gov/std/Hpv/STDFact-HPV-vaccine.htm#hpvvac. Accessed November 14, 2008.

[43] Kim JJ, Goldie SJ. Health and economic implications of HPV vaccination in the United States. N Engl J Med 2008;359:821–32.

[44] Monk BJ, Wiley DJ. Will widespread human papillomavirus prophylactic vaccination change sexual practices of adolescent and young adult women in America? Obstet Gynecol 2006;108:420–4.

[45] Bloack SL, Nolan T, Sattler C, et al. Comparison of the immunogenicity and reactogenicity of a prophylactic quadrivalent human papillomavirus (types 6, 11, 16 and 18) L1 virus like particle vaccine in male and female adolescents and young adult women. Pediatrics 2006;118:2135–45.

[46] Giuliano AR. Human papillomavirus vaccination in males. Gynecol Oncol 2007;107:S24–6.

[47] FDA. Information from CDC and FDA on the safety of Gardasil vaccine. Available at: http://www.fda.gov/cber/safety/gardasil071408.htm. Accessed November 14, 2008.

[48] FDA. Rotarix product approval information. Available at: http://www.fda.gov/cber/products/rotarix.htm. Accessed November 17, 2008.

[49] CDC. ACIP provisional recommendations for the prevention of rotavirus gastroenteritis among infants and children. Available at: http://www.cdc.gov/vaccines/recs/provisional/downloads/roto-7-1-08-508.pdf. Accessed November 21, 2008.

[50] Vesikari T, Matson DO, Dennehy P, et al. Safety and efficacy of a pentavalent human bovine (WC3) reassortant rotavirus vaccine. N Engl J Med 2006;354:23–33.

[51] Ruiz-Palacios GM, Perez-Schael I, Velázquez FR, et al. Safety and efficacy of an attenuated vaccine against severe rotavirus gastroenteritis. N Engl J Med 2006;354:11–22.

[52] Haber P, Patel M, Izurieta HS, et al. Postlicensure monitoring of intussusceptions after Rota-teq vaccination in the United States. Pediatrics 2008;121:1206–12.

[53] CDC. Delayed onset and diminished magnitude of rotavirus activity—United States. MMWR Morb Mortal Wkly Rep 2008;57:697–700.

[54] Daskalaki I, Wood SJ, Inumerable YM, et al. Epidemiology of rotavirus associated hospitaliza-tions pre and post implementation of immunization: North Philadelphia 2000–2008. Presen-tation G1-432, Annual Meeting of the IDSA/ICAAC. Washington, DC, October 25-28, 2008.

[55] Harrison CJ, Jackson M, Olson-Burgess C, et al. Fewer 2008 hospitalizations for rotavirus (RV) in Kansas City, two years post RV vaccine. Presentation G1-435. Annual Meeting of the IDSA/ICAAC. Washington, DC October 25–28, 2008.

[56] Hatch S, Fontechio S, Gibson L, et al. Rapid decline in pediatric rotavirus cases following introduction of rotavirus vaccine. Presentation G1-436. Annual Meeting of the IDSA/ICAAC. Washington, DC October 25–28, 2008.

[57] Liebermann JM, Huang X, Koski E, et al. Decline in rotavirus cases in the US after licensure of a live, oral rotavirus vaccine. Presentation G1-437. Annual Meeting of the IDSA/ICAAC. Washington, DC, October 25–28, 2008.

[58] CDC. Prevention and control of influenza. Recommendations of the ACIP. MMWR Morb Mortal Wkly Rep 2008;57:1–60.

[59] Zaman K, Roy E, Arifeen SE, et al. Effectiveness of maternal influenza immunization in mothers and infants. N Engl J Med 2008;359:1555–64.

[60] Eisenberg CW, Szilagyi PG, Fairbrother G, et al. Vaccine effectiveness against laboratory-confirmed influenza in children 6 to 59 months of age during the 2003–2004 and 2004–2005 influenza seasons. Pediatrics 2008;122:911–9.

[61] Poehling KA, Edwards KM, Weinberg GA, et al. The underrecognized burden of influenza in young children. N Engl J Med 2006;355:31–40.

[62] Elveback LR, Fox JP, Ackerman E, et al. An influenza simulation model for immunization studies. Am J Epidemiol 1976;103:152–65.

[63] Piedra PA, Gaglani MJ, Kozinetz CA, et al. Herd immunity in adults against influenza related illnesses with use of the trivalent-live attenuated influenza vaccine (CAIV-T) in chil-dren. Vaccine 2005;23:1540–8.

[64] Davis MM, King JC, Moag L, et al. Countrywide school-based influenza immunization: direct and indirect impact on student absenteeism. Pediatrics 2008;122:e260–5.

[65] Neuzil KM, Hohlbein C, Zhu Y. Illness amongst school children during influenza season: effect of school absenteeism, parental absenteeism from work, and secondary illness in families. Arch Pediatr Adolesc Med 2002;156:986–91.

[66] CDC. 2008-2009 Influenza prevention and control recommendations: Influenza vaccina-tion coverage levels. Available at: http://www.cdc.gov/flu/professionals/acip/coveragelevels.htm Accessed November 24, 2008.

[67] Harper SA, Fuduka K, Uyeki TM, et al. Prevention and control of influenza: recommenda-tions of the Advisory Committee on Immunization Practices (ACIP). MMWR Recomm Rep 2004;53:1–40.

[68] FDA. Kinrix product information. Available at: http://www.fda.gov/cber/products/kinrix.htm. Accessed November 14, 2008.

[69] FDA. Pentacel product information. Available at: http://www.fda.gov/CbER/products/pentacel.htm. Accessed November 24, 2008.

[70] CDC. Hib vaccine shortage. Available at: http://www.cdc.gov/vaccines/vac-gen/short-ages/downloads/hib-flyer-042308.pdf. Accessed November 24, 2008.

[71] CDC. ACIP, VFC Program. Vaccines to prevent poliomyelitis. Available at: http://www.cdc.gov/vaccines/programs/vfc/downloads/resolutions/0608polio.pdf. Accessed November 24, 2008.

[72] CDC. Update: recommendations from the Advisory Committee on Immunization Practices (ACIP) regarding administration of combination MMRV vaccine. MMWR Morb Mortal Wkly Rep 2008;57:258–60.

[73] CDC. Update: prevention of hepatitis A after exposure to hepatitis A vaccine and in international travelers. Updated recommendations of the ACIP. MMWR Morb Mortal Wkly Rep 2007;56:1080–4.

[74] Gavi Alliance. Available at: http://www.gavialliance.org/vision/strategy/vaccine_investment/index.php. Accessed November 14, 2008.

[75] Orenstein W. NVAC Vaccine Financing workgroup white paper. Presented at the NVAC meeting, June 3–4, 2008, Washington, DC.

[76] CDC. Update: measles—United States. MMWR Morb Mortal Wkly Rep 2008;57:893–6.

[77] AAP. New immunization alliance issues national call to action. Available at: http://www.aap.org/advocacy/releases/sept08Immunizationalliance.htm. Accessed January 15, 2008.

[78] Gust DA, Darling N, Kennedy A, et al. Parents with doubts about vaccines: which vaccines and reasons why. Pediatrics 2008;122:718–25.

Advances in Pediatrics 56 (2009) 47–73

ELSEVIER
MOSBY

ADVANCES IN PEDIATRICS

Severe Childhood Respiratory Viral Infections

Kam-Lun Hon, MD (CUHK)[a,*],
Alexander K.C. Leung, MBBS, FRCPC, FRCP(UK&Irel),
FRCPCH, FAAP[b]

[a]Department of Paediatrics, Prince of Wales Hospital, The Chinese University of Hong Kong,
Shatin, New Territories, Hong Kong
[b]Department of Pediatrics, The Alberta Children's Hospital, University of Calgary, # 200, 233-
16th Avenue NW, Calgary, AB T2M 0H5, Canada

R espiratory viruses cause significant morbidity and mortality worldwide. The usual clinical manifestations are described as symptomatology of "common cold." Although diseases caused by these viruses are usually trivial and lasting only a few days, these viruses can cause diseases that are severe and at time fatal. Common respiratory viruses include influenza and parainfluenza viruses, respiratory syncytial virus (RSV), adenovirus, and rhinovirus. This review describes severe viral infections caused by the various respiratory viruses. Specific entities of childhood respiratory infections of the upper airway, lower airway, and lung parenchyma are described.

EPIDEMIOLOGY

Epidemiologic data on respiratory viral infections are available in many nations, and many factors have been studied in predicting outcome and guiding national policy on management of these infections. Respiratory viral infections cause significant morbidity and misery, affecting millions of children annually worldwide.

Although most infections are short-lived and managed by the general practitioner, some children are seriously affected and require hospitalization [1–11]. These viruses account for a large workload in many pediatric departments and are responsible for upper respiratory infections, croup, bronchiolitis, and pneumonia.

In a study of nearly 100,000 pediatric admissions, the commonest childhood hospital admissions were associated with respiratory viral infections [2]. Chiu and colleagues [8] also described that influenza infections were the commonest. Assessing disease burden of respiratory disorders in Hong Kong children with hospital discharge data and linked laboratory data, Nelson and colleagues [3]

*Corresponding author. E-mail address: ehon@cuhk.edu.hk (K-L. Hon).

0065-3101/09/$ – see front matter
doi:10.1016/j.yapd.2009.08.019

found that a primary diagnosis of a respiratory disorder was common (upper respiratory 30.1%, tonsillitis/pharyngitis 10.5%, croup/laryngitis 2.3%, acute otitis media 2.7%, bronchitis/chest infection 2.6%, bronchiolitis 10.2%, pneumonia 20.9%, influenza 4%, asthma and allergic rhinitis 16.5%). In a recent study, viral and atypical bacterial pathogens in children hospitalized with acute respiratory infections were identified by using a broad-capture, rapid, and sensitive method (multiplex polymerase chain reaction [PCR] assay) to detect 20 different respiratory pathogens from respiratory specimens of 475 children hospitalized over a 12-month period for acute respiratory tract infections, including influenza A subtypes H1, H3, and H5; influenza B; parainfluenza types 1, 2, 3, and 4; RSV groups A and B; adenoviruses; human rhinoviruses; enteroviruses; human metapneumoviruses; human coronaviruses OC43, 229E, and SARS-CoV; *Chlamydophila pneumoniae; Legionella pneumophila;* and *Mycoplasma pneumoniae* [12]. The overall positive rate (47%) was about 2 times higher than previous reports based on conventional methods. Influenza A, parainfluenza, and RSV accounted for 51%, and noncultivable viruses accounted for 30% of positive cases. Influenza A peaked in March and June. Influenza B was detected in January, February, and April. Parainfluenza was prevalent throughout the year except from April to June. Most RSV infections were found between February and September. Adenovirus had multiple peaks, whereas rhinovirus and coronavirus OC43 were detected mainly in winter and early spring. RSV infection was associated with bronchiolitis, and parainfluenza was associated with croup; otherwise the clinical manifestations were largely nonspecific. In general, children infected with influenza A, adenovirus, and mixed viruses had higher temperatures. In view of the increasing concern about unexpected outbreaks of severe viral infections, a rapid multiplex PCR assay is a valuable tool to enhance the management of hospitalized patients, and for the surveillance for viral infections circulating in the community.

Among hospital admissions, a small percentage of children would require pediatric intensive care unit (PICU) support [13–16]. Hon and colleagues [17] reported the clinical pattern and outcome of all children with a laboratory-proven diagnosis of respiratory virus infection admitted to the PICU of a teaching hospital. Three respiratory virus species, RSV (n = 17), influenza (n = 13), and parainfluenza (n = 12), accounted for 86% of cases. PICU admissions due to influenza A were more common than influenza B, whereas parainfluenza type 3 was the commonest subtype of parainfluenza infection. Comparing these 3 common viruses, the mean age of children admitted with RSV was lower than with influenza or parainfluenza. Preexisting conditions such as prematurity and chronic lung disease were only present in children with RSV infection. These respiratory viruses caused both upper (croup) and lower respiratory tract diseases (bronchiolitis, pneumonia). Extrapulmonary presentations were less prevalent and included encephalitis, seizures, cardiac arrest, coexisting diabetes ketoacidosis, and acute lymphoblastic leukemia. One patient with RSV and another with influenza A died during their PICU stay. Nearly half of these patients required ventilatory support or received systemic corticosteroids, and 88% received initial broad-spectrum antibiotic coverage. Approximately 1 in 5 of them had nebulized adrenaline, airway endoscopies, or bacterial coinfections. Adenovirus was isolated in 4 patients, and 2 (both with adenovirus type 3) died during the PICU stay. Similar findings in PICU were reported [14,15]. In particular, influenza infection causes significant morbidity and mortality in young children [15]. Immunizations are recommended for all children aged 6 months to 18 years. Although severe forms of influenza are rare in children, the disease may be life-threatening and most occur in children with underlying disease [16]. During the 2003 influenza season there was an increased number of children with influenza A infection admitted to an Australian PICU, and an increased number of deaths compared with previous years [16]. The cost of influenza-related hospitalizations in children is high [13]. In a United States study, high-risk patients had higher mean total costs than low-risk patients, and cardiac, metabolic, and neurologic/neuromuscular diseases and age of 18 to 21 years were independently associated with the highest hospitalization costs [13].

THE VIRUSES
Influenza viruses
The influenza viruses are RNA viruses of the family *Orthomyxoviridae*. Influenzavirus A, Influenzavirus B, and Influenzavirus C are the genera that affect humans [18]. Influenzavirus A has one species, influenza A virus. The type A viruses are the most virulent human pathogens among the 3 influenza types and cause the most severe disease [19]. The influenza A virus has different serotypes based on the antibody response to these viruses [20]. Influenzavirus B also has only one species. The virus almost exclusively infects humans [20], and is less common than influenza A. This virus mutates at a lower rate than type A and consequently is less genetically diverse, with only one influenza B serotype [20,21]. This reduced rate of antigenic change, combined with its limited host range, ensures that pandemics of influenza B do not occur [18,22]. Influenzavirus C has only one species. Influenza C virus causes mild disease in children [23,24]. Indeed, seroepidemiological studies have revealed that influenza C virus is widely distributed globally. Nevertheless, because the isolation of this virus is difficult, there have been few reports on its clinical features [23]. Severe illness and local epidemics from influenza C have been reported [19,23,25]. Hay and colleagues [20] summarized the evolution of influenza viruses, which results in recurrent annual epidemics of disease that are caused by progressive antigenic drift of influenza A and B viruses due to the mutability of the RNA genome, and infrequent but severe pandemics caused by the emergence of novel influenza A subtypes to which the population has little immunity. The latter characteristic is a consequence of the wide antigenic diversity and peculiar host range of influenza A viruses, and the ability of their segmented RNA genomes to undergo frequent genetic reassortment (recombination) during mixed infections. Contrasting features of the evolution of recently circulating influenza AH1N1, AH3N2, and B viruses include the rapid

drift of AH3N2 viruses as a single lineage, the slow replacement of successive antigenic variants of AH1N1 viruses, and the cocirculation over some 25 years of antigenically and genetically distinct lineages of influenza B viruses. Constant monitoring of changes in the circulating viruses is important for maintaining the efficacy of influenza vaccines in combating disease.

The diagnosis of influenza based on clinical impression is problematic. In a prospective study, children 13 years old or younger with respiratory infections were examined [26]. At each visit, a nasal swab specimen was obtained for the detection of influenza, and the physician recorded his or her opinion on whether the child had influenza. Among 2288 infections, the overall sensitivity of the clinical diagnosis of influenza was 38% and the positive predictive value was 32%.

The transmission of influenza can be mathematically modeled to help predicting how the virus will spread in a population [27,28]. People who contract influenza are most infectious between the second and third days after infection, and infectivity lasts for around 10 days [27]. Children are much more infectious than adults, and shed virus from just before they develop symptoms until 2 weeks after infection [27,29]. For influenza control it is very important to investigate viral shedding and resistant viruses [29]. According to Mitamura and colleagues [29], viral loads are decreased after the start of antiviral agents, but resistant viruses are detected in some patients. Influenza can be spread by direct transmission when an infected person sneezes mucus into the eyes, nose, or mouth of another person; through people inhaling the aerosols produced by infected people with coughing, sneezing, and spitting; and through hand-to-mouth transmission from contaminated surfaces or direct personal contact [30,31]. The relative importance of airborne, droplet, and contact transmission of influenza A virus and the efficiency of control measures depends on the inactivation of viruses in different environmental media. Weber and colleagues [31] systematically reviewed information on the environmental inactivation of influenza A viruses and modes of transmission. The airborne route is a potentially important transmission pathway for influenza in indoor environments. The importance of droplet transmission has to be reassessed. Contact transmission can be limited by fast inactivation of influenza virus on hands, and is more dependent on behavioral parameters than airborne transmission. However, the potentially large inocula deposited in the environment through sneezing and the protective effect of nasal mucus on virus survival could make contact transmission a key transmission mode. In the airborne route, it has been demonstrated that the inhalation of just one inhalable droplet (0.5–5 μm in diameter) might be enough to cause an infection [31]. Although a single sneeze releases up to 40,000 droplets [32], most of these droplets are large and will quickly settle out of the air [31]. The influenza virus can also be transmitted by contaminated surfaces. Successful control of a viral disease requires knowledge of the different vectors that could promote its transmission among hosts. Thomas and colleagues [33] assessed the survival of human influenza viruses on banknotes, given that billions of these notes are exchanged daily worldwide. Banknotes were experimentally contaminated with representative influenza virus subtypes at various concentrations, and survival was tested after different time periods. Influenza A viruses tested by cell culture survived up to 3 days when they were inoculated at high concentrations. The same inoculum in the presence of respiratory mucus showed a striking increase in survival time (up to 17 days). B/Hong Kong/335/2001 virus was still infectious after 1 day when it was mixed with respiratory mucus. When nasopharyngeal secretions of naturally infected children were used, influenza virus survived for at least 48 h in one-third of the cases. The investigators concluded that unexpected stability of influenza virus in this nonbiological environment suggests that unusual environmental contamination should be considered in the setting of pandemic preparedness [33]. Bean and colleagues investigated the transmission of influenza viruses via hands and environmental surfaces; the survival of laboratory-grown influenza A and influenza B viruses on various surfaces was studied. Both influenza A and B viruses survived for 24 to 48 hours on hard, nonporous surfaces such as stainless steel and plastic, but survived for less than 8 to 12 hours on cloth, paper, and tissues. Measurable quantities of influenza A virus were transferred from stainless steel surfaces to hands for 24 hours and from tissues to hands for up to 15 minutes. Virus survived on hands for up to 5 minutes after transfer from the environmental surfaces. Their observations suggest that the transmission of virus from donors who are shedding large amounts could occur for 2 to 8 hours via stainless steel surfaces and for a few minutes via paper tissues. The investigators concluded that the transmission of influenza virus via fomites may be possible under conditions of heavy environmental contamination [34]. However, if the virus is present in mucus, the virus can survive for longer periods [31].

New influenza viruses are constantly evolving by mutation or by reassortment [20]. Definitive means of prophylaxis is by vaccination. In particular, high-risk patients may develop life-threatening primary viral pneumonia or complications such as bacterial pneumonia [35]. Vaccination against influenza with an influenza vaccine is recommended for all children 6 months to 18 years old. Due to the high mutation rate of the virus, a particular influenza vaccine usually confers protection for no more than a few years. The World Health Organization annually predicts which viral strains are most likely to be circulating in the next year, allowing pharmaceutical companies to develop vaccines that will provide the best immunity against these strains [35]. The vaccine is reformulated each season for a few specific flu strains. Hence, it is possible to be vaccinated and still get influenza.

In an influenza pandemic, the benefit of vaccines and antiviral medications are often constrained by limitations on supplies and effectiveness. Nonpharmaceutical public health interventions are vital in curtailing disease spread. Good personal health and hygiene habits, such as hand washing, avoiding spitting, and covering the nose and mouth when sneezing or coughing, are reasonably effective in reducing influenza transmission [36]. In particular, hand washing with soap and water or with alcohol-based hand rubs is effective in inactivating influenza viruses [37]. These simple personal hygiene precautions are recommended as the main way of reducing infections during pandemics [36,37]. Surface sanitizing may also help prevent influenza and respiratory viral infections [38]. Alcohol is an effective sanitizer against influenza viruses. Quaternary ammonium compounds can also be used with alcohol so that the sanitizing effect lasts for longer [39]. A wide variety of active chemical agents (biocides) are found in these sanitizing products, many of which have been used for hundreds of years, including alcohols, phenols, iodine, and chlorine [39]. In hospitals, quaternary ammonium compounds and bleach are used to sanitize rooms that have been occupied by or equipment used for patients with influenza symptoms [39].

It is uncertain if reducing public gatherings, by for example closing schools and workplaces, will reduce transmission because people with influenza may just be moved from one area to another; such measures would also be difficult to enforce and are often unpopular [36]. When small numbers of people are infected, isolating the sick might reduce the risk of transmission [36]. Influenza infects many animal species, and transfer of viral strains between species can occur. Birds are thought to be the principal animal reservoirs of influenza viruses [40]. Phylogenetic analysis showed that nucleoprotein genes have evolved into 5 host-specific lineages, including (i) Equine/Prague/56 (EQPR56), (ii) recent equine strains, (iii) classic swine (H1N1 swine, eg, A/Swine/Iowa/15/30) and human strains, (iv) gull H13 viruses, and (v) avian strains (including North American, Australian, and Old World subgroups). The presence of avian and human nucleoproteins in some swine isolates demonstrates the susceptibility of swine to different viral strains, and supports the hypothesis that swine may serve as intermediates for the introduction of avian influenza virus genes into the human virus gene pool [40]. Some strains are highly virulent to poultry, and may cause more severe symptoms and significant mortality [41,42]. An avian-adapted, highly pathogenic strain of H5N1 (called HPAI A[H5N1], for "highly pathogenic avian influenza virus of type A of subtype H5N1") causes H5N1 flu (or "avian influenza"), which is endemic in many bird populations, especially in Southeast Asia. This Asian lineage strain of HPAI A (H5N1) is spreading globally. At present, there is no evidence suggesting efficient human-to-human transmission of HPAI A (H5N1). Nevertheless, H5N1 may mutate or reassort into a strain capable of efficient human-to-human transmission. The exact changes that are required for this to happen are not well understood, and there is a need to find better predictors of both seasonal and potentially pandemic influenza [43].

Outbreaks in pigs are common and do not cause severe mortality [44]. In 2009 an outbreak of influenza A virus subtype H1N1 occurred in Mexico. The virus is being commonly referred to as "swine flu," but there is no evidence of transmission from pigs to people; instead the virus is spreading from person to person. This strain is a reassortment of several strains of H1N1 that are usually found separately, in humans, birds, and pigs [45].

Parainfluenza viruses

Parainfluenza viruses belong to the RNA *paramyxovirus* family, and are a common cause of respiratory infections in children [46–48]. These viruses are the second most common cause of lower respiratory tract infection in younger children [48]. Human parainfluenza viruses (HPIVs) are second to RSV as a common cause of lower respiratory tract disease in young children. Similar to RSV, HPIVs can cause repeated upper respiratory tract infections throughout life. HPIVs can also cause serious lower respiratory tract disease with recurrent infection (eg, pneumonia, bronchitis, and bronchiolitis) [48]. Each of the 4 HPIVs has different clinical and epidemiologic features. The most distinctive clinical feature of HPIV-1 and HPIV-2 is croup (ie, laryngotracheobronchitis); HPIV-1 is the leading cause of croup in children, whereas HPIV-2 is less frequently detected. Both HPIV-1 and HPIV-2 can cause other upper and lower respiratory tract illnesses. HPIV-3 is more often associated with bronchiolitis and pneumonia. HPIV-4 is infrequently detected, possibly because it is less likely to cause severe disease. The incubation period for HPIVs is generally from 1 to 7 days [49]. The virion is unstable in the environment (surviving a few hours on environmental surfaces), and is readily inactivated with soap and water. HPIVs spread from respiratory secretions through close contact with infected persons, or contact with contaminated surfaces or objects. Infection can occur when infectious material contacts mucous membranes of the eyes, mouth, or nose, and possibly through the inhalation of droplets generated by a sneeze or cough. HPIVs can remain infectious in aerosols for over an hour. HPIVs are ubiquitous and infect most people during childhood. The highest rates of serious HPIV illnesses occur among young children. Serologic surveys have shown that 90% to 100% of children aged 5 years and older have antibodies to HPIV-3, and about 75% have antibodies to HPIV-1 and -2. The different HPIV serotypes differ in their clinical features and seasonality. HPIV-1 causes biennial outbreaks of croup in the fall (presently in the United States during odd-numbered years). HPIV-2 causes annual or biennial fall outbreaks. HPIV-3 peak activity occurs during the spring and early summer months each year, but the virus can be isolated throughout the year. Infection with HPIVs can be confirmed either by isolation and identification of the virus in cell culture or by direct detection of the virus in respiratory secretions (usually collected within 1 week of onset of symptoms) using immunofluorescence, enzyme immunoassay, or PCR assay, or by demonstration of a significant increase in specific IgG antibodies between appropriately collected paired serum specimens or specific IgM antibodies in a single serum specimen. In particular, the multiplex reverse transcription-PCR (RT-PCR) assay can be used as a rapid and sensitive diagnostic method for the viruses [50]. Accumulating knowledge on the molecular structure and mechanisms of replication of HPIVs has accelerated research on prevention and treatment. Several strategies for vaccine development, such as the use of live attenuated, inactivated, recombinant, and subunit vaccines, have been investigated, and it may become possible to prevent HPIV infections in the near future.

Nevertheless, no vaccine is currently available to protect against infection caused by any of the HPIVs [51]. Passively acquired maternal antibodies may play a role in protection from HPIV types 1 and 2 in the first few months of life, highlighting the importance of breastfeeding. Strict attention to infection-control practices should decrease or prevent spread of infection. Frequent hand washing and not sharing items such as cups, glasses, and utensils with an infected person should decrease the spread of virus to others. Excluding children with colds or other respiratory illnesses (without fever) who are well enough to attend child care or school settings will probably not decrease the spread of HPIVs, because the viruses are often spread in the early stages of illness. In a hospital setting, spread of HPIVs can and should be prevented by strict attention to contact precautions, such as hand washing and wearing of protective gowns and gloves.

Rhinovirus

Rhinoviruses (RVs) are nonenveloped single-strand RNA viruses that belong to the *Picornaviridae* family. The virus is most frequently associated with common cold. Rhinovirus plays a significant role in the pathogenesis of otitis media and asthma exacerbations [52,53]. Current evidence indicates that viral, and not bacterial, infections are the most important respiratory illnesses that increase the severity of asthma [52]. The most significant risk factor for the development of preschool childhood wheezing is the occurrence of symptomatic rhinovirus illnesses during infancy, which are clinically and prognostically informative based on their seasonal nature [54]. RVs have proven to be the virus most often found in association with increased asthma severity [52]. With the use of sensitive RT-PCR methods, respiratory viruses are found in approximately 80% of wheezing episodes in children and in approximately one-half of such episodes in adults [53]. In one study, RV RNA was detectable in more than 40% of asthmatic children 6 weeks after an acute exacerbation [55]. Asthma exacerbations were more severe in patients with persistence of RV RNA, suggesting that the severity of acute asthma might be linked to prolonged and possibly more severe RV infections. Most cases of RV infection are mild and self-limited despite its high incidence and prevalence. Nasopharyngitis, croup, and pneumonia are occasionally caused by RV. RVs can be transmitted by aerosol or direct contact. The primary site of inoculation is the nasal mucosa. The conjunctiva may be involved to a lesser extent. RV attaches to respiratory epithelium and spreads locally. RV does not efficiently replicate at body temperature. The optimal temperature for RV replication is 33 to 35°C. This fact may explain why RV replicates well in the nasal passages and upper tracheobronchial tree, but less well in the lower respiratory tract. The incubation period is approximately 2 to 4 days [49]. RV is shed in large amounts, with as many as 1 million infectious virions present per milliliter of nasal washings, but viremia is uncommon. Viral shedding can occur a few days before cold symptoms are recognized by the patient, peaks on days 2 to 7 of the illness, and may last as long as 3 to 4 weeks. A local inflammatory response to the virus in the respiratory tract can lead to nasal discharge, nasal congestion, sneezing, and throat irritation.

RV possesses various transmission modes and can infect a huge population at any given time. Aerosol transmission is the most common transmission mode for respiratory tract infections. Transmission occurs when small airborne particles are inhaled or large droplets are directly touched. Direct hand contact with infected secretions or indirect contact with fomites is also important. Patients then infect themselves by touching their noses or conjunctivae. Highly contagious behavior includes nose blowing, sneezing, and physically transferring infected secretions onto environmental surfaces or paper tissue. Contrary to popular belief, behaviors such as kissing, talking, coughing, or even drooling do not contribute highly to the spread of disease. Infection rates approximate 50% within the household and range from 0% to 50% within schools, which indicates that transmission requires long-term contact with infected individuals. Brief exposures to others in places such as movie theaters, shopping malls, friends' houses, or doctors' offices incur low risk of transmission.

Pleconaril is an orally bioavailable antiviral drug being developed for the treatment of infections caused by picornaviruses [56]. This drug acts by binding to a hydrophobic pocket in VP1, and stabilizes the protein capsid to such an extent that the virus cannot release its RNA genome into the target cell. When tested in volunteers, during the clinical trials this drug caused a significant decrease in mucus secretions and illness-associated symptoms [57]. However, the Food and Drug Administration has not approved this drug for treatment of common cold, and the gastrointestinal side effects are not insignificant.

Coronavirus and severe acute respiratory syndrome

Coronavirus is a genus of animal virus belonging to the family *Coronaviridae*, and the virus is enveloped with a positive-sense single-stranded RNA genome and a helical symmetry [58]. Human coronaviruses are difficult to grow in the laboratory. Coronaviruses primarily infect the upper respiratory and gastrointestinal tract of mammals and birds. The most publicized human coronavirus, SARS-CoV, which causes severe acute respiratory syndrome (SARS), has a unique pathogenesis because it causes both upper and lower respiratory tract infections and can also cause gastroenteritis. Coronaviruses are believed to cause a significant percentage of all common colds in human adults, primarily in the winter and early spring seasons [49].

In 2003, following the outbreak of SARS that had begun in the previous year in Asia, and secondary cases elsewhere in the world, the World Health Organization issued a press release stating that a novel coronavirus identified by several laboratories was the causative agent for SARS [59]. The virus was officially named the SARS coronavirus (SARS-CoV). The genome of SARS-CoV is 29,727 nucleotides in length and has 11 open reading frames, and its genome organization is similar to that of other coronaviruses. Phylogenetic analyses and sequence comparisons show that SARS-CoV is not closely related to any of the previously characterized coronaviruses [60] The SARS epidemic resulted in more than 8000 infections, about 10% of which resulted in death [61]. Following the high-profile publicity of SARS outbreaks, there has been a renewed interest in coronaviruses. For many years, scientists knew only about the existence of 2 human coronaviruses (HCoV-229E and HCoV-OC43). The discovery of SARS-CoV added another human coronavirus to the list. By the end of 2004, 3 independent research laboratories reported the discovery of a fourth human coronavirus, named NL63, NL, or the New Haven coronavirus by the different research groups [62]. Screening of clinical specimens from individuals suffering from respiratory illness identified additional HCoV-NL63–infected individuals, indicating that the virus was widely spread within the human population [62].

Adenovirus

Adenovirus infections most commonly cause illness of the respiratory system as well as various other illnesses, such as gastroenteritis, conjunctivitis, and cystitis. Symptoms caused by adenovirus infection range from the common cold syndrome to pneumonia, croup, and bronchitis [49,63]. Patients with compromised immune systems are especially susceptible to severe complications of adenovirus infection. Adenoviruses are transmitted by direct contact, fecal-oral transmission, and occasionally waterborne transmission. Some types are capable of establishing persistent asymptomatic infections in tonsils, adenoids, and intestines of infected hosts, and shedding can occur for months or years. Adenovirus infections can occur throughout the year but outbreaks of adenovirus-associated respiratory disease are more common in the late winter, spring, and early summer. Antigen detection, PCR assay, virus isolation, and serology can be used to identify adenovirus infections. Because adenovirus can be excreted for prolonged periods, the presence of virus does not necessarily mean it is associated with disease. Most infections are mild and require either no therapy or only symptomatic treatment. Because there is no virus-specific therapy, serious adenovirus illness can be managed only by treating symptoms and complications of the infection. Deaths are rare but have been reported [17]. Strict attention to good infection control practices is effective for stopping nosocomial outbreaks of adenovirus-associated disease, such as epidemic keratoconjunctivitis. Maintaining adequate levels of chlorination is necessary for preventing swimming pool associated outbreaks of adenovirus conjunctivitis.

Human metapneumovirus

Human metapneumovirus (hMPV) was first isolated in 2001 in the Netherlands by using the RNA arbitrarily primed PCR (RAP-PCR) technique for identification of unknown viruses growing in cultured cells [64,65]. Serologic studies showed that by the age of 5 years, virtually all children in the Netherlands have been exposed to human metapneumovirus, and that the virus has been circulating in humans for at least 50 years [64]. hMPV is a negative single-stranded RNA virus of the family *Paramyxoviridae*, and is closely related to the avian metapneumovirus (AMPV) subgroup C. hMPV may be the second most common cause (after the RSV) of lower respiratory infection in young children, although infection with hMPV tends to occur in slightly older children and to produce disease that is less severe [63,66–68]. Coinfection with both viruses can occur, and is generally associated with worse disease [69]. hMPV has been shown to have worldwide circulation, with nearly universal infection by age 5 years. Similar to influenza and RSV, activity is greatest during the winter in temperate climates [63,66,67]. Most of the available data on the clinical manifestations of hMPV infection are from studies of children in whom the virus causes upper respiratory tract infections, bronchiolitis, and pneumonia [63,66,67]. Reinfections with hMPV occur throughout adult life, and hMPV infection has been documented in 1% to 9% of adults each year using RT-PCR and serology for diagnosis. Illness is generally mild in young adults, with serologic evidence of asymptomatic infection in many cases [65]. Human metapneumovirus accounts for approximately 10% of respiratory tract infections that are not related to previously known causative agents [70]. The virus seems to be distributed worldwide and to have a seasonal distribution, with its incidence comparable to that of the influenza viruses during winter [63,64,67,71]. Serologic studies have shown that by the age of 5 years virtually all children have been exposed to the virus, and reinfections are common. Human metapneumovirus usually causes mild respiratory tract infection, although small children and immunocompromised individuals are at risk of severe disease and hospitalization [64]. The identification of hMPV has predominantly relied on RT-PCR technology to amplify directly from RNA extracted from respiratory specimens. Treatment is symptomatic. No effective treatment or vaccine for hMPV is currently available, but ribavirin has shown effectiveness in an animal model [70,72].

MAJOR CATEGORIES OF VIRAL INFECTIONS OF THE RESPIRATORY TRACT

All the aforementioned viruses can lead to infections of different parts of the respiratory systems, with distinctive symptomatology. These parts can be divided into the upper airway syndrome, the lower airway, and the lung parenchyma.

Common cold, upper respiratory tract infection, and flu

The symptoms of common cold or upper respiratory tract infection resemble symptoms of influenza disease except that they are usually milder. Symptoms of influenza can start abruptly 1 to 2 days after infection [73]. Usually the first symptoms are chills or a chilly sensation, and fever with body temperatures ranging from 38 to 39°C [74,75]. Suzuki and colleagues [74] studied the natural course of fever during influenza virus infection in children, and found that fever was most prominent in A/H3N2 and young children. Secondary fever was observed frequently at 72 to 132 hours in all types. The duration of fever was associated negatively with the age of the child and positively with the maximal temperature [74]. Symptoms of influenza may also include aches, especially joints and throat, extreme coldness, fatigue, headache, irritated watering eyes, and reddened eyes, face, mouth, throat, and nose [73]. It is difficult to distinguish between the common cold and influenza in the early stages of these infections [73,75], but flu can be identified by a high fever with a sudden onset and extreme fatigue [75]. In the subtropics, influenza is an important cause of hospitalization among children, with rates exceeding those reported for temperate regions [8] and influenza-related hospitalizations among children in Hong Kong [7]. The influenza viruses are significant human respiratory pathogens that cause both seasonal, endemic infections and periodic, unpredictable pandemics. The worst pandemic on record, in 1918, killed approximately 50 million people worldwide. It is striking that the spectrum of pathologic changes described in the 1918 influenza pandemic is not significantly different from the histopathology observed in other less lethal pandemics or even in deaths occurring during seasonal influenza outbreaks [19]. Coronaviruses, parainfluenza, and RSV are important viruses that can cause the clinical syndrome of common colds. Other viruses such as adenoviruses and influenza viruses can cause common colds, but are more likely to cause acute nasopharyngitis and more severe respiratory infections.

Several studies demonstrate the incidence of the common cold to be highest in preschool and elementary school-aged children. An average of 3 to 8 colds per year is observed in this age group, with an even higher incidence in children who attend daycare centers. Because of the numerous viral agents involved and the many serotypes of several viruses (especially RV), it is not unusual for younger children to have new colds each month during the winter season. Adults and adolescents typically have 2 to 4 colds per year. A seasonal increase in incidence during the winter months is observed worldwide. The most common manifestation of RV, the common cold, is mild and self-limited. Common colds, by definition, do not have objective evidence of pharyngeal irritation, and RV is an uncommon cause of acute nasopharyngitis. However, severe respiratory disease, including bronchiolitis, asthma exacerbations, and pneumonia can occur in infants and young children [76]. Indeed, RV may be associated with more severe lower respiratory tract infection in children than previously reported, particularly in the noninfluenza, RSV season [76]. Because antibodies to viral serotypes develop over time, the highest incidence is found in infants and young children. In addition, young children are more likely to have the frequent, close, personal contact necessary to transmit rhinovirus.

Children with common cold are usually afebrile, although temperatures of 38 to 39°C may occur in younger children. Profuse nasal discharge can be clear and watery or mucopurulent. Purulent secretions are common after the first few days of illness, and do not imply bacterial sinusitis unless symptoms and signs of an upper respiratory infection persist for more than 10 days without appreciable improvement [77]. Despite sore throat, the pharynx has a normal appearance, without any erythema, exudate, or ulceration. Infection occurs rapidly, with the virus adhering to surface receptors within 15 minutes of entering the respiratory tract. RVs preferentially grow at 32°C as opposed to the body temperature of 37°C, and hence infect mainly the upper respiratory tract.

Influenza can cause pneumonia, which can be fatal particularly for the young and the elderly. Although it is often confused with other influenza-like viral infections such as the common cold, influenza is generally a more severe disease [73]. Influenza is typically transmitted through airborne aerosols created by coughing or sneezing. Infections also occur through contact with infected body fluids or with contaminated surfaces. Influenza viruses can be inactivated by sunlight, disinfectants, and detergents [78].

Vaccinations against influenza are available [79,80]. The most common human vaccine is the trivalent influenza vaccine (TIV) that contains purified and inactivated material from 3 viral strains. This vaccine typically includes material from 2 influenza A virus subtypes and 1 influenza B virus strain. The TIV carries no risk of transmitting the disease, and it has very low reactivity. A vaccine formulated for 1 year may be ineffective in the following year, because the influenza virus evolves rapidly and new strains quickly replace the older ones. Most people will recover completely in about 1 to 2 weeks, but some will develop life-threatening complications. Young children, people with chronic medical conditions, and pregnant women are at risk for complications from influenza [81,82]. Guillain-Barré syndrome can be a rare side effect of influenza vaccines, with an incidence of about 1 case per million vaccinations [83]. Adverse event reporting rates have been reasonably constant over time, and no new safety concerns emerged after review of 15 years of postlicensure surveillance data [83].

Patients with flu are advised to get plenty of rest, drink plenty of liquids, avoid using alcohol and tobacco and, if necessary, take medications such as paracetamol (acetaminophen) to relieve the fever and muscle aches associated with the flu. Children and teenagers with flu symptoms (particularly fever) should avoid taking aspirin during an influenza infection (especially influenza type B), because of the risk of Reye syndrome [84]. Antibiotics have no effect on the infection; unless prescribed for secondary infections such as bacterial pneumonia. The 2 classes of antiviral drugs used against influenza are neuraminidase inhibitors and M2 protein inhibitors (adamantane derivatives) [85]. Neuraminidase inhibitors are currently preferred for flu virus infections because they are less toxic and more effective [35]. Antiviral drugs such as oseltamivir (trade name Tamiflu) and zanamivir (trade name Relenza) are neuraminidase inhibitors that are designed to halt the spread of the virus in the body [86]. These drugs are often effective against both influenza A and B [87]. The Cochrane Collaboration reviewed these drugs and concluded that they reduce symptoms and complications [88]. All the aforementioned antiviral drugs shorten the course of influenza disease by approximately 1 day and relieve symptoms to some extent [89]. Different strains of influenza viruses have differing degrees of resistance against these antivirals, and it is impossible to predict what degree of resistance a future pandemic strain might have [90]. The increase in influenza vaccinations among young children, together with the routine therapeutic use of neuraminidase inhibitors, has led to a decrease in the influenza-associated mortality rate [91]. To determine the interventions most likely to curtail an influenza pandemic, Carrat and colleagues [27] and Grassly and colleagues [28] mathematically modeled the transmission of influenza to predict how the virus will spread in a population. These results support the stockpiling of antiviral drugs and accelerated vaccine development. Nevertheless, neuraminidase inhibitors should not be used in routine seasonal influenza control. In a serious epidemic or pandemic, neuraminidase inhibitors should be used with other public health measures. [88].

Acute viral infections producing upper airway obstruction (Croup)

The most common syndrome that often affects infants and children younger than 6 years is laryngotracheobronchitis [92]. The condition is commonly known as croup due to the characteristic croupy cough associated with infection and inflammatory of the subglottic region [92]. Croup is characterized by a barking cough, varying degrees of inspiratory stridor, and hoarseness as a result of laryngeal or tracheal obstruction [93]. The condition may be mild, moderate, or severe, and even fatal. Croup is most often caused by parainfluenza virus, with types 1 and 2 responsible for the majority of cases [92,93]. However, other viral infections can also cause it [17]. Croup is most common in the fall and winter but can occur year-round, with a slight predilection for males [92]. The respiratory distress is caused by an inflammatory response to the infection rather than by the infection itself. Respiratory distress usually occurs in young children as their airways are smaller and differently shaped to those of adults, making them more susceptible. The treatment of croup depends on the severity of symptoms. It is important to maintain a calm atmosphere for the parents and child. Most children can be managed effectively at home. Antipyretics should be given if the child is febrile. Adequate hydration should be maintained. Corticosteroids are the mainstay of therapy [93]. Corticosteroids have potent vasoconstrictive and anti-inflammatory properties, and can reduce airway inflammation, vascular permeability, and mucosal edema [93]. Good evidence now exists to support the use of corticosteroid in the management of severe, moderate, or even mild croup [94]. Dexamethasone is often used due to its prolonged physiologic effects. The severe form requires emergency medical treatment in the intensive care unit. Nebulized epinephrine should be considered for children with moderate to severe croup, and should be used with caution in children who have tachycardia or ventricular outlet obstruction. Racemic epinephrine works by stimulation of the α-adrenergic receptors in the airway with resultant mucosal vasoconstriction and decreased subglottic edema, and by stimulation of the β-adrenergic receptors with resultant relaxation of the bronchial smooth muscle. Randomized studies comparing racemic epinephrine with either placebo or no treatment have shown significant improvements in croup scores in the treated patients over controls [95]. The simultaneous use of corticosteroid helps to reduce the rebound phenomenon associated with the use of epinephrine and obviates the need for hospitalization [93]. Children who have moderate or severe croup with blood oxygen saturation of less than 92% should receive oxygen. Antibiotics have no value. Children with moderate to severe croup are hospitalized for observation. Intubation is rarely needed [17].

Lower airway diseases: wheezy bronchitis and asthma

Bronchitis is a common disease in the adult population but is less frequently described in children. Bronchitis is usually due to common viral infections, but can occasionally be complicated by secondary bacterial infections. Jartti and colleagues [96] detected metapneumovirus by PCR in 10 (8%) of 132 consecutive children admitted to Turku Hospital, Finland, for acute expiratory wheezing (median age 7 months, range 4–25 months). The mean duration of hospital stay was 2.5 days (standard deviation 1.6) and mean duration of respiratory symptoms was 19 days. The white blood cell count, C-reactive protein, and RANTES (Regulated on Activation, Normal T-Expressed and Secreted cytokine) concentrations in nasal secretion remained low, whereas interleukin-8 concentrations in nasal secretion were high. Human metapneumovirus is a clinically important causative agent of acute wheezing in young children [96]. Smuts and colleagues [97] evaluated the role of the novel respiratory viruses, such as human metapneumovirus (hMPV), human coronavirus NL63 (HCoV NL63), and human bocavirus (HBoV) in wheezing illness in children. Consecutive children presenting with acute wheezing to a pediatric hospital from May 2004 to November 2005 were prospectively studied. A nasal swab was taken for RT-PCR and PCR for hMPV, HCoV NL63, and HBoV; when positive, the genes were sequenced. Shell vial culture for RSV, influenza A and B viruses, adenovirus, and parainfluenza viruses 1, 2, and 3 was performed on every fifth sample. Two hundred and forty-two nasal swabs were collected from 238 children (median age 12.4 months). A novel respiratory virus was found in 44 of 242 (18.2%). hMPV, HBoV, and HCoV NL63 was found in 20 (8.3%), 18 (7.4%), and 6 (2.4%) of samples, respectively. Fifteen of 59 (25%) samples were positive for other respiratory viruses. Viral coinfections occurred in 6 of 242 (2.5%). Viruses are an important cause of wheezing in preschool children; hMPV, HCoV NL63, and HBoV are less common than the usual respiratory pathogens [97].

Bronchiolitis

The term usually refers to acute viral bronchiolitis of infancy. In temperate climates, bronchiolitis is most frequently seen during winter and early spring. In tropical countries, the disease occurs more frequently during the rainy season [98]. Bronchiolitis is most commonly caused by RSV (or human pneumovirus) [1,4]. Other common respiratory viruses that may also cause the same clinical entity include metapneumovirus, influenza, parainfluenza, coronavirus, adenovirus, and rhinovirus [66]. Coryza, mild cough, fever, lethargy, and decreased appetite are common at the onset of illness; this then progresses to noisy, raspy breathing and wheezy cough. Physical examination is character-ized by prolonged expiratory phase, wheezing, tachypnea, dyspnea, intercostal retractions, hyperresonance on chest percussion, and tachycardia [98]. The diagnosis is usually made by clinical examination in ambulatory settings. Chest radiography is not routinely indicated, but may sometimes be useful to exclude pneumonia. Testing for specific viral cause such as RSV by nasopharyngeal aspirate can be performed, but the testing usually has little effect on manage-ment. Identification of RSV-positive patients can be helpful for disease surveil-lance, patient cohorts in hospital wards to prevent cross-infection, and reducing the need for other unnecessary diagnostic procedures.

Respiratory complications are common in infants with severe RSV bronchio-litis, which include apnea and hypoxemia [98]. Children with RSV bronchioli-tis in early life are at increased risk of developing asthma later in childhood, although the association is lost by 13 years of age [99,100].

There is no effective specific treatment for bronchiolitis. Therapy is primarily supportive. Frequent small feeds are encouraged to maintain hydra-tion as evidenced by good urine output, and sometimes oxygen may be required to maintain blood oxygen levels. Suction of the nasopharynx to re-move excessive secretions is often performed to maintain a clear airway. In severe cases, nasogastric tube feeding or intravenous fluids are required. In extreme cases, mechanical ventilation might be necessary. Kellner and colleagues [101,102] performed a meta-analysis of bronchodilator therapy in infants with bronchiolitis, and reported that bronchodilators produced a modest short-term improvement in clinical scores. The rate and duration of hospitali-zation, however, were not affected by bronchodilator therapy. The investiga-tors concluded that routine use of bronchodilators in those who wheeze for the first time is not justified, given the modest short-term clinical improvement along with the high cost of the medication. In theory, epinephrine has an added advantage over β_2-adrenergic selective bronchodilators because its α-adrenergic component may diminish catarrhal secretions and mucosal edema of the airway. A meta-analysis of 14 randomized, controlled trials that included inhaled or systemic epinephrine as one of the bronchodilators showed that epinephrine may be favorable to salbutamol and placebo among outpatients with bronchiolitis [103]. However, there is insufficient evidence to support its use for the treatment of bronchiolitis among inpatients. Because some children will respond to bronchodilators, if bronchodilators are to be tried, careful clin-ical evaluation of the response to the first few doses must be made in order for a decision to be made about continuance or discontinuance of the medication. A recent multicenter, double-blind, placebo-controlled trial that included 800 infants with bronchiolitis seen in the emergency department suggests that combined therapy with dexamethasone and epinephrine may significantly reduce the rate of hospital admission [104]. The use of ribavirin in treating RSV infection is controversial. Ribavirin is used sometimes for infants with pre-existing lung, heart, or immune disease [105–108]. The American Academy of Pediatrics has recommended that decisions about ribavirin administration should be made based on the particular clinical circumstances and physicians' experience [109]. Antibiotics are usually not indicated in uncomplicated bronchiolitis [110,111]. Nevertheless, Thorburn and colleagues [112] found that up to 40% of children with severe RSV bronchiolitis requiring admission to the PICU were infected with bacteria in their lower airways and were at increased risk for bacterial pneumonia. In general, prevention of bronchiolitis relies on measures to reduce the spread of the viruses that cause respiratory infections, such as hand washing and avoiding exposure to those symptomatic with respiratory infections.

Premature infants, and others with certain major cardiac and respiratory disorders, may benefit from passive immunization with Palivizumab (a monoclonal antibody against RSV). Palivizumab is administered intramuscularly at a dosage of 15 mg/kg monthly, beginning just before the onset of the RSV season for a total of 5 months, as recommended by the American Academy of Pediatrics for prophylaxis in high-risk children [109,113]. The use of Palivizumab in Asian cities with no winter or definite seasonality is controversial.

Risk factors for bronchiolitis deaths in the United States have been described, and multiple cause-of-death and linked birth/infant death data for 1996 through 1998 were used to examine bronchiolitis-related infant deaths [114]. Risk factors were assessed by comparing infants who died with bronchiolitis and surviving infants. During 1996 through 1998 there were 229 bronchiolitis-related infant deaths, resulting in an average annual infant mortality rate of 2.0 per 100,000 live births. The majority (55%) of infant deaths occurred among infants younger than 3 months. The bronchiolitis mortality rate was highest among infants weighing less than 1500 g at birth (very low birth weight; VLBW) as compared with infants weighing 1500 to 2499 g (low birth weight; LBW) and 2500 g or heavier at birth (29.8, 6.4, and 1.3 per 100 000 live births, respectively). VLBW and LBW infants remained at an increased risk of dying of bronchiolitis after controlling for other risk factors. Other risk factors included increasing birth order, low 5-minute Apgar score, young maternal age, unmarried mother, and tobacco use during pregnancy. The investigators concluded that VLBW and LBW infants are at increased risk of dying of bronchiolitis [114].

Leader and colleagues [115] provide current estimates of the incidence, associated risk factors, and costs of severe RSV infections among infants in the United States, defined as emergency department visits, hospitalization, and death. Between 1997 and 2000, there were 718,008 emergency department visits by infants with lower respiratory infection diagnoses during the RSV season (22.8/1000), and 29% were admitted. Costs of emergency department visits were approximately US$202 million. RSV bronchiolitis was the leading cause of infant hospitalization annually. Total hospital charges for RSV-coded primary diagnoses during the 4 years were more than $2.6 billion. An estimated 390 RSV-associated postneonatal deaths occurred in 1999. Low birth weight and prematurity significantly increased RSV-associated mortality rates. The investigators concluded that RSV is a major cause of infant morbidity and mortality. Severe RSV is highest among infants of black mothers and Medicaid-insured infants. Prematurity and low birth weight significantly increase RSV mortality rates.

Admission criteria for bronchiolitis can be derived based on the severity of the disease [116]. A clinical score is useful in the evaluation and grading of bronchiolitis severity [117]. Clinical deterioration requiring PICU admission is an uncommon occurrence in previously healthy infants admitted to a general pediatric inpatient unit with RSV infection. Extreme tachypnea and hypoxemia are both associated with subsequent deterioration; however, only a small proportion of patients who clinically deteriorate present in this way. The clinical usefulness of these parameters, therefore, is limited [118]. Adequate oxygen saturations should be maintained to avoid hypoxia [119]. Chest physiotherapy using vibration and percussion techniques does not reduce length of hospital stay, oxygen requirements, or improve the severity clinical score in infants with acute bronchiolitis [120,121]. The course of RSV disease is variable. In an East Denmark study, the clinical course was milder than reported elsewhere, possibly as a result of the low prevalence of bronchopulmonary dysplasia in Denmark [5]. However, RSV constitutes a considerable burden to the Danish pediatric health care system, and the investigators suggest that prophylaxis against RSV is desirable [5].

Viral pneumonia

Severe forms of respiratory viral infections are rare in children but may lead to life-threatening conditions, such as severe pneumonia necessitating PICU admission and occasionally resulting in death [17,122]. Community-acquired pneumonia (CAP) is a significant cause of childhood morbidity and mortality worldwide. Viral etiology is most common in young children [68,122–129]. In CAP, viral coinfection (especially RSV, human bocavirus, rhinovirus, human metapneumovirus, and parainfluenza viruses) ranges between 28.2% and 68.8%. Children with viral coinfection more frequently require hospital admission than those with single viral infection. Suffice to say, viral coinfections are frequent in children younger than 3 years with CAP, and can be a poor prognostic factor [130]. Although a possible microbial cause is identified in less than half of the patients, clinical findings and results of blood cultures, chest radiographs, and white blood cell and differential counts usually do not distinguish patients with a defined cause from those without a known cause for pneumonia [124,128,129,131,132]. Children with typical bacterial or mixed bacterial/viral infections have the greatest inflammation and disease severity. Michelow and colleagues [133] evaluated consecutive immunocompetent children hospitalized with radiographically confirmed lower respiratory infections from January 1999 through March 2000. One hundred and fifty-four hospitalized children with lower respiratory infections were enrolled. Median age was 33 months (range: 2 months to 17 years). A pathogen was identified in 79% of children. Typical respiratory bacteria were identified in 60% (of which 73% were *Streptococcus pneumoniae*), viruses in 45%, *Mycoplasma pneumoniae* in 14%, *Chlamydia pneumoniae* in 9%, and mixed bacterial/viral infections in 23%. Multivariate logistic-regression analyses revealed that high temperature (≥38.4°C) within 72 hours after admission and the presence of pleural effusion were significantly associated with bacterial pneumonia [133].

Oxygen therapy is life-saving and should be given when oxygen saturation is less than 92% [127]. Antimicrobials are often used to cover for possible coinfections with bacteria [124,128,134,135]. Mechanical ventilation is often required for respiratory failure [17,125]. Death is uncommon [17,125,136].

PREVENTION AND PROGNOSIS

Hand hygiene through washing with soap and water or alcohol-based hand rub is highly effective in reducing influenza A virus on human hands [37]. Appropriate hand hygiene may be an important public health initiative to reduce pandemic and influenza transmission. Influenza immunization can be given to children as young as 6 months. There is no vaccine available for parainfluenza, adenovirus, rhinovirus, or metapneumovirus. RSV prophylaxis is available but expensive.

One of the clinical problems facing pediatric intensivists is the differentiation between viral and bacterial infections when an acutely ill child, with or without respiratory manifestations, is admitted. An empirical course of antibiotics is often used in the initial management to avoid missing any treatable bacterial coinfections [17]. A low threshold for negative-pressure reverse isolation should be considered whenever possible so that other critically ill patients are not put at risk. Rapid diagnosis of respiratory viral infections in children is important, as prompt diagnosis results in significantly reduced hospital stays, antibiotic use, and laboratory use [137].

Upper airway obstruction in croup is usually caused by the parainfluenza virus. However, influenza may be more common than parainfluenza in causing croup in the PICU [17]. In lower respiratory disease such as bronchiolitis and pneumonia, radiographic abnormalities are often present, rendering differentiation from bacterial infections and coinfections difficult [10]. Sometimes parenchymal involvement as evidenced by abnormal radiography is more common with RSV than influenza infection [17]. As it is often difficult to delineate viral from bacterial infection in the acute setting, initial broad-spectrum antibiotics are used in the majority of patients to cover for pneumonia and sepsis [138,139]. Antibiotics can be discontinued when viral studies are positive and the patients have stabilized.

In one study, the mortality potentially attributable to the 4 respiratory viruses (RSV, influenza, parainfluenza, and adenovirus) was low during the PICU stay [17]. Adenovirus was notorious in its preponderance in causing severe diseases like encephalitis, bronchiolitis obliterans, and myocarditis. In the series of Hon and colleagues [17], 2 of the 4 patients with adenovirus died during their PICU stay. Three of the patients had the serotype 3, which is known to be able to cause severe respiratory infection [140]. Bacterial coinfections were often present and included various gram-positive and gram-negative bacteria cultured in the tracheal aspirate, urine, or blood [17]. The most common organism was *Streptococcus pneumoniae*.

Extrapulmonary manifestations of viral infection are an important cause of morbidity, and range from seizures to cardiac arrest [141–143].

Age is an important demographic factor. Among the 3 respiratory viruses, RSV infections in particular can cause significant morbidity and mortality in young children. Chronic lung disease and prematurity have been found to be associated with infection with the RSV virus [144–147].

Monthly intramuscular injection of Palivizumab has been advocated in patients vulnerable to RSV infections [5,148,149]. Universal influenza vaccination of children older than 6 months may help prevent infection by influenza, and is now recommended in the United States [11,15].

SUMMARY

Respiratory viral infections leading to PICU admissions may lead to significant morbidity and mortality [17]. Presentation can be pulmonary and extrapulmonary. Prompt diagnosis will ensure that the appropriate treatment (such as corticosteroid for croup) can be instituted as soon as possible. Vaccination of the high-risk groups may help to prevent infection and ICU admission.

The causes of severe childhood respiratory virus infections are heterogeneous, and the infections may at time be life-threatening. Many of these respiratory viral infections share similar symptomatology, and occasionally cause outbreaks and severe respiratory disease. The misleading abbreviation "SARS" was coined in 2003 [150]. The diagnosis of Severe Acute Respiratory Syndrome was based on a clinical definition in that patients who had fever, respiratory symptoms (not necessarily severe), and with an epidemiologic link were considered to have SARS. Patients clinically diagnosed to have SARS may or may not have SARS-CoV [150,151]. Overdiagnosis may lead to stigmatization and inconvenience in the workplace or at school. In contrast, underdiagnosing the condition may lead to the disease being unrecognized and the potential for the pathogen to spread in the community. Imprecise definition therefore carries serious public health consequences. In fact, the clinical features of many patients with SARS were neither "severe" nor "respiratory" in nature [150]. Many new surveillance guidelines and confusing abbreviations appeared. A new abbreviation "ILI" was introduced to mean influenza-like illness. The definitions for many of these abbreviations are nearly identical, if not the same as the clinical definition of SARS (ie, contact + fever + respiratory symptomatology ± other symptoms); this can cause unnecessary confusion. Indeed, the only difference between ILI, influenza, avian flu, swine flu, and SARS is the virus. Applying the initial clinical definition of SARS to avian or swine influenza, these patients all had SARS, because their symptoms and epidemiologic links were just like SARS [150,152]. However, the term SARS is no longer used unless SARS-CoV is isolated from the patient, regardless of whether "severe respiratory" symptoms and epidemiologic links are present. Outbreaks of severe acute respiratory infections with epidemiologic links will occur from time to time. Although SARS-CoV is out and may never come back, the SARS concept of index surveillance, and epidemiologic and prognostication studies for severe respiratory viral infections is here to stay. SARS is very much alive among us [150,152].

References

[1] Sung RY, Chan RC, Tam JS, et al. Epidemiology and aetiology of acute bronchiolitis in Hong Kong infants. Epidemiol Infect 1992;108(1):147–54.

[2] Hon KL, Nelson EA. Gender disparity in paediatric hospital admissions. Ann Acad Med Singap 2006;35(12):882–8.

[3] Nelson EAS, Tam JS, Yu LM, et al. Assessing disease burden of respiratory disorders in Hong Kong children with hospital discharge data and linked laboratory data. Hong Kong Med J 2007;13(2):114–21.

[4] O'Kelly EA, Hillary IB. Epidemiology of respiratory syncytial virus infection among infants over three winter seasons. Ir J Med Sci 1991;160(1):12–6.

[5] Kristensen K, Dahm T, Frederiksen PS, et al. Epidemiology of respiratory syncytial virus infection requiring hospitalization in East Denmark. Pediatr Infect Dis J 1998;17(11): 996–1000.

[6] Chan PK, Sung RY, Fung KS, et al. Epidemiology of respiratory syncytial virus infection among paediatric patients in Hong Kong: seasonality and disease impact. Epidemiol Infect 1999;123(2):257–62.

[7] Chiu SS, Tse CY, Lau YL, et al. Influenza A infection is an important cause of febrile seizures [see comment]. Pediatrics 2001;108(4):E63.

[8] Chiu SS, Lau YL, Chan KH, et al. Influenza-related hospitalizations among children in Hong Kong [see comment]. N Engl J Med 2002;347(26):2097–103.

[9] Nicholson KG, McNally T, Silverman M, et al. Influenza-related hospitalizations among young children in Leicestershire. Pediatr Infect Dis J 2003;22(10 Suppl):S228–30.

[10] van Woensel JB, van Aalderen WM, Kimpen JL. Viral lower respiratory tract infection in infants and young children. BMJ 2003;327(7405):36–40.

[11] Rojo JC, Ruiz-Contreras J, Fernandez MB, et al. Influenza-related hospitalizations in children younger than three years of age. Pediatr Infect Dis J 2006;25(7):596–601.

[12] Sung RY, Chan PK, Tsen T, et al. Identification of viral and atypical bacterial pathogens in children hospitalized with acute respiratory infections in Hong Kong by multiplex PCR assays. J Med Virol 2009;81(1):153–9.

[13] Keren R, Zaoutis TE, Saddlemire S, et al. Direct medical cost of influenza-related hospitalizations in children. Pediatrics 2006;118(5):e1321–7.

[14] Straliotto SM, Siqueira MM, Machado V, et al. Respiratory viruses in the pediatric intensive care unit: prevalence and clinical aspects. Mem Inst Oswaldo Cruz 2004;99(8):883–7.

[15] Milne BG, Williams S, May ML, et al. Influenza A associated morbidity and mortality in a paediatric intensive care unit. Commun Dis Intell 2004;28(4):504–9.

[16] Richard N, Hackme C, Stamm D, et al. [Influenza in pediatric intensive cure unit]. Arch Pediatr 2004;11(7):879–84 [in French].

[17] Hon KL, Hung E, Tang J, et al. Premorbid factors and outcome associated with respiratory virus infections in a pediatric intensive care unit. Pediatr Pulmonol 2008;43(3):275–80.

[18] Zambon MC. Epidemiology and pathogenesis of influenza. J Antimicrob Chemother 1999;44(Suppl B):3–9.

[19] Taubenberger JK, Morens DM. The pathology of influenza virus infections. Annu Rev Pathol 2008;3:499–522.

[20] Hay AJ, Gregory V, Douglas AR, et al. The evolution of human influenza viruses. Philos Trans R Soc Lond B Biol Sci 2001;356(1416):1861–70.

[21] Nobusawa E, Sato K. Comparison of the mutation rates of human influenza A and B viruses. J Virol 2006;80(7):3675–8.

[22] Grist NR. Epidemiology and pathogenesis of influenza. BMJ 1970;3(5718):344–5.

[23] Matsuzaki Y, Katsushima N, Nagai Y, et al. Clinical features of influenza C virus infection in children. J Infect Dis 2006;193(9):1229–35.

[24] Katagiri S, Ohizumi A, Homma M. An outbreak of type C influenza in a children's home. J Infect Dis 1983;148(1):51–6.

[25] Matsuzaki Y, Sugawara K, Mizuta K, et al. Antigenic and genetic characterization of influenza C viruses which caused two outbreaks in Yamagata City, Japan, in 1996 and 1998. J Clin Microbiol 2002;40(2):422–9.

[26] Peltola V, Reunanen T, Ziegler T, et al. Accuracy of clinical diagnosis of influenza in outpatient children. Clin Infect Dis 2005;41(8):1198–200.

[27] Carrat F, Luong J, Lao H, et al. A 'small-world-like' model for comparing interventions aimed at preventing and controlling influenza pandemics. BMC Med 2006;4:26.

[28] Grassly NC, Fraser C. Mathematical models of infectious disease transmission Microbiology. Natl Rev 2008;6(6):477–87.

[29] Mitamura K, Sugaya N. [Diagnosis and treatment of influenza—clinical investigation on viral shedding in children with influenza]. Uirusu 2006;56(1):109–16 [in Japanese].

[30] Hall CB. The spread of influenza and other respiratory viruses: complexities and conjectures [see comment]. Clin Infect Dis 2007;45(3):353–9.

[31] Weber TP, Stilianakis NI. Inactivation of influenza A viruses in the environment and modes of transmission: a critical review. J Infect 2008;57(5):361–73.

[32] Cole EC, Cook CE. Characterization of infectious aerosols in health care facilities: an aid to effective engineering controls and preventive strategies. Am J Infect Control 1998;26(4):453–64.

[33] Thomas Y, Vogel G, Wunderli W, et al. Survival of influenza virus on banknotes. Appl Environ Microbiol 2008;74(10):3002–7.

[34] Bean B, Moore BM, Sterner B, et al. Survival of influenza viruses on environmental surfaces. J Infect Dis 1982;146(1):47–51.

[35] Beigel J, Bray M. Current and future antiviral therapy of severe seasonal and avian influenza. Antiviral Res 2008;78(1):91–102.

[36] Aledort JE, Lurie N, Wasserman J, et al. Non-pharmaceutical public health interventions for pandemic influenza: an evaluation of the evidence base. BMC Public Health 2007;7:208.

[37] Grayson ML, Melvani S, Druce J, et al. Efficacy of soap and water and alcohol-based handrub preparations against live H1N1 influenza virus on the hands of human volunteers. Clin Infect Dis 2009;48(3):285–91.

[38] Hota B. Contamination, disinfection, and cross-colonization: are hospital surfaces reservoirs for nosocomial infection? Clin Infect Dis 2004;39(8):1182–9.

[39] McDonnell G, Russell AD. Antiseptics and disinfectants: activity, action, and resistance [Erratum appears in Clin Microbiol Rev 2001 Jan;14(1):227]. Clin Microbiol Rev 1999;12(1):147–79.

[40] Gorman OT, Bean WJ, Kawaoka Y, et al. Evolution of the nucleoprotein gene of influenza A virus. J Virol 1990;64(4):1487–97.

[41] Bano S, Naeem K, Malik SA. Evaluation of pathogenic potential of avian influenza virus serotype H9N2 in chickens. Avian Dis 2003;47(3 Suppl):817–22.

[42] Nguyen T, Davis CT, Stembridge W, et al. Characterization of a highly pathogenic avian influenza H5N1 virus sublineage in poultry seized at ports of entry into Vietnam. Virology 2009;387(2):250–6.

[43] Salomon R, Webster RG. The influenza virus enigma. Cell 2009;136(3):402–10.

[44] Webster RG, Bean WJ, Gorman OT, et al. Evolution and ecology of influenza A viruses. Microbiol Rev 1992;56(1):152–79.

[45] Zimmer SM, Burke DS. Historical perspective-emergence of influenza A (H1N1) viruses. N Engl J Med 2009;361(3):279–85.

[46] Vainionpaa R, Hyypia T. Biology of parainfluenza viruses. Clin Microbiol Rev 1994;7(2):265–75.

[47] Hall CB. Respiratory syncytial virus and parainfluenza virus [see comment]. N Engl J Med 2001;344(25):1917–28.

[48] Lee MS, Walker RE, Mendelman PM. Medical burden of respiratory syncytial virus and parainfluenza virus type 3 infection among US children. Implications for design of vaccine trials. Hum Vaccin 2005;1(1):6–11.

[49] Lessler J, Reich NG, Brookmeyer R, et al. Incubation periods of acute respiratory viral infections: a systematic review. Lancet Infect Dis 2009;9(5):291–300.

[50] Osiowy C. Direct detection of respiratory syncytial virus, parainfluenza virus, and adenovirus in clinical respiratory specimens by a multiplex reverse transcription-PCR assay. J Clin Microbiol 1998;36(11):3149–54.

[51] Sato M, Wright PF. Current status of vaccines for parainfluenza virus infections. Pediatr Infect Dis J 2008;27(10 Suppl):S123–5.

[52] Busse WW, Gern JE, Dick EC. The role of respiratory viruses in asthma. Ciba Found Symp 1997;206:208–13.

[53] Friedlander SL, Busse WW. The role of rhinovirus in asthma exacerbations. J Allergy Clin Immunol 2005;116(2):267–73.

[54] Lemanske RF Jr, Jackson DJ, Gangnon RE, et al. Rhinovirus illnesses during infancy predict subsequent childhood wheezing [see comment]. J Allergy Clin Immunol 2005;116(3):571–7.

[55] Kling S, Donninger H, Williams Z, et al. Persistence of rhinovirus RNA after asthma exacerbation in children. Clin Exp Allergy 2005;35(5):672–8.

[56] Pevear DC, Tull TM, Seipel ME, et al. Activity of pleconaril against enteroviruses. Antimicrobial Agents Chemother 1999;43(9):2109–15.

[57] Fleischer R, Laessig K. Safety and efficacy evaluation of pleconaril for treatment of the common cold [comment]. Clin Infect Dis 2003;37(12):1722.

[58] de Haan CA, Rottier PJ. Molecular interactions in the assembly of coronaviruses. Adv Virus Res 2005;64:165–230.

[59] Ksiazek TG, Erdman D, Goldsmith CS, et al. A novel coronavirus associated with severe acute respiratory syndrome [see comment]. N Engl J Med 2003;348(20):1953–66.

[60] Rota PA, Oberste MS, Monroe SS, et al. Characterization of a novel coronavirus associated with severe acute respiratory syndrome [see comment]. Science 2003;300(5624):1394–9.

[61] Li F, Li W, Farzan M, et al. Structure of SARS coronavirus spike receptor-binding domain complexed with receptor [see comment]. Science 2005;309(5742):1864–8.

[62] van der HL, Pyrc K, Jebbink MF, et al. Identification of a new human coronavirus. Nat Med 2004;10(4):368–73.

[63] Garcia-Garcia ML, Calvo C, Martin F, et al. Human metapneumovirus infections in hospitalised infants in Spain. Arch Dis Child 2006;91(4):290–5.

[64] van den Hoogen BG, de Jong JC, Groen J, et al. A newly discovered human pneumovirus isolated from young children with respiratory tract disease. Nat Med 2001;7(6):719–24.

[65] Falsey AR. Human metapneumovirus infection in adults. Pediatr Infect Dis J 2008;27(10):S80–3.

[66] Boivin G, De Serres G, Cote S, et al. Human metapneumovirus infections in hospitalized children. Emerg Infect Dis 2003;9(6):634–40.

[67] Nissen MD, Siebert DJ, Mackay IM, et al. Evidence of human metapneumovirus in Australian children. Med J Aust 2002;176(4):188.

[68] Lin PY, Lin TY, Huang YC, et al. Human metapneumovirus and community-acquired pneumonia in children. Chang Gung Med J 2005;28(10):683–8.

[69] Semple MG, Cowell A, Dove W, et al. Dual infection of infants by human metapneumovirus and human respiratory syncytial virus is strongly associated with severe bronchiolitis. J Infect Dis 2005;191(3):382–6.

[70] Deffrasnes C, Hamelin ME, Boivin G. Human metapneumovirus. Semin Respir Crit Care Med 2007;28(2):213–21.

[71] Pelletier G, Dery P, Abed Y, et al. Respiratory tract reinfections by the new human meta-pneumovirus in an immunocompromised child. Emerg Infect Dis 2002;8(9):976–8.

[72] Bao X, Liu T, Shan Y, et al. Human metapneumovirus glycoprotein G inhibits innate immune responses. PLoS Pathog 2008;4(5):e1000077.

[73] Eccles R. Understanding the symptoms of the common cold and influenza. Lancet Infect Dis 2005;5(11):718–25.

[74] Suzuki E, Ichihara K, Johnson AM. Natural course of fever during influenza virus infection in children. Clin Pediatr 2007;46(1):76–9.

[75] Call SA, Vollenweider MA, Hornung CA, et al. Does this patient have influenza? [see comment]. JAMA 2005;293(8):987–97.

[76] Louie JK, Roy-Burman A, Guardia-Labar L, et al. Rhinovirus associated with severe lower respiratory tract infections in children. Pediatr Infect Dis J 2009;28(4):337–9.

[77] Leung AK, Kellner JD. Acute sinusitis in children: diagnosis and management. J Pediatr Health Care 2004;18(2):72–6.

[78] Suarez DL, Spackman E, Senne DA, et al. The effect of various disinfectants on detection of avian influenza virus by real time RT-PCR. Avian Dis 2003;47(3 Suppl):1091–5.

[79] Villegas P. Viral diseases of the respiratory system. Poult Sci 1998;77(8):1143–5.

[80] Horwood F, Macfarlane J. Pneumococcal and influenza vaccination: current situation and future prospects. Thorax 2002;57(Suppl 2):II24–30.

[81] Hilleman MR. Realities and enigmas of human viral influenza: pathogenesis, epidemi-ology and control. Vaccine 2002;20(25–26):3068–87.

[82] Whitley RJ, Monto AS. Prevention and treatment of influenza in high-risk groups: children, pregnant women, immunocompromised hosts, and nursing home residents. J Infect Dis 2006;194(Suppl 2):S133–8.

[83] Vellozzi C, Burwen DR, Dobardzic A, et al. Safety of trivalent inactivated influenza vaccines in adults: background for pandemic influenza vaccine safety monitoring. Vaccine 2009;27(15):2114–20.

[84] Glasgow JF, Middleton B. Reye syndrome-insights on causation and prognosis. Arch Dis Child 2001;85(5):351–3.

[85] Colman PM. A novel approach to antiviral therapy for influenza. J Antimicrob Chemother 1999;44(Suppl B):17–22.

[86] Moscona A. Neuraminidase inhibitors for influenza. N Engl J Med 2005;353(13): 1363–73.

[87] Stephenson I, Nicholson KG. Chemotherapeutic control of influenza. J Antimicrob Chemo-ther 1999;44(1):6–10.

[88] Jefferson TO, Demicheli V, Di Pietrantonj C, et al. Neuraminidase inhibitors for preventing and treating influenza in healthy adults. Cochrane Database Syst Rev 2006;(3): CD001265.

[89] Schmidt AC. Antiviral therapy for influenza: a clinical and economic comparative review. Drugs 2004;64(18):2031–46.

[90] Webster RG, Govorkova EA. H5N1 influenza-continuing evolution and spread [see comment]. N Engl J Med 2006;355(21):2174–7.

[91] Sugaya N, Takeuchi Y. Mass vaccination of schoolchildren against influenza and its impact on the influenza-associated mortality rate among children in Japan. Clin Infect Dis 2005;41(7):939–47.

[92] Cherry JD. Clinical practice. Croup. N Engl J Med 2008;358(4):384–91.

[93] Leung AK, Kellner JD, Johnson DW. Viral croup: a current perspective. J Pediatr Health Care 2004;18(6):297–301.

[94] Bjornson CL, Klassen TP, Williamson J, et al. A randomized trial of a single dose of oral dexamethasone for mild croup [see comment]. N Engl J Med 2004;351(13):1306–13.

[95] Ledwith CA, Shea LM, Mauro RD. Safety and efficacy of nebulized racemic epinephrine in conjunction with oral dexamethasone and mist in the outpatient treatment of croup. Ann Emerg Med 1995;25(3):331–7.

[96] Jartti T, van den HB, Garofalo RP, et al. Metapneumovirus and acute wheezing in children. Lancet 2002;360(9343):1393–4.

[97] Smuts H, Workman L, Zar HJ. Role of human metapneumovirus, human coronavirus NL63 and human bocavirus in infants and young children with acute wheezing. J Med Virol 2008;80(5):906–12.

[98] Leung AK, Kellner JD, Davies HD. Respiratory syncytial virus bronchiolitis. J Natl Med Assoc 2005;97(12):1708–13.

[99] Openshaw PJ, Dean GS, Culley FJ. Links between respiratory syncytial virus bronchiolitis and childhood asthma: clinical and research approaches. Pediatr Infect Dis J 2003;22(2 Suppl):S58–64.

[100] Kneyber MCJ, Steyerberg EW, de Groot R, et al. Long-term effects of respiratory syncytial virus (RSV) bronchiolitis in infants and young children: a quantitative review. Acta Paediatr 2000;89(6):654–60.

[101] Kellner JD, Ohlsson A, Gadomski AM, et al. Efficacy of bronchodilator therapy in bronchiolitis. A meta-analysis. Arch Pediatr Adolesc Med 1996;150(11):1166–72.

[102] Kellner JD, Ohlsson A, Gadomski AM, et al. Bronchodilators for bronchiolitis [see comment] [update in Cochrane Database Syst Rev. 2006;3:CD001266; PMID: 16855963]. Cochrane Database Syst Rev 2000;(2):CD001266.

[103] Hartling L, Wiebe N, Russell K, et al. Epinephrine for bronchiolitis. Cochrane Database Syst Rev 2004;(1):CD003123.

[104] Plint AC, Johnson DW, Patel H, et al. Epinephrine and dexamethasone in children with bronchiolitis [see comment]. N Engl J Med 2009;360(20):2079–89.

[105] Randolph AG, Wang EE. Ribavirin for respiratory syncytial virus lower respiratory tract infection. A systematic overview. Arch Pediatr Adolesc Med 1996;150(9): 942–7.

[106] Ventre K, Randolph A. Ribavirin for respiratory syncytial virus infection of the lower respiratory tract in infants and young children [update in Cochrane Database Syst Rev. 2007;(1):CD000181; PMID: 17253446] [update of Cochrane Database Syst Rev. 2000;(2):CD000181; PMID: 10796503]. Cochrane Database Syst Rev 2004;(4): CD000181.

[107] Ventre K, Randolph AG. Ribavirin for respiratory syncytial virus infection of the lower respiratory tract in infants and young children [update of Cochrane Database Syst Rev. 2004;(4):CD000181; PMID: 15494991]. Cochrane Database Syst Rev 2007;(1):CD000181.

[108] Chen CH, Lin YT, Yang YH, et al. Ribavirin for respiratory syncytial virus bronchiolitis reduced the risk of asthma and allergen sensitization. Pediatr Allergy Immunol 2008;19(2):166–72.

[109] Faber TE, Kimpen JL, Bont LJ. Respiratory syncytial virus bronchiolitis: prevention and treatment. Expert Opin Pharmacother 2008;9(14):2451–8.

[110] Titus MO, Wright SW. Prevalence of serious bacterial infections in febrile infants with respiratory syncytial virus infection. Pediatrics 2003;112(2):282–4.

[111] Randolph AG, Reder L, Englund JA. Risk of bacterial infection in previously healthy respiratory syncytial virus-infected young children admitted to the intensive care unit. Pediatr Infect Dis J 2004;23(11):990–4.

[112] Thorburn K, Harigopal S, Reddy V, et al. High incidence of pulmonary bacterial co-infection in children with severe respiratory syncytial virus (RSV) bronchiolitis [see comment]. Thorax 2006;61(7):611–5.

[113] American Academy of Pediatrics Committee on Infectious Diseases and Committee on Fetus and Newborn. Revised indications for the use of palivizumab and respiratory syncytial virus immune globulin intravenous for the prevention of respiratory syncytial virus infections. Pediatrics 2003;112(6 Pt 1):1442–6.

[114] Holman RC, Shay DK, Curns AT, et al. Risk factors for bronchiolitis-associated deaths among infants in the United States. Pediatr Infect Dis J 2003;22(6):483–90.

[115] Leader S, Kohlhase K. Recent trends in severe respiratory syncytial virus (RSV) among US infants, 1997 to 2000. J Pediatr 2003;143(5 Suppl):S127–32.

[116] Lind I, Gill JH, Calabretta N, et al. Clinical inquiries. What are hospital admission criteria for infants with bronchiolitis? J Fam Pract 2006;55(1):67–9.

[117] Wood DW, Downes JJ, Lecks HI. A clinical scoring system for the diagnosis of respiratory failure. Preliminary report on childhood status asthmaticus. Am J Dis Child 1972;123(3): 227–8.

[118] Brooks AM, McBride JT, McConnochie KM, et al. Predicting deterioration in previously healthy infants hospitalized with respiratory syncytial virus infection. Pediatrics 1999;104(3 Pt 1):463–7.

[119] Black CP. Systematic review of the biology and medical management of respiratory syncytial virus infection. Respir Care 2003;48(3):209–31.

[120] Perrotta C, Ortiz Z, Roque M. Chest physiotherapy for acute bronchiolitis in paediatric patients between 0 and 24 months old [update in Cochrane Database Syst Rev. 2007;(1):CD004873; PMID: 17253527]. Cochrane Database Syst Rev 2005;(2):CD004873.

[121] Perrotta C, Ortiz Z, Roque M. Chest physiotherapy for acute bronchiolitis in paediatric patients between 0 and 24 months old [update of Cochrane Database Syst Rev. 2005;(2):CD004873; PMID: 15846736]. Cochrane Database Syst Rev 2007;(1):CD004873.

[122] Gimenez SF, Sanchez MA, Battles Garrido JM, et al. [Clinicoepidemiological characteristics of community-acquired pneumonia in children aged less than 6 years old]. Ann Pediatr 2007;66(6):578–84 [in Spanish].

[123] Wijnands GJ. Diagnosis and interventions in lower respiratory tract infections. Am J Med 1992;92(4A):91S–7S.

[124] Sandora TJ, Harper MB. Pneumonia in hospitalized children. Pediatr Clin North Am 2005;52(4):1059–81.

[125] Delport SD, Brisley T. Aetiology and outcome of severe community-acquired pneumonia in children admitted to a paediatric intensive care unit Suid-Afrikaanse Tydskrif Vir Geneeskunde. S Afr Med J 2002;92(11):907–11.

[126] McIntosh K. Community-acquired pneumonia in children [see comment]. N Engl J Med 2002;346(6):429–37.

[127] Chetty K, Thomson AH. Management of community-acquired pneumonia in children. Paediatr Drugs 2007;9(6):401–11.

[128] Malek E, Lebecque P. [Etiology and treatment of community acquired pneumonia in children]. J Pharm Belg 2007;62(1):21–4 [in French].

[129] Patwari AK, Bisht S, Srinivasan A, et al. Aetiology of pneumonia in hospitalized children. J Trop Pediatr 1996;42(1):15–20.

[130] Cilla G, Onate E, Perez-Yarza EG, et al. Viruses in community-acquired pneumonia in children aged less than 3 years old: high rate of viral coinfection. J Med Virol 2008;80(10):1843–9.

[131] Lucero MG, Tupasi TE, Gomez ML, et al. Respiratory rate greater than 50 per minute as a clinical indicator of pneumonia in Filipino children with cough. Rev Infect Dis 1990;12(Suppl 8):S1081–3.

[132] Albaum MN, Hill LC, Murphy M, et al. Interobserver reliability of the chest radiograph in community-acquired pneumonia. PORT Investigators. Chest 1996;110(2): 343–50.

[133] Michelow IC, Olsen K, Lozano J, et al. Epidemiology and clinical characteristics of community-acquired pneumonia in hospitalized children [see comment]. Pediatrics 2004;113(4):701–7.

[134] Harris JA, Kolokathis A, Campbell M, et al. Safety and efficacy of azithromycin in the treatment of community-acquired pneumonia in children. Pediatr Infect Dis J 1998;17(10): 865–71.

[135] Kabra SK, Lodha R, Pandey RM. Antibiotics for community acquired pneumonia in children. Cochrane Database Syst Rev 2006;(3):CD004874.

[136] Dowell SF, Kupronis BA, Zell ER, et al. Mortality from pneumonia in children in the United States, 1939 through 1996. N Engl J Med 2000;342(19):1399–407.

[137] Woo PC, Chiu SS, Seto WH, et al. Cost-effectiveness of rapid diagnosis of viral respiratory tract infections in pediatric patients. J Clin Microbiol 1997;35(6):1579–81.

[138] van Woensel JB, von Rosenstiel IA, Kimpen JL, et al. Antibiotic use in pediatric intensive care patients with lower respiratory tract infection due to respiratory syncytial virus. Intensive Care Med 2001;27(8):1436.

[139] Bloomfield P, Dalton D, Karleka A, et al. Bacteraemia and antibiotic use in respiratory syncytial virus infections. Arch Dis Child 2004;89(4):363–7.

[140] Lin KH, Lin YC, Chen HL, et al. A two decade survey of respiratory adenovirus in Taiwan: the reemergence of adenovirus types 7 and 4. J Med Virol 2004;73(2):274–9.

[141] Dominguez O, Rojo P, de Las HS, et al. Clinical presentation and characteristics of pharyngeal adenovirus infections. Pediatr Infect Dis J 2005;24(8):733–4.

[142] Castro-Rodriguez JA, Daszenies C, Garcia M, et al. Adenovirus pneumonia in infants and factors for developing bronchiolitis obliterans: a 5-year follow-up. Pediatr Pulmonol 2006;41(10):947–53.

[143] Kim Y-P, Hong J-Y, Lee H-J, et al. Genome type analysis of adenovirus types 3 and 7 isolated during successive outbreaks of lower respiratory tract infections in children. J Clin Microbiol 2003;41(10):4594–9.

[144] Stevens TP, Sinkin RA, Hall CB, et al. Respiratory syncytial virus and premature infants born at 32 weeks' gestation or earlier: hospitalization and economic implications of prophylaxis [see comment]. Arch Pediatr Adolesc Med 2000;154(1):55–61.

[145] McCormick J, Tubman R. Readmission with respiratory syncytial virus (RSV) infection among graduates from a neonatal intensive care unit. Pediatr Pulmonol 2002;34(4):262–6.

[146] Liese JG, Grill E, Fischer B, et al. Incidence and risk factors of respiratory syncytial virus-related hospitalizations in premature infants in Germany. Eur J Pediatr 2003;162(4):230–6.

[147] Pedersen O, Herskind AM, Kamper J, et al. Rehospitalization for respiratory syncytial virus infection in infants with extremely low gestational age or birthweight in Denmark. Acta Paediatr 2003;92(2):240–2.

[148] Vogel AM, Lennon DR, Broadbent R, et al. Palivizumab prophylaxis of respiratory syncytial virus infection in high-risk infants [see comment]. J Paediatr Child Health 2002;38(6):550–4.

[149] Feltes TF, Cabalka AK, Meissner HC, et al. Palivizumab prophylaxis reduces hospitalization due to respiratory syncytial virus in young children with hemodynamically significant congenital heart disease [see comment]. J Pediatr 2003;143(4):532–40.

[150] Hon KL, Li AM, Cheng FW, et al. Personal view of SARS: confusing definition, confusing diagnoses. Lancet 2003;361(9373):1984–5.

[151] Li AM. Severe acute respiratory syndrome: 'SARS' or 'not SARS'. J Paediatr Child Health 2004;40(1–2):63–5.

[152] Hon KL. Just like SARS. Pediatri Pulmonol, in press.

Advances in Pediatrics 56 (2009) 75–86

ELSEVIER
MOSBY

ADVANCES IN PEDIATRICS

Lymphocytic Choriomeningitis Virus: A Prenatal and Postnatal Threat

Daniel J. Bonthius, MD, PhD

Department of Pediatrics, University of Iowa Hospital, 2504 JCP, 200 Hawkins Drive, Iowa City, IA 52242, USA

Lymphocytic choriomeningitis virus (LCMV) is not as well known to pediatricians and neurologists as it ought to be. A prevalent human pathogen, LCMV is an important cause of meningitis in children and adults, and of encephalopathy and neurologic birth defects in newborns. Acquired and congenital LCMV infections are underrecognized by pediatricians and neurologists, and are probably responsible for far more cases of meningitis and congenital brain and retinal dysfunction than is generally realized [1].

HISTORICAL NOTE

LCMV was first isolated in 1933 from the cerebrospinal fluid of a woman with a severe case of meningo-encephalitis, from which she died. The virus was named lymphocytic choriomeningitis virus, for the pathologic changes that it induced in the choroid plexus and meninges of experimentally infected mice and monkeys [2].

After its initial discovery, LCMV was subsequently isolated from cerebrospinal fluid of many patients with aseptic meningitis. It was soon firmly established that LCMV was an important etiologic agent of aseptic meningitis in man. Subsequent clinical and etiologic studies identified LCMV as one of the most frequent infectious causes of aseptic meningitis [3].

The first recognized case of congenital LCMV infection was reported in England in 1955 [4]. In the decades that followed, multiple cases of congenital infection with the virus were reported throughout Europe. Although LCMV has been recognized as an important cause of aseptic meningitis in the United States for many decades, the first cases of congenital LCMV infection were not reported in the United States until 1993 [5,6].

Although LCMV was discovered in 1933, the virus was not classified until the late 1960s, when it was placed in the newly formed *Arenaviridae* family of viruses. The arenaviruses are enveloped, single-stranded, RNA viruses. The name of the arenaviruses is derived from *arenosus*, the Latin word for "sandy,"

E-mail address: daniel-bonthius@uiowa.edu

0065-3101/09/$ – see front matter
doi:10.1016/j.yapd.2009.08.007

because of the fine granularities observed within the virion on ultrathin electron microscopic sections [7].

THE ECOLOGY OF LYMPHOCYTIC CHORIOMENINGITIS VIRUS

LCMV, like all arenaviruses, uses rodents as its principal reservoir. The common house mouse, *Mus musculus*, is both the natural host and reservoir for the virus, which is transferred vertically from one generation to the next within the mouse population by intrauterine infection. Hamsters are also competent reservoirs. Although they may be heavily infected with LCMV, rodents that acquire the virus transplacentally often remain asymptomatic because congenital infection provides rodents with immunologic tolerance for the virus. Mice and hamsters infected with LCMV shed the virus in large quantities in nasal secretions, saliva, milk, semen, urine, and feces throughout their lives [7].

Postnatal humans typically acquire LCMV by contacting fomites contaminated with infectious virus or by inhalation of aerosolized virus. Postnatal humans can also acquire the virus via organ transplantation [8,9]. Congenital LCMV infection occurs when a woman acquires a primary LCMV infection during pregnancy. The virus passes through the placenta to the fetus during maternal viremia. The fetus may also acquire the virus during passage through the birth canal, due to exposure to infected vaginal secretions [4].

CLINICAL MANIFESTATIONS

The clinical manifestations of LCMV infection depend on the developmental stage of the patient at the time of infection [10]. In particular, clinical signs and symptoms depend on whether the infection occurs prenatally or postnatally. Congenital infection of a human with LCMV is unique, as it involves both the postnatal infection of a pregnant woman and the prenatal infection of a fetus.

Acquired (postnatal) lymphocytic choriomeningitis virus infection

LCMV infection during postnatal life (during childhood or adulthood) usually consists of a brief febrile illness, from which the patient has a full recovery. Classic LCMV infection includes 2 clinical phases. In the first phase, the patient's symptoms are those of a nonspecific viral syndrome and include myalgia, fever, malaise, headache, anorexia, nausea, and vomiting. These symptoms typically begin to resolve after several days, only to be followed by a second phase, consisting of central nervous system (CNS) disease. The symptoms of this CNS phase of the disease are usually those of aseptic meningitis, including fever, headache, nuchal rigidity, photophobia, and vomiting. The entire course of the biphasic disease is usually 1 to 3 weeks [11].

Laboratory abnormalities commonly observed during the initial febrile phase include thrombocytopenia, leukopenia, and mild elevations of liver enzymes. In many cases, infiltrates appear on chest radiographs. The hallmark laboratory abnormality during the second CNS phase of the disease is a cerebrospinal fluid (CSF) pleocytosis. The CSF typically contains hundreds to thousands of white blood cells, almost all of which are lymphocytes. However, CSF eosinophilia has also been reported [12]. Mild elevations of CSF protein and hypoglycorrhachia can also occur.

Whereas the typical acquired LCMV infection is a biphasic illness, the clinical spectrum is broad. As many as one-third of postnatal infections are asymptomatic. Other patients develop extraneural disease that extends beyond the usual symptoms and may include orchitis, pneumonitis, myocarditis, parotitis, dermatitis, and pharyngitis [13]. In some patients the neurologic disease may be considerably more severe than usual, and may include transverse myelitis, Guillain-Barré syndrome, hydrocephalus, and encephalitis. Although recovery is usually complete, fatalities from acquired LCMV infection occasionally occur [3].

Those who acquire LCMV infection via solid organ transplantation always have severe disease. Recipients of infected organs typically develop fever, leucopenia, and lethargy several weeks after transplantation. Following these nonspecific symptoms, the patients rapidly progress to multiorgan system failure and shock. These cases are almost always fatal [8,9].

Congenital lymphocytic choriomeningitis virus infection

Infection with LCMV during pregnancy can kill the fetus and induce spontaneous abortion [14]. Among those fetuses that survive, the 2 hallmark signs of congenital LCMV infection are (1) vision impairment and (2) brain dysfunction [15].

The vision impairment in congenital LCMV infection is due principally to chorioretinitis and the subsequent formation of chorioretinal scars (Fig. 1). The chorioretinal scarring is usually bilateral and is most commonly located in the periphery of the fundus, but scarring of the macula is also common [16]. Other ocular abnormalities induced by congenital LCMV infection may include optic atrophy, nystagmus, vitreitis, strabismus, microphthalmos, and cataract [17].

Although the ocular effects of congenital LCMV infection are often severe, it is the effect of LCMV on the developing fetal *brain* that causes the greatest disability. Prenatal infection with LCMV commonly induces either macrocephaly or microcephaly. Macrocephaly following this infection is almost invariably due to a noncommunicating hydrocephalus, whereas microcephaly is attributable to virus-induced failure of brain growth. In addition to disturbances of head size, periventricular calcifications are also cardinal features of congenital LCMV infection (Fig. 2) [18,19].

Although hydrocephalus, microencephaly, and periventricular calcifications are by far the most commonly observed abnormalities of the brain in congenital LCMV, other forms of neuropathology, alone or in combination, can also occur. These forms include periventricular cysts, porencephalic cysts, encephalomalacia, intraparenchymal calcifications, cerebellar hypoplasia, and neuronal migration disturbances [19].

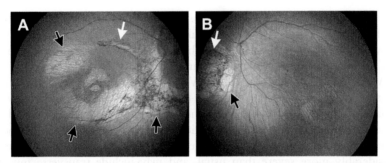

Fig. 1. Optic fundi of a child with congenital LCMV infection. (*A*) The right fundus has a large chorioretinal scar (*black arrows*) that includes the macula and surrounds the optic disk. In many places, the chorioretinal scar is surrounded by abnormal pigmentation (*white arrows*). (*B*) The left fundus has a chorioretinal scar (*black arrow*) inferonasal to the optic disk with adjacent abnormal pigmentation (*white arrow*). (*Courtesy of* Dr. Susannah Longmuir, Iowa City, IA.)

In children with congenital LCMV infection, brain function is often severely and permanently impaired. Mental retardation, cerebral palsy, ataxia, epilepsy, and blindness are common neurologic sequelae [20]. However, the outcome of children with congenital LCMV infection is diverse [19]. All children with the combination of microencephaly and periventricular calcifications are

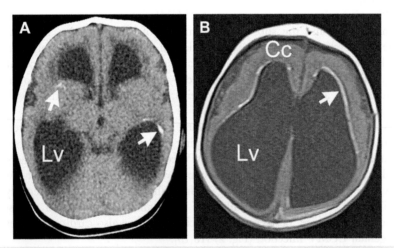

Fig. 2. Neuroimaging studies obtained during early infancy on a microcephalic patient with congenital LCMV infection. (*A*) The head computed tomography scan reveals ventriculomegaly with enlargement of the lateral ventricles (Lv) and periventricular mineralizations (*white arrows*). (*B*) Brain magnetic resonance imaging scan reveals enlarged lateral ventricles (Lv) and periventricular mineralizations (*white arrow*). In addition, the gyral pattern of the cerebral cortex (Cc) is smooth and featureless, suggestive of a cortical neuronal migration disturbance.

profoundly neurologically impaired. Blindness, medically refractory epilepsy, spastic quadriparesis, and mental retardation are typical of this group. However, other children with congenital LCMV infection, who do not have the combination of microencephaly and periventricular calcifications, often have a more favorable outcome with less severe motor, mental, and vision impairments. Children with isolated cerebellar hypoplasia may be ataxic, but have only mild or moderate mental retardation and vision loss [19]. The differences in outcome among children with congenital LCMV infection likely reflect differences in the gestational timing of infection [21].

Within the fetus, LCMV has a strong tropism for the brain. Thus, unlike many other congenital infections, LCMV usually does not induce systemic manifestations. Birth weight is typically appropriate for gestational age. Rashes and thrombocytopenia, which are common in several other prominent congenital infections, are unusual in congenital LCMV infection. Hepatosplenomegaly is only rarely observed, and serum liver enzyme levels are usually normal. Auditory deficits are unusual.

PATHOGENESIS

LCMV is not a cytolytic virus. Thus, unlike herpes and several other pathogens that directly induce brain damage by killing host brain cells, LCMV pathogenesis involves other underlying mechanisms. Furthermore, the pathogenic mechanisms are different in postnatal (acquired) infection than in prenatal (congenital) infection. A critical difference in the pathogenesis of postnatal versus prenatal infection is that the virus infects brain parenchyma in the case of prenatal infection, but is restricted to the meninges and choroid plexus in postnatal cases [10,19,21].

In children and adults (postnatal infections), LCMV replicates to high titers in the choroid plexus and meninges. Viral antigen within these infected tissues becomes the target of an acute mononuclear cell infiltration driven by CD8+ T lymphocytes. The presence of these T lymphocytes in large numbers within the meninges and CSF leads to the symptoms of meningitis that mark acquired LCMV infection. As the T cells clear the virus from the meninges and CSF, the density of T cells declines and the symptoms of meningitis resolve. Thus, symptoms of acquired (postnatal) LCMV infection are essentially immune-mediated and are due to the presence of large numbers of lymphocytes [7].

As is true for postnatal infections, prenatal infection also leads to inflammation of the tissues surrounding the brain parenchyma and to some of the signs of congenital LCMV. In particular, congenital LCMV infection often leads to ependymal inflammation within the ventricular system [21]. This inflammation of the ependyma may block the egress of CSF, especially at the cerebral aqueduct, and lead to hydrocephalus.

However, unlike postnatal cases, prenatal infection with LCMV includes infection of the substance of the brain, rather than just the meninges or ependyma. This infection of brain parenchyma leads to the substantial neuropathologic changes typically accompanying congenital LCMV infection. In particular, LCMV infects the mitotically active neuroblasts, located at periventricular sites [22]. Through an unknown mechanism, presence of the virus kills these periventricular cells, leading to periventricular calcifications, a radiographic hallmark of this disorder. Within the fetal brain, LCMV infection of neurons and glial cells also disrupts neuronal migration, leading to abnormal gyral patterns, and interferes with neuronal mitosis, leading to microcephaly and cerebellar hypoplasia [19,21,22].

Animal models of congenital LCMV infection have shown that the effect of LCMV on the developing brain depends critically on the developmental stage of the fetus at the time of infection [23]. The cellular targets of infection, peak viral titers in tissues, and the nature and severity of neuropathology all depend strongly on gestational age of the fetus. All of the various neuropathologic changes evident in humans with congenital LCMV infection can be recapitulated in animal models by infecting the experimental animals at different developmental stages. These findings suggest that the variability in outcome among children with congenital LCMV infection is due to differences in the gestational timing of infection [19,21].

EPIDEMIOLOGY
Acquired LCMV infections can occur at any time of the year; however, most occur during the late autumn and winter months, probably reflecting seasonal variations in the cohabitation of humans with mice. During the cold months of autumn and winter, wild mice are driven indoors, carrying LCMV with them and increasing the likelihood of a human infection.

The prevalence and incidence of congenital LCMV infection are unknown. Whereas the published case reports of LCMV infection during pregnancy make it clear that LCMV can be a severe neuroteratogen, it is not known whether the profoundly affected infants described in the case reports represent the typical outcome of gestational LCMV infection or whether they represent only the most severely affected cases. Prospective epidemiologic or clinical studies of congenital LCMV infection have not been conducted. Information regarding the incidence and spectrum of LCMV-induced teratogenicity is further limited by LCMV not being one of the infectious agents for which infants with a suspected congenital infection are routinely checked. Therefore, it is possible that congenital LCMV infection, like many other congenital infections, produces a spectrum of pathologic effects that range from minimal to profound [24].

Although the incidence of gestational LCMV infection is unknown, it is known that LCMV is prevalent in the environment, has a great geographic range, and infects large numbers of humans. LCMV is endemic in wild mice throughout temperate regions [25,26] and probably occurs wherever the genus *Mus* has been introduced (every continent but Antarctica). An epidemiologic study has demonstrated that 9% of the house mice in urban Baltimore, Maryland are infected with LCMV, and that significant clustering occurs where the prevalence is higher [27]. Serologic studies have found that 4.7% of adults in

Baltimore and 5.1% of healthy black women in Birmingham, Alabama possess antibodies to LCMV, indicating prior exposure and infection [27–29]. Together, these data suggest that congenital LCMV infection is an underdiagnosed disease, and that the virus is responsible for more cases of congenital neurologic and vision dysfunction than has previously been recognized [11,16,17].

PREVENTION

No vaccine exists to prevent LCMV infection. However, measures can be taken to reduce the risk of infection. Because rodents, especially house mice, are the principal reservoir of LCMV, people can reduce their risk of contracting LCMV by minimizing their exposure to the secretions and excretions of mice. This precaution can be accomplished most effectively by eliminating cohabitation with mice. Congenital LCMV infection will not occur unless a woman contracts a primary infection with LCMV during pregnancy. Thus, women should be especially careful to avoid contact or cohabitation with mice during pregnancy. Pregnant women should also avoid contact with pet rodents, especially mice and hamsters. Laboratory personnel who work with rodents have an increased risk of infection with LCMV. Pregnant women who work in animal care facilities or research laboratories should wear gloves, gowns, and face masks to avoid potential aerosolized or secreted LCMV.

Because congenitally infected mice can secrete large quantities of LCMV and remain essentially asymptomatic, LCMV may be rampant within animal colonies at research institutions, thus putting laboratory workers, and especially pregnant women and their fetuses, at risk. Therefore, all animal colonies should be tested periodically for LCMV [27].

Acquisition of LCMV from solid organ transplantation represents a substantial risk to the life of the organ recipient. Prospective donors with LCMV meningitis or encephalitis pose a clear risk for transmitting a fatal infection to recipients. Health care providers, transplant centers, and organ procurement organizations should be aware of the risks posed by LCMV, and should consider LCMV in any potential donor with signs of aseptic meningitis, but no identified infectious agent. The risks and benefits of offering and receiving organs from donors with possible LCMV infection should be carefully weighed [9].

DIFFERENTIAL DIAGNOSIS

For acquired (postnatal) LCMV infection, the principal items in the differential diagnosis are the other infectious agents that can induce meningitis. These agents include bacteria, fungi, viruses, and some other forms of pathogens. The most common viral causes of meningitis are the enteroviruses, including Coxsackie viruses and echoviruses, and the arboviruses, including LaCross encephalitis virus and equine encephalitis virus. Unlike LCMV, which is most common in winter, the enteroviruses and arboviruses are most commonly acquired in summer and early fall.

The principal items in the differential diagnosis of congenital LCMV infection are the other infectious pathogens that can cross the placenta and damage the developing fetus. These infectious agents are linked by the acronym "TORCHS" and include *Toxoplasma gondii*, rubella virus, cytomegalovirus, herpes simplex virus, and syphilis. Cytomegalovirus and toxoplasmosis are particularly difficult to differentiate from LCMV because infection with any of these 3 infectious agents can produce microcephaly, intracerebral mineralization, and chorioretinitis [30]. Although clinical clues may aid in distinguishing one congenital infection from another, definitive identification of the causative infectious agent usually requires laboratory data, including cultures and serologic studies.

Symptomatic congenital cytomegalovirus infection is usually associated with several systemic signs that are not observed in congenital LCMV infection. These indications include hepatosplenomegaly, jaundice, anemia, intrauterine growth retardation, and a petechial or purpuric rash. Hearing deficits are common in infants infected with cytomegalovirus but are unusual in congenital LCMV infection. The diagnosis of congenital cytomegalovirus infection is best established by isolating the virus from urine or saliva within the first 3 weeks of life. Detection beyond this time point may reflect postnatal acquisition of the virus [30].

Of all of the congenital infections, toxoplasmosis most closely resembles congenital LCMV infection. Microencephaly, hydrocephalus, chorioretinitis, and intracranial calcifications are hallmarks of both congenital infections. Approximately 10% of newborns infected with *T. gondii* exhibit hepatosplenomegaly, jaundice, and rash [31]. These systemic signs are usually absent in congenital LCMV infection. The 2 infections also tend to differ neuroradiographically. In cases of congenital toxoplasmosis, the intracranial mineralization tends to be diffuse within the brain parenchyma. In contrast, in congenital LCMV infection the mineralizations are typically periventricular. Congenital infection with toxoplasmosis and LCMV are so clinically similar, however, that differentiating between them requires laboratory testing. The diagnosis of congenital toxoplasmosis can be established by serologic studies and confirmed by detecting the infectious organisms in tissues, blood, or CSF.

The differential diagnosis of congenital LCMV infection also includes several noninfectious entities. Chromosomal abnormalities are prominent causes of microencephaly. However, abnormalities in the structure or number of chromosomes commonly induce dysmorphic features (especially of the hands, feet, and facies) or structural abnormalities (especially of the heart or genitourinary system) that are not observed in congenital LCMV infection.

Several genetic disorders can mimic congenital LCMV infection [32]. In particular, Aicardi-Goutieres syndrome is an autosomal recessive disorder that often presents as neonatal encephalopathy and intracranial calcifications [33]. However, its progressive course and identifiable mutations in the TREX1 and RNASEH2 genes distinguish it from congenital LCMV infection.

A second disorder that mimics congenital LCMV and that may be genetic in etiology is pseudo-TORCH syndrome [34]. In this disorder, infants have many of the classic features of the common congenital infections that gave rise to the TORCH acronym [35]. However, in pseudo-TORCH syndrome, no serologic or microbiologic evidence of a congenital infection is ever identified. Because multiple siblings may be similarly affected, pseudo-TORCH syndrome is presumed to be a genetic disorder [36]. However, no genetic locus for pseudo-TORCH syndrome has been identified. The possibility exists that pseudo-TORCH syndrome is actually an unidentified congenital infection. Congenital LCMV infection can be distinguished from pseudo-TORCH syndrome in several ways. First, most mothers of infants with congenital LCMV infection have a history of exposure to wild mice and have experienced a definite "flulike" illness during the pregnancy. These historical factors are typically absent in pseudo-TORCH syndrome. Most importantly, chorioretinitis is present in virtually all cases of congenital LCMV infection and absent in all cases of pseudo-TORCH syndrome [24].

DIAGNOSTIC WORKUP

Acute human LCMV infections can be diagnosed by isolating the virus from CSF. However, by the time of birth a baby prenatally infected with LCMV may no longer harbor the virus. Thus, congenital LCMV infection is usually diagnosed by serologic testing. The immunofluorescent antibody test detects both IgM and IgG, and has greater sensitivity than the more widely available complement fixation method [37]. The immunofluorescent antibody test is commercially available, and its specificity and sensitivity make it an acceptable diagnostic tool. A more sensitive test for detecting congenital LCMV infection is the enzyme-linked immunosorbent assay, which measures titers of LCMV IgG and IgM, and is performed at the Centers for Disease Control and Prevention. The polymerase chain reaction (PCR) has also been used to detect LCMV RNA in an infected infant [1]. The use of PCR offers exciting possibilities for both prenatal and postnatal detection of LCMV infection. However, LCMV is not known to induce persistent infections in humans, and the time course of viral clearance from an infected human fetus is unknown. A fetus may sustain substantial brain damage from LCMV but effectively clear the virus, and may have no LCMV RNA to be detected by PCR in the postnatal period.

PROGNOSIS AND COMPLICATIONS

The prognosis for children and adults who acquire LCMV postnatally is generally excellent. Most are symptomatic for only several weeks and suffer no long-term consequences. Hydrocephalus has occurred in some patients who acquire LCMV during childhood [6]. On rare occasions an otherwise healthy individual who acquires LCMV postnatally dies from the infection.

The prognosis for children with congenital LCMV infection is generally poor. A meta-analysis of all reported cases of congenital LCMV infection revealed a mortality rate of 35% by age 21 months [18]. Of those that survive, most have severe neurodevelopmental disorders, including substantial mental retardation, microcephaly, poor somatic growth, profound vision impairment, severe seizure disorders, and spastic weakness [19]. However, some of these children have only moderate neurologic and mental disabilities, and a few have been described as having a normal outcome [20]. Hearing is nearly always spared in children with congenital LCMV infection, and developmental regression is virtually absent.

Complications in children with congenital LCMV infection are nonspecific and include the medical problems that commonly arise in scenarios involving ventriculoperitoneal shunts, severe seizure disorders, and static encephalopathy. These complications include shunt failure or infection, aspiration pneumonia, injuries from falls, and joint contractures.

MANAGEMENT

There is no specific treatment for acquired or congenital LCMV infection. An effective antiviral therapy for LCMV infection has not yet been developed. Children with hydrocephalus due to congenital LCMV infection often require placement of a ventriculoperitoneal shunt during infancy. Seizures often begin during early postnatal life, are often difficult to control, and require administration of multiple antiepileptic medications. The mental retardation induced by congenital LCMV infection is often profound. In most cases, affected children should be referred for educational intervention during early life. The spasticity accompanying congenital LCMV infection is often severe. Although physical therapy can help to maintain range of motion and minimize painful spasms and contractures, implantation of a baclofen pump is often necessary and helpful.

References

[1] Enders G, Varho-Gobel M, Lohler J, et al. Congenital lymphocytic choriomeningitis virus infection: an underdiagnosed disease. Pediatr Infect Dis J 1999;18:652–5.

[2] Armstrong C, Lillie RD. Experimental lymphocytic choriomeningitis of monkeys and mice produced by a virus encountered in studies of the 1933 St. Louis encephalitis epidemic. Public Health Rep 1934;49:1019–22.

[3] Meyer HM Jr, Johnson RT, Crawford IP, et al. Central nervous system syndromes of "viral" etiology: a study of 713 cases. Am J Med 1960;29:334–47.

[4] Komrower GM, Williams BL, Stones PB. Lymphocytic choriomeningitis in the newborn. Probable transplacental infection. Lancet 1955;1:697–8.

[5] Barton LL, Budd SC, Morfitt WS, et al. Congenital lymphocytic choriomeningitis virus infection in twins. Pediatr Infect Dis J 1993;12:942–6.

[6] Larsen PD, Chartrand SA, Tomashek KM, et al. Hydrocephalus complicating lymphocytic choriomeningitis virus infection. Pediatr Infect Dis J 1993;12:528–31.

[7] Buchmeier MJ, Zajac AJ. Lymphocytic choriomeningitis virus. In: Ahmed R, Chen I, editors. Persistent viral infections. New York: Wiley; 1999. p. 575–605.

[8] Fischer SA, Graham MB, Kuehnert M, et al. Transmission of lymphocytic choriomeningitis virus by organ transplantation. N Engl J Med 2006;354:2235–49.

[9] Barry A, Gunn J, Tormey P, et al. Lymphocytic choriomeningitis virus transmitted through solid organ transplantation—Massachusetts, 2008. MMWR 2008;57(29):799–801.

[10] Bonthius DJ, Karacay B. Meningitis and encephalitis in children: an update. Neurol Clin 2002;20:1013–38.

[11] Jahrling PB, Peters CJ. Lymphocytic choriomeningitis virus: a neglected pathogen of man. Arch Pathol Lab Med 1992;116:486–8.

[12] Chesney PJ, Katcher ML, Nelson DB, et al. CSF eosinophilia and chronic lymphocytic choriomeningitis virus meningitis. J Pediatr 1979;94:750–2.

[13] Lewis JM, Utz JP. Orchitis, parotitis and meningoencephalitis due to lymphocytic choriomeningitis virus. N Engl J Med 1961;265:776–80.

[14] Biggar R, Woodall J, Walter P, et al. Lymphocytic choriomeningitis outbreak associated with pet hamsters: fifty seven cases from New York state. JAMA 1975;232:494.

[15] Barton LL, Peters CJ, Ksiazek TG. Lymphocytic choriomeningitis virus: an unrecognized teratogenic pathogen. Emerg Infect Dis 1995;1:152–3.

[16] Mets MB, Barton LL, Khan AS, et al. Lymphocytic choriomeningitis virus: an underdiagnosed cause of congenital chorioretinitis. Am J Ophthalmol 2000;130:209–15.

[17] Barton LL, Mets MB. Congenital lymphocytic choriomeningitis virus infection: decade of rediscovery. Clin Infect Dis 2001;33:370–4.

[18] Wright R, Johnson D, Neumann M, et al. Congenital lymphocytic choriomeningitis virus syndrome: a disease that mimics congenital toxoplasmosis or cytomegalovirus infection. Pediatrics 1997;100:1–6.

[19] Bonthius DJ, Wright R, Tseng B, et al. Congenital lymphocytic choriomeningitis virus infection: spectrum of disease. Ann Neurol 2007b;62:347–55.

[20] Larsen PD, Wright R. Early clinical manifestations and long-term outcome in children with symptomatic congenital lymphocytic choriomeningitis virus infection. Neurology 2001;56:A39–40.

[21] Bonthius DJ, Nichols B, Harb H, et al. Lymphocytic choriomeningitis virus infection of the developing brain: critical role of host age. Ann Neurol 2007;62:356–74.

[22] Bonthius DJ, Mahoney JC, Buchmeier MJ, et al. Critical role for glial cells in the propagation and spread of lymphocytic choriomeningitis virus in the developing rat brain. J Virol 2002;76(13):6618–35.

[23] Bonthius DJ, Perlman S. Congenital viral infections of the brain: lessons learned from lymphocytic choriomeningitis virus in the neonatal rat. PLoS Pathog 2007;3:1541–50. Available at: www.plospathogens.org. Accessed June 1, 2009.

[24] Bonthius DJ. Diagnosed cases of congenital LCMV infection: tip of the iceberg? Ann Neurol 2008;64:356.

[25] Lehmann-Grube F. Portraits of viruses: arenaviruses. Intervirology 1984;22:121–45.

[26] Ambrosio AM, Feuillade MR, Gamboa GS, et al. Prevalence of lymphocytic choriomeningitis virus infection in a human population of Argentina. Am J Trop Med Hyg 1994;50:381–6.

[27] Childs JE, Glass GE, Korch GW, et al. Lymphocytic choriomeningitis virus infection and house mouse (Mus musculus) distribution in urban Baltimore. Am J Trop Med Hyg 1992;47:27–34.

[28] Stephensen CB, Blount SR, Lanford RE, et al. Prevalence of serum antibodies against lymphocytic choriomeningitis virus in selected populations from two U.S. cities. J Med Virol 1992;38:27–31.

[29] Dykewicz CA, Dato VM, Fisher-Hoch SP. Lymphocytic choriomeningitis outbreak associated with nude mice in a research institute. JAMA 1992;267:1349–53.

[30] Bale JF, Murph JR. Congenital infections and the nervous system. Pediatr Clin North Am 1992;39:669–90.

[31] Koppe JG, Loewer-Sieger DH, De Roever-Bonnet H. Results of 20-year follow-up of congenital toxoplasmosis. Lancet 1986;1:254.

[32] Sanchis A, Cervero L, Bataller A, et al. Genetic syndromes mimic congenital infections. J Pediatr 2005;146:701–5.

[33] Rice G, Patrick T, Parmar R, et al. Clinical and molecular phenotype of Aicardi-Goutieres syndrome. Am J Hum Genet 2007;81:713–25.

[34] Vivarelli R, Grosso S, Cioni M, et al. Pseudo-TORCH syndrome or Baraitser-Reardon syndrome: diagnostic criteria. Brain Dev 2001;23:18–23.

[35] Farmer M, Sebire G. Genetic mimics of congenital lymphocytic choriomeningitis virus encephalitis. Ann Neurol 2008;64:353–5.

[36] Knoblauch H, Tennstedt C, Brueck W, et al. Two brothers with findings resembling congenital intrauterine infection-like syndrome (pseudo-TORCH syndrome). Am J Med Genet 2003;120:261–5.

[37] Lehmann-Grube F, Kallay M, Ibscher B, et al. Serologic diagnosis of human infections with lymphocytic choriomeningitis virus: comparative evaluation of seven methods. J Med Virol 1979;4:125–36.

ELSEVIER
MOSBY

Advances in Pediatrics 56 (2009) 87–106

ADVANCES IN PEDIATRICS

Sexually Transmitted Diseases in Adolescents

Diane M. Straub, MD, MPH

Division of Adolescent Medicine, University of South Florida, 2 Tampa General Circle, Suite 500, Tampa, FL 33606, USA

S exually transmitted infections (STIs) have reached crisis proportions in United States adolescents today. There are 19 million STIs annually, almost half of which occur among young people aged 15 to 24 years [1,2]. The rates of many STIs are highest among adolescents and young adults. Data from the National Health and Nutrition Examination Survey (NHANES) 2003 to 2004 estimated that approximately 1 in 4 adolescent females in the United States has an STI. Among those that are sexually active, the numbers were even more dramatic, reaching 40% [3]. It is not hard to see why this crisis has occurred. When one looks at the most recent data from the Youth Risk Behavior Surveillance Survey (YRBS), one can see how youth are putting themselves at risk. Nationwide, 47.8% of students report having ever had sexual intercourse, 7.1% report intercourse before the age of 13 years, 14.9% report having had 4 or more partners lifetime, and among the 35.0% who are currently sexually active, only 65.1% report condom use at last intercourse [4].

PREVALENCE AND TRENDS

Chlamydia is the most commonly reported STI, with more than 1 million cases reported in 2007. Continued increases are likely, partially due to increased screening and availability of more sensitive diagnostic tests; even so, the Centers for Disease Control and Prevention (CDC) estimates that more than half of cases remain undiagnosed and unreported. In 2007, adolescent females (15–19 years old) had the highest rates of any population or risk group. Gonorrhea is the second most commonly reported STI, with 355, 991 new cases in 2007. Rates vary by region, with the South having the highest rates. Gonorrhea has become more difficult to treat with increasing fluoroquinolone resistance, discussed further later in this article. Although syphilis rates decreased steadily in the United States during 1990 to 2000, rates have been increasing since 2001; rates vary geographically, with the highest in the South, and by population, with men who have sex with men accounting for the majority of cases [2].

E-mail address: dstraub@health.usf.edu

0065-3101/09/$ – see front matter
doi:10.1016/j.yapd.2009.08.015

In terms of viral STIs, a recently published study of women aged 14 to 65 years receiving routine cervical screening found an overall high-risk human papilloma virus (HPV) prevalence of 23%, with prevalence highest (35%) among those aged 14 to 19 years [5]. An estimated 50 million people in the United States have genital herpes, with 1 million new infections per year [6]. From United States National Health and Nutrition Examination Surveys data from 1999 to 2004, Xu and colleagues [7] found a seroprevalence of 1.6% among 14- to 19-year-olds. Finally, the CDC estimates that there were about 56,300 new cases of human immunodeficiency virus (HIV) in 2006. It is thought that at least half of new infections occur among people younger than 25 years old. About a quarter of those infected are unaware of their status [8].

The CDC's 2007 disease profile highlighted racial disparities. Some sobering statistics include that, despite African Americans comprising only 12% of the population, they account for 70% of gonorrhea cases and almost half of Chlamydia and syphilis. These rates are 19, 8, and 7 times higher than the rates in whites, respectively [2]. In addition, almost half of all HIV/AIDS cases diagnosed in 2006 in the 33 states with name-based reporting occurred among African Americans [8]. The 2008 CDC study looking at multiple STIs showed that almost half of African American adolescent girls has an STI [3].

CONFIDENTIAL HEALTH CARE OF ADOLESCENTS

Before considering the issue of STIs in adolescents, it is important to take into consideration the issue of confidential health care. Multiple studies demonstrate that lack of confidential health care impedes adolescents' access to needed health care, and numerous laws now protect adolescents' rights to confidential health care. It is important for providers to familiarize themselves with such laws in order to diagnose and treat STIs in adolescence [9]. Resources for such information include the Guttmacher Institute (http://www.guttmacher.org/statecenter/spibs/spib_MASS.pdf) and Physicians for Reproductive Choice and Healthcare (http://www.prch.org/resources-minors-access-cards).

COMMON SEXUALLY TRANSMITTED INFECTIONS

Unless otherwise stated, all treatment recommendations in this article are the CDC sexually transmitted disease (STD) treatment recommendations, which can be found at the following user-friendly, evidence-based, and frequently updated Web site: http://www.cdc.gov/std/treatment.

Herpes simplex virus

There are 2 serotypes of herpes simplex virus (HSV) called, appropriately, 1 and 2. Although type 2 previously caused the most genital herpes, type 1 now causes up to 50% of first clinical episodes, and generally has a milder course with less frequent recurrences than type 2. Of note, most HSV is not diagnosed, and most genital herpes is transmitted by persons unaware of their infection or asymptomatic when transmission occurs. Other presentations

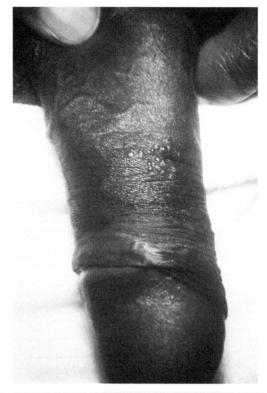

Fig. 1. Herpetic rash (vesicles). (*Courtesy of* the Centers for Disease Control and Prevention.)

include painful or itchy blisters (Fig. 1) and ulcers (Fig. 2), vaginal or penile discharge, and tender inguinal lymphadenopathy. Many patients initially develop mild symptoms, which can later become severe or prolonged, and occasionally systemic, flulike symptoms can result in hospitalization.

In terms of diagnosis, several methods of varying utility are available. Visualization is very nonspecific. Viral culture is the gold standard and preferred method. However, sensitivity declines rapidly as lesions heal, usually within days of onset, and as the lesions progress from vesicles to ulcers to crusted lesions. Polymerase chain reaction (PCR) assays are more sensitive, but are not Food and Drug Administration (FDA)-approved except for testing spinal fluid for central nervous system infections. The Tzanck preparation relies on cytologic detection of cellular changes in genital lesions. This method is insensitive and nonspecific, and is not recommended. Of note, lack of detection of HSV does not necessarily indicate absence of infection, as shedding is intermittent. Serum testing for type-specific antibodies can aid in diagnosis and management. Because almost all HSV-2 infections are sexually acquired, the presence of HSV-2 antibodies indicates anogenital infection, but the presence of HSV-1 antibodies does not distinguish anogenital from orolabial infections. As one

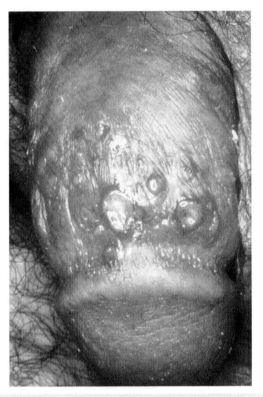

Fig. 2. Herpetic rash (ulcers). (*Courtesy of* the Centers for Disease Control and Prevention.)

would expect, serum antibody testing will lag behind the clinical presentation in first episodes but can be used to confirm clinical diagnosis.

Differential diagnosis includes syphilis, which is less common in adolescents, and chancroid, which is also less common in United States adolescents. HSV classically has grouped vesicles and painful, shallow ulcers accompanied by tender inguinal lymphadenopathy. The classic chancre of primary syphilis is usually solitary and painless (Figs. 3 and 4), has indurated, well-defined borders, and the lymphadenopathy is not as tender. Finally, chancroid also usually has multiple, painful ulcers, but they usually have ragged edges, and the accompanying tender lymphadenopathy is often suppurative (termed "buboes"). Testing for chancroid is by culturing for *Haemophilius ducreyi*, which is not widely available and is only about 80% sensitive. The clinician should consider empirical treatment for chancroid if the presentation is of a painful ulcer or ulcers and tender inguinal lymphadenopathy, and workup is negative for HSV and syphilis. Very rare STIs in the United States that can be confused with HSV include Donovanosis, or granuloma inguinale, which is caused by a gram-negative bacteria called *Calymmatobacterium granulomatis*, and lympho-granuloma venereum, which is caused by *Chlamydia trachomatis* serovars.

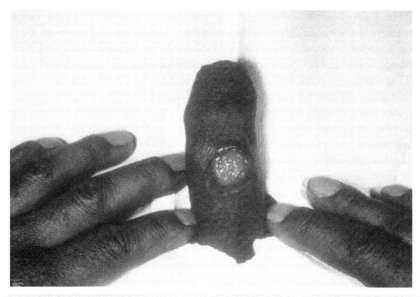

Fig. 3. Primary syphilis ("chancre"). (*Courtesy of* the Centers for Disease Control and Prevention.)

Accepted treatment regimens for the first clinical episode of genital herpes include the following: acyclovir, 200 mg by mouth, three times a day for 7 to 10 days; acyclovir, 200 mg by mouth, four times a day for 7 to 10 days; famciclovir, 250 mg by mouth, twice daily for 7 to 10 days; or valacyclovir, 1.0 g by mouth, twice daily for 7 to 10 days. Note that treatment does not eradicate the latent virus or affect the risk, frequency, or severity of reoccurrences after the drug is discontinued. Approximately 50% of patients with recurrent episodes experience a prodrome, which results in tingling or pain 30 minutes to 48 hours before and at the site of the eruption. Effective episodic treatment must begin within 24 hours of lesion onset, or during the prodrome. The patient should be provided with a prescription and instructions to self-initiate treatment as appropriate. Accepted episodic treatment recommendations include: acyclovir, 400 mg by mouth three times a day *or* 800 mg twice a day for 5 days; acyclovir, 200 mg three times a day for two days; famciclovir, 1000 mg two times a day for one day; valacyclovir, 500 mg by mouth twice a day for 3 or 1 g daily for 5 days. Patients desiring to prevent reoccurrences can be offered suppressive therapy comprising once- or twice-a-day dosing of the antiviral drug. Studies have also shown decreased transmission with suppressive treatment. Of note, the natural history of genital herpes is of decreasing frequency and severity of outbreaks over time and improved psychological adjustment to these outbreaks, so periodic reassessment of therapy is recommended.

The CDC has the following recommendations related to genital herpes: routinely use viral culture or other tests for HSV in the diagnosis of genital ulcers, use only type-specific tests for HSV serologic diagnosis and case finding, consider offering HSV serologic testing when patients request comprehensive STI screening, and advise patients whenever STI evaluation does not include this testing. When counseling patients, advise of the following: the natural history of the disease, including the potential for recurrent episodes, asymptomatic shedding, and risks of sexual transmission; the availability of effective suppressive and episodic antiviral therapy; latex condoms can decrease the risk of transmission; abstain from sexual activity during outbreaks (including the prodrome); inform current and future sexual partners of genital herpes and that it is frequently asymptomatic; and the risk of neonatal HSV.

Human papilloma virus

There are over 100 types of HPV that infect humans, about 40 of which are through sexual contact. "High-risk" oncogenic types include 16, 18, 31, 33, 35, 39, 45, 51, 52, 56, and 58, and can result in low-grade cervical abnormalities (cervical intraepithelial neoplasia [CIN] type 1), cancer precursors (CIN 2 and 3), and genital cancers. "Low-risk" types include 6, 11, 42, 43, and 44, and can result in low-grade cervical abnormalities (CIN 1), genital warts, and respiratory papillomas.

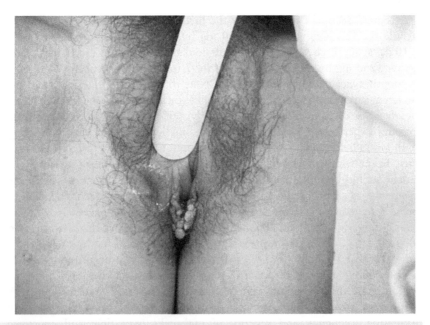

Fig. 4. Primary syphilis ("chancre") and condyloma accuminata (human papilloma virus). (*Courtesy of* the Centers for Disease Control and Prevention.)

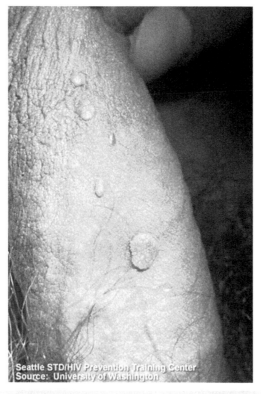

Fig. 5. Condyloma accuminata. (*Courtesy of* the Seattle STD/HIV Prevention Training Center at the University of Washington.)

Condyloma accuminata (Figs. 4 and 5), or genital warts, can occur on any genital surface. These warts are usually diagnosed by visual inspection, although the clinical presentation can be very similar to condyloma lata (Fig. 6), a presentation of syphilis, which should be a reminder to consider this in one's differential diagnosis. Other considerations include pearly pink papules (a normal variant found on the corona of the penis and a cause of great concern in young men thinking they have an STI), molluscum contagiosum, and scabies.

The natural history of genital warts includes spontaneous resolution, no change, or increased number and size. Therefore, the goal of treatment should be to remove symptomatic warts. It is important to advise patients that treatment will not eradicate HPV or eliminate infectivity, that condoms are only partially protective (they may not cover the infected skin), and that the strains that cause warts do not cause cervical cancer. There are multiple treatments available, both provider- and patient-applied. Treatment may result in considerable discomfort, erythema, epithelial erosion, ulceration, depigmentation,

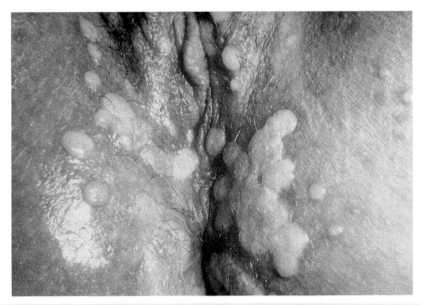

Fig. 6. Condyloma lata (secondary syphilis). (*Courtesy of* the Centers for Disease Control and Prevention.)

and scarring, and duration of therapy may be lengthy. A commonly used provider-applied therapy includes trichloroacetic acid, which is applied weekly until resolution. A commonly used patient-applied therapy is imiquimod, which is applied 3 times per week for 6 to 10 hours overnight for up to 16 weeks. In addition, an acceptable alternative is to forgo treatment and await spontaneous resolution.

Subclinical genital HPV infection is a term used to refer to manifestations of infection in the absence of genital warts. This infection occurs more frequently than visible genital warts among both men and women. Subclinical genital HPV is most commonly diagnosed by Papanicolou smear of the cervix with detection of squamous intraepithelial lesions, and is also diagnosed by colposcopy or biopsy. The application of 3% to 5% acetic acid usually turns HPV-infected genital mucosa a whitish color, but it is neither a sensitive nor specific screening procedure.

HPV screening recommendations for adolescents have changed in recent years, based on new research findings. Persistent infection is the primary risk factor in progression of infection to serious disease [10,11]. Yet, in adolescents, HPV infections usually do not persist. Moscicki and colleagues [10,12] found that among women 13 to 22 years old, most HPV infections are transient, with approximately 70% regression of high-risk HPV types and more than 90% regression of low-risk HPV types within 3 years. Furthermore, in adolescents most infections result in no symptoms or cellular changes, or low-grade intraepithelial lesions (LSILs), and 95% of LSILs resolve within 3 years. The purpose of screening is to detect cervical cancer precursors and remove high-grade lesions, and thus prevent potential progression to cervical carcinoma. To this end, recommendations from the American Cancer Society and the American College of Obstetrics and Gynecologists recommend that screening with Papanicolou smear begin approximately 3 years after the onset of vaginal intercourse, but no later than 21 years of age, and should continue yearly (American Cancer Society [ACS], American College of Obstetricians and Gynecologists) or every other year with liquid-based Papanicolou smears (ACS) [13,14].

Subclinical HPV should only be treated in the presence of coexisting squamous intraepithelial lesions, and management is determined by histopathology. The reader is referred to current guidelines [15] for management at the following URL: http://www.asccp.org.

A final point on HPV relates to vaccination. The American Academy of Pediatrics recommends that all girls aged 11 to 12 years should routinely be immunized with 3 doses of quadrivalent HPV vaccine. The vaccine can be given to girls as young as 9 years old, and adolescents and young women aged 13 to 26 years who have not been immunized or who have not completed the series should receive the vaccine. Vaccinated females should continue to have routine cervical cancer screening as recommended [16].

Chlamydia

Chlamydia trachomatis is an obligate intracellular parasite. Incidence varies from 2% to 35% in adolescents, depending on the location and subgroup. Clinical presentation is usually asymptomatic; approximately 75% of female and 50% of male genital Chlamydia infections are detected by testing asymptomatic persons. Other presentations can include dysuria, vaginal or penile discharge, abdominal or back pain, and irregular menstrual bleeding. Clinical syndromes include cervicitis, urethritis, Bartholinitis, pelvic inflammatory disease (PID), perihepatitis, epididymitis, and proctitis. Sequelae include PID, chronic pelvic pain, ectopic pregnancy, infertility, and perinatal transmission.

For diagnosis, low-cost nonamplified tests have lower sensitivity and specificity than the nucleic acid amplification tests. However, nucleic acid amplification tests (NAATs) can be used on urine specimens, and have recently been approved for use in self-collected vaginal swabs, which are more easily obtainable (and certainly patient preferred) than penile or endocervical specimens. Culture is indicated in cases of suspected sexual abuse or rape; specificity is 100%, but sensitivity is lower.

Recommended treatment of uncomplicated cervicitis/urethritis includes azithromycin, 1 g by mouth in one dose, or doxycycline, 100 mg by mouth, twice a day for 7 days. Azithromycin is the treatment of choice during pregnancy. Of note, the 2 recommended regimens are equally efficacious, but azithromycin should be available for patients in whom compliance is a question for directly observed therapy. Patients should be instructed to abstain from sexual activity for 7 days after starting treatment, regardless of which therapy is used, and until 7 days after all sexual partners are treated. All sexual contacts within the 60 days preceding the onset of symptoms should receive a full STI evaluation and be empirically treated. Treatment of sex partners helps prevent reinfection. The CDC recommends expedited partner therapy for Chlamydia, or dispensing medication (and information and instructions on its use) to index patients to distribute to their partner(s). However this is still illegal in many states, due to mandates requiring a formal doctor-patient relationship prior to prescription of medication and liability issues. A recent innovative idea to facilitate treating of partners is e-mail notification, which has proved to be of some success [17] (for further information, see the Web site at http://www.inkspot.org). Test of cure is not recommended except during pregnancy. However, test for reinfection is recommended, due to the high rates of Chlamydia reinfection rates among females by untreated partners. Providers should retest all females treated for chlamydial infection whenever they next seek medical care within the following 3 to 12 months, regardless of whether the patient believes that her sex partners were treated.

In terms of routine screening, the 2007 United States Preventative Services Task Force (USPSTF) recommended yearly screening of sexually active females younger than 25 years, with the rationale that such screening reduces the incidence of PID. For males, due to "critical gaps in knowledge," they did not make the same recommendation, with the caveat that although it would likely be beneficial if it leads to decreased incidence in females, there is little direct benefit to males [18].

Gonorrhea

Among men most infections produce symptoms causing them to seek medical care prior to any serious sequelae, although not soon enough to prevent transmission. Unfortunately, women often do not have recognizable symptoms until complications like PID have occurred. Clinical syndromes include urethritis, cervicitis, pharyngitis, proctitis, Bartholinitis, PID, and conjunctivitis. Sequelae include PID, Bartholin abscess, lymphangitis, arthritis, disseminated gonococcal infection (meningitis, endocarditis), and neonatal infections. Of note, some strains that cause disseminated gonococcal infection may cause minimal genital inflammation.

Diagnosis is similar to Chlamydia, with amplified testing providing good sensitivity and specificity. However, product inserts for each NAAT should be carefully checked, as FDA-approved specimen types for each may vary.

Current treatment options for uncomplicated gonorrhea infection include ceftriaxone, 125 mg intramuscularly (IM) and cefixime, 400 mg by mouth, which has recently become available again after being taken off the market in 2002. The Gonococcal Isolate Surveillance Project (GISP) (a sentinel surveillance project located in 28 STD clinics nationwide) demonstrated fluoroquinolone resistance in 14% of isolates collected in 2006, compared with 9% in 2005; these data prompted the CDC to revise its guidelines in 2007 such that floroquinolones are no longer recommended for treatment of gonorrhea [19]. Chlamydial infection accompanies up to 46% of gonococcal infections [20], so routine cotreatment against Chlamydia is recommended. In addition, most gonococci in the United States are sensitive to azithromycin and doxycycline, so routine dual therapy hinders the development of resistance. Due to the high sensitivity of NAATs, treatment of Chlamydia is not recommended if the NAAT result is negative for Chlamydia at the time of treatment of gonorrhea. Treatment of sex partners is identical to Chlamydia, including all partners within the previous 60 days prior to diagnosis or onset of symptoms, or the most recent sexual partner if contact was longer than 60 days prior. Test of cure is not recommended, although screening for reinfection again is. Routine screening is recommended by the USPSTF for all sexually active adolescent females [21].

HIV

A thorough discussion of HIV is beyond the scope of this article, but mention of HIV should be part of any discussion of STIs in adolescence. Over half of all HIV infections occur in youth younger than 25 years, and about a quarter of those infected are not aware of their status. Symptoms of acute antiretroviral syndrome include many manifestations of common ailments seen during adolescence: fever (>80%–90% of patients), fatigue (>70%–90%), rash (>40%–80%), headache (32%–70%), lymphadenopathy (40%–70%), pharyngitis (50%–70%), myalgias/arthralgias (50%–70%), nausea/vomiting or diarrhea (30%–60%), night sweats (50%), aseptic meningitis (24%), oral ulcers (10%–20%), genital ulcers (5%–15%), thrombocytopenia (45%), leukopenia (40%), and elevated liver enzymes (21%) [22]. Providers should consider acute antiretroviral syndrome in their differential diagnosis in sexually active adolescents who demonstrate constellations of these symptoms. Furthermore, the most recent CDC testing recommendations [23] are a somewhat radical departure from previous risk-based paradigms advocating thorough counseling and consent procedures, and include the following:

- HIV screening is recommended for patients in all health care settings after the patient is notified that testing will be performed unless the patient declines (opt-out screening).
- Persons at high risk for HIV infection should be screened for HIV at least annually.
- Separate written consent for HIV testing should not be required; general consent for medical care should be considered sufficient to encompass consent for HIV testing.
- Prevention counseling should not be required with HIV diagnostic testing or as part of HIV screening programs in health care settings.

These recommendations are often at odds with state mandates related to HIV testing, and implementation has been slow. Clinicians should always remember to consider HIV in cases of possible acute antiretroviral syndrome, in any STI evaluations in adolescents, and as part of routine medical care. In addition, using saliva-based tests to avoid phlebotomy and rapid tests to ensure that results are delivered are useful strategies when dealing with adolescents.

Syphilis

Although syphilis is less of a problem in adolescents, relative to adults and relative to the other STIs discussed in this article, it deserves some mention. Patients might present to care for signs or symptoms of primary infection (the "chancre", discussed above, see Figs 3 and 4), secondary infection (ie, rash) (Fig. 7), "copper penny" rash on hands and feet (Fig. 8), mucocutaneous lesions, lymphadenopathy, condyloma lata (see Fig. 6), or tertiary infection (cardiac or ophthalmic manifestations, auditory abnormalities, gummatous lesions), or might be asymptomatic (latent syphilis, detected by serologic testing). The clinician should remember to consider syphilis in the differential diagnosis, and should check regional epidemiology when considering screening.

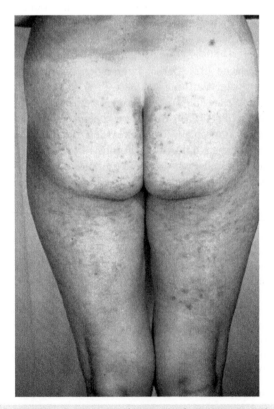

Fig. 7. Secondary syphilis rash. (*Courtesy of* the Centers for Disease Control and Prevention.)

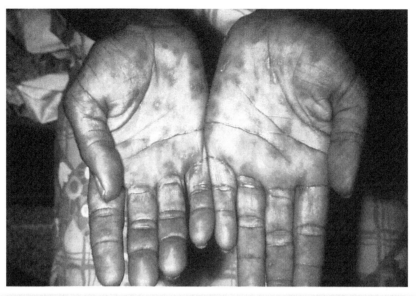

Fig. 8. "Copper penny" rash (secondary syphilis). (*Courtesy of* the Centers for Disease Control and Prevention.)

CLINICAL SYNDROMES

Urethritis

Urethritis is urethral discharge of mucopurulent or purulent material plus or minus dysuria or urethral pruritus. The principal pathogens are *Gonococcus* and *Chlamydia*, which comprises 15% to 55% of nongonococcal urethritis. Other agents sometimes implicated include *Ureaplasma*, *Mycoplasma*, *Trichomonas*, and HSV. Confirmed urethritis can be diagnosed by visualization of discharge; Gram stain showing 5 white blood cells or more per high-powered field (wbc/hpf), with added evidence of noting any intracellular gram-negative diplococci; or by a positive leukocyte esterase test or 10 wbc/hpf or more on first-void urine. Testing for specific etiology is recommended because both gonorrhea and Chlamydia are reportable conditions, and a specific diagnosis may enhance partner notification and improve compliance with treatment, especially in the exposed partner. NAATs are recommended, especially if Gram stain capabilities are not available. Empirical treatment of confirmed urethritis should include coverage for both gonorrhea and Chlamydia; if unconfirmed, treatment should only be given for those patients unlikely to return for follow-up.

Cervicitis

Cervicitis can present asymptomatically or as vaginal discharge, dyspareunia, irregular menstrual bleeding, back pain, or abdominal pain. Confirmed diagnosis is by visualization of purulent or mucopurulent endocervical exudate in the endocervical canal or on a swab, plus or minus sustained endocervical bleeding with cotton swab, or positive tests for gonorrhea or Chlamydia. Causative organisms/etiologies are gonorrhea or Chlamydia, and less commonly *Trichomonas*, HSV, or bacterial vaginosis. However, in most cases it is never determined. As with urethritis, testing for gonorrhea and Chlamydia is recommended. Also, empirical treatment of both is recommended if the likelihood of infection is high and the patient may be difficult to locate for treatment. Partners should be notified, evaluated, and treated for the suspected STI.

Pelvic inflammatory disease

PID is a spectrum of inflammatory disorders of the upper genital tract, including any combination of endometritis, salpingitis, tubo-ovarian abscess (TOA), and pelvic peritonitis. Causative organisms include gonorrhea, Chlamydia, and vaginal flora, including anaerobes, Garnerella, *Haemophilus influenzae*, enteric G-rods, and *Streptococcus agalactiae*. Clinical diagnosis has a positive predictive value of only 65% to 90%, depending on the clinical setting, compared with laparoscopy. However, laparoscopy cannot detect endometritis or subtle salpingitis, so it is a questionable gold standard. There is basically no combination of clinical guidelines that has both high sensitivity and specificity. PID is often undiagnosed and has serious sequelae, so providers should have a low threshold for diagnosis. Empirical treatment should be given to any sexually active young woman experiencing pelvic or abdominal pain, the presence of uterine, adnexal, or cervical motion tenderness, and when no other cause(s) can be identified. Most adolescents with PID can be managed as an outpatient, but one should consider hospitalization in the following scenarios: if possible surgical emergency, such as appendicitis, cannot be ruled out; pregnancy; failed outpatient therapy; inability to follow or tolerate outpatient therapy; severe illness, nausea or vomiting, or high fever; and TOA. Multiple treatment recommendations are discussed in the guidelines, and they include empirical, broad-spectrum antibiotics that are effective against gonorrhea and Chlamydia. Parenteral regimens include: (A) cefotetan, 2 g intravenously (IV) every 12 hours, *or* cefoxitin, 2 g IV every 6 hours PLUS doxycycline, 100 mg by mouth or IV every 12 hours; and (B) clindamycin, 900 mg IV every 8 hours PLUS gentamicin loading dose IV or IM (2 mg/kg of body weight), followed by a maintenance dose (1.5 mg/kg) every 8 hours. Outpatient therapy recommendations include ceftriaxone, 250 mg IM as a single dose, cefoxitin, 2 g IM and probenecid, 1 g by mouth as concurrent singles doses, *or* other parenteral third-generation cephalosporin as a single dose, PLUS doxycycline, 100 mg by mouth twice a day for 14 days, WITH or WITHOUT metronidazole, 500 mg by mouth twice a day for 14 days. For inpatient care, IV antibiotics should continue until 24 hours after clinical improvement, and outpatient care should include an IM cephalosporin; both situations should include 14 days of therapy with doxycycline. Follow-up should be within 72 hours to ensure appropriate response to therapy.

Vaginitis

Vaginitis often presents clinically as vaginal discharge, vulvar itching/irritation, and variably vaginal odor. Diagnosis is primarily by presentation, vaginal pH, and microscopic examination of the discharge. The basic differential includes physiologic leukorrhea, bacterial vaginosis, vulvovaginal candidiasis, and trichomoniasis. Of note, only trichomoniasis is considered an STI; the others are sexually associated. Also, the presence of objective signs of external vulvar inflammation in the absence of vaginal pathogens, along with a minimal amount of discharge, suggests the possibility of mechanical, chemical, allergic, or other noninfectious irritation of the vulva. One should always ask patients about bubble baths, vulvar use of soap, and douching.

Physiologic leukorrhea

Physiologic leukorrhea presents as thick, white, mucous discharge, with a normal pH (<4.5). Microscopic examination reveals numerous epithelial cells without evidence of inflammation. Treatment, which may or may not improve the discharge, includes local hygiene, sitz baths, cotton underwear, and loose clothing. Again, asking about and warning against bubble baths, vulvar soap, and douching is recommended.

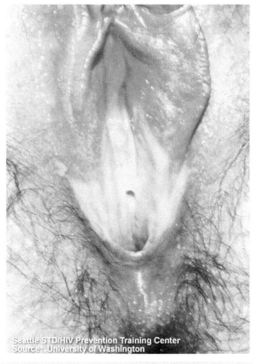

Fig. 9. Bacterial vaginosis. (*Courtesy of* the Seattle STD/HIV Prevention Training Center at the University of Washington.)

Bacterial vaginosis

Bacterial vaginosis (BV) is a clinical syndrome resulting from replacement of the normal H_2O_2-producing *Lactobacillus* sp in the vagina, with high concentrations of anaerobic bacteria, *Gardnerella vaginalis*, and *Mycoplasma hominis*. BV is the most prevalent cause of vaginal discharge or malodor, but up

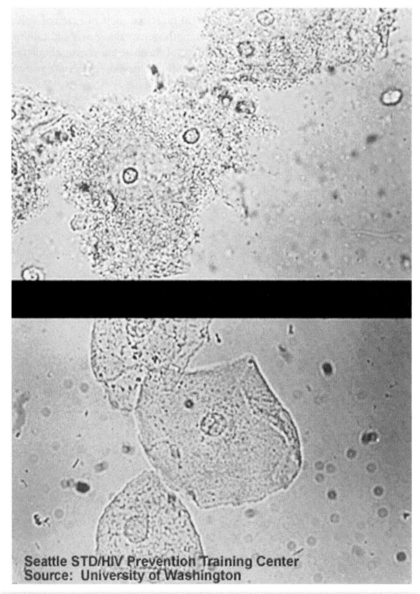

Seattle STD/HIV Prevention Training Center
Source: University of Washington

Fig. 10. Vaginal saline prep: normal (*below*); clue cells (*above*). (*Courtesy of* the Seattle STD/HIV Prevention Training Center at the University of Washington.)

to 50% of women with BV may not report symptoms of BV. BV is associated with multiple sex partners, douching, and lack of lactobacilli; it is unclear whether BV results from acquisition of a sexually transmitted pathogen. However, it rarely affects women who have never been sexually active. Diagnosis can be made by the presence of 3 of the 4 following clinical criteria: (1) homogeneous, gray-white, noninflammatory discharge that smoothly coats vaginal walls (Fig. 9); (2) more than 20% clue cells on microscopic examination (Fig. 10); (3) pH greater than 4.5; and (4) fishy odor ± 10% KOH ("whiff test"). Gold standard for diagnosis is Gram stain for relative concentrations of vaginal flora. Other potential diagnostic modalities include a DNA probe-based test, and card tests that detect elevated pH/ trimethylamine and prolineaminopeptidase. Treatment should be initiated if the patient is symptomatic or pregnant, or before a therapeutic abortion, and regimens include the following: metronidazole, 500 mg by mouth twice a day for 7 days, metronidazole gel (0.75%), 5 g intravaginally every bedtime for 5 days, or clindamycin cream (2%), 5 g intravaginally every bedtime for 7 days.

Vulvovaginal candidiasis

Vulvovaginal candidiasis (VVC) presents as pruritus and vaginal discharge, vaginal soreness, vulvar burning, dyspareunia, or external dysuria. The cause is usually *Candida albicans*, but occasionally is due to other *Candida* species or yeasts. In terms of epidemiology, 75% of women experience 1 episode or more, 40% to 45% have 2 episodes or more, and 10% to 20% of cases are considered "complicated," implying other diagnostic considerations (ie, diabetes, immunocompromise). Inspection reveals thick, cheesy, white, clingy

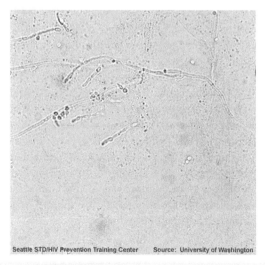

Seattle STD/HIV Prevention Training Center   Source: University of Washington

Fig. 11. Yeast seen in 10% KOH wet mount. (*Courtesy of* the Seattle STD/HIV Prevention Training Center at the University of Washington.)

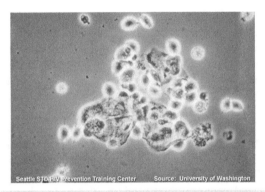

Seattle STD/HIV Prevention Training Center   Source: University of Washington

Fig. 12. *Trichomonas vaginalis* motile organisms seen in web mount prep. (*Courtesy of* the Seattle STD/HIV Prevention Training Center at the University of Washington.)

discharge with a normal pH (<4.5). Microscopic examination reveals yeast or pseudohyphae (more readily apparent on a slide using 10% KOH) (Fig. 11). Recommended treatment includes an intravaginal azole or fluconazole, 150 mg by mouth. Most of the intravaginal azoles are over-the-counter (OTC) medicines. However, self-medication with OTC preparations should only be advised for women who have been diagnosed with VVC currently or previously, with recurrence of the same symptoms. Unnecessary or inappropriate use of OTC preparations is common, and can lead to delay in the treatment of other causes of vulvovaginitis that could result in adverse clinical outcomes. Partners may need treatment in recurrent cases; a minority may have balanitis.

Trichomoniasis
Trichomoniasis is not a reportable STI, but is thought to be very common. Many women with trichomoniasis have diffuse, bubbly, malodorous, yellow-green discharge with vulvar irritation; however, some women have minimal or no symptoms. pH of vaginal discharge will be elevated (>4.5). Microscopic examination (Fig. 12) reveals lively, flagellated organisms, which obviously has a specificity of 100%. However, this method has a sensitivity of only about 60% to 70%, probably much less so with the standard practice of completing a bimanual examination before evaluation of cervical specimens. Other diagnostic tools include rapid tests (not widely available), amplified tests (including self-collected vaginal specimens), and culture. In men, microscopy is insensitive, and no PCR testing is FDA-approved in the United States. Treatment recommendations include metronidazole, 2 g by mouth, or tinidazole, 2 g in a single dose. Sex partners should be treated.

SUMMARY
STIs among adolescents in the United States have reached epidemic proportions, and should always be considered when dealing with this population.

The clinician should remember to consider newer tests for screening and diagnosis, including urine and self-collected vaginal specimens; have a low threshold for treatment; offer HIV counseling and testing; remember case-reporting and partner treatment strategies; and take all opportunities to counsel regarding prevention and safer sexuality.

References

[1] Weinstock H, et al. Sexually transmitted diseases among American youth: incidence and prevalence estimates, 2000. Perspectives on Sexual and Reproductive Health 2004;36: 6–10.

[2] Eaton DK, Kann L, Kinchen S, et al. Centers for Disease Control and Prevention. Youth risk behavior surveillance–United States, 2007. MMWR Surveill Summ 2008;57:1–131.

[3] Available at: http://cdc.confex.com/cdc/std2008/webprogram/Paper14888.html.

[4] Centers for Disease Control and Prevention. Youth risk behavior surveillance—United States, 2007. MMWR Surveill Summ 2008;57(4).

[5] Datta SD, Koutsky LA, Ratelle S, et al. Human papillomavirus infection and cervical cytology in women screened for cervical cancer in the United States, 2003-2005. Ann Intern Med 2008;148(7):493–500.

[6] Leone P. Reducing the risk of transmitting genital herpes: advances in understanding and therapy. Curr Med Res Opin 2005;21(10):1577–82.

[7] Xu F, Sternberg MR, Kottiri BJ, et al. Trends in herpes simplex virus type 1 and type 2 seroprevalence in the United States. JAMA 2006;296(8):964–73.

[8] Centers for Disease Control and Prevention. National center for HIV/AIDS, viral hepatitis, STD, and TB prevention. 2006 disease profile, 2008: 1–72. Available at: http://www.cdc.gov/std/stats06.

[9] Morreale MC, et al. Access to health care for adolescents and young adults: position paper of the society for adolescent medicine. J Ariz Hist 2004;35:342–4.

[10] Moscicki AB, et al. The natural history of human papillomavirus infection as measured by repeated DNA testing in adolescent and young women. J Pediatr 1998;132(2):277–84.

[11] Schlect NF, et al. Persistent human papillomavirus infection as a predictor of cervical intra-epithelial neoplasia. JAMA 2001;286(24):3106–14.

[12] Moscicki AB, et al. Regression of low-grade squamous intra-epithelial lesions in young women. Lancet 2004;364(9446):1642–4.

[13] Saslow D, et al. American Cancer Society Guideline for the early detection of cervical neoplasia and cancer. CA Cancer J Clin 2002;52:342–62. Available at: http://caonline.amcancersoc.org/cgi/content/full/52/6/342.

[14] ACOG. Cervical cytology screening. ACOG practice bulletin no. 45. ACOG 2003;102: 417–27. Available at: http://www.acog.org/from_home/publications/press_releases/nr07-31-03-1.cfm.

[15] Wright TC, et al. 2006 consensus guidelines for the management of women with cervical intraepithelial neoplasia or adenocarcinoma in situ. Am J Obstet Gynecol 2007;340–5.

[16] Markowitz LE, et al. Quadrivalent human papillomavirus vaccine: recommendations of the Advisory Committee on Immunization Practices early release. MMWR Recomm Rep 2007;56:1–24.

[17] Levine D, Woodruff AJ, Mocello AR, et al. inSPOT: the first online STD partner notification system using electronic postcards. PLoS Med 2008;5(10):e213, doi:10.1371/journal.pmed.0050213.

[18] Available at: http://www.ahrq.gov/clinic/uspstf/uspschlm.htm.

[19] Centers for Disease Control and Prevention (CDC). Update to CDC's sexually transmitted diseases treatment guidelines, 2006: fluoroquinolones no longer recommended for treatment of gonococcal infections. MMWR Morb Mortal Wkly Rep 2007;56(14):332–6.

[20] Datta SD, Sternberg M, Johnson RE, et al. Gonorrhea and chlamydia in the United States among persons 14 to 39 years of age, 1999 to 2002. Ann Intern Med 2007;147(2):89–96.

[21] US Preventive Services Task Force. Screening for gonorrhea: recommendation statement. Ann Fam Med 2005;3:263–7.

[22] Kahn JO, Walker BD. Acute human immunodeficiency virus type 1 infection. N Engl J Med 1998;339(1):33–9.

[23] Branson BM, Handsfield HH, Lampe MA, et al. Revised recommendations for HIV testing of adults, adolescents, and pregnant women in health-care settings. MMWR Recomm Rep 2006;55(RR14):1–17.

Advances in Pediatrics 56 (2009) 107–133

ADVANCES IN PEDIATRICS

ELSEVIER
MOSBY

Opportunities for the Primary Prevention of Obesity during Infancy

Ian M. Paul, MD, MSc[a],*, Cynthia J. Bartok, PhD[b],
Danielle S. Downs, PhD[b], Cynthia A. Stifter, PhD[b],
Alison K. Ventura, PhD[c], Leann L. Birch, PhD[b]

[a]Pediatrics, Penn State College of Medicine, HS83, 500 University Drive, Hershey, PA 17033, USA
[b]Penn State College of Health and Human Development, University Park, PA, USA
[c]Monell Chemical Senses Center, Philadelphia, PA, USA

WEIGHT GAIN DURING INFANCY AND LONG-TERM EFFECTS

Are chubby babies healthy babies? Whereas most seem well during infancy, evidence is increasing that heavier babies have a poorer long-term health trajectory than their trimmer counterparts. Data have emerged over the past 2 decades that early life growth patterns and behaviors play an important role in the etiology of obesity, yet there has been very little focus on the primary prevention of obesity during infancy by the medical, behavioral health, and public health communities. A recent report from the National Health and Nutrition Examination Survey (NHANES) highlighted the need for very early intervention when it revealed that between 2003 and 2006, a staggering 24.4% of children aged 2 to 5 years *already* were overweight or obese (body mass index [BMI; calculated as the weight in kilograms divided by height in meters squared] 85th–94th and ≥95th percentiles, respectively) [1]. NHANES data also have described obesity (weight-for-length/height ≥95th percentile) among infants younger than 2 years (Fig. 1). Between the late 1970s and 2000, the prevalence of obesity among infants 6 to 23 months old increased by more than 60% [2]. Reports from the Centers for Disease Control and Prevention (CDC) Pediatric Nutrition Surveillance System [3] and a Massachusetts Health Maintenance Organization [4] similarly showed significant increases in the prevalence of overweight for infants and toddlers for all age groups since the 1980s.

The Institute of Medicine publication, "Preventing Childhood Obesity: Health in the Balance," stated that the prevention of obesity in children should

This work was supported by grants DK72996 and DK075867 from the National Institute of Diabetes and Digestive and Kidney Diseases (NIDDK). Additional support was received from the Penn State Children, Youth and Families Consortium. Financial Disclosure and Conflicts of Interest: None.

*Corresponding author. E-mail address: ipaul@psu.edu (I.M. Paul).

0065-3101/09/$ – see front matter
doi:10.1016/j.yapd.2009.08.012

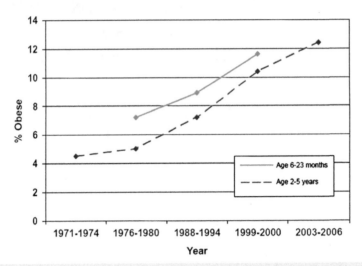

Fig. 1. Trends in infant (weight-for-length ≥95th percentile) and toddler (BMI ≥95th percentile) obesity. (*Data from* Ogden CL, Carroll MD, Flegal KM. High body mass index for age among US children and adolescents, 2003–2006. JAMA 2008;299:2401–05; Ogden CL, Flegal KM, Carroll MD, et al. Prevalence and trends in overweight among US children and adolescents, 1999–2000. JAMA 2002;288:1728–32; and Koplan JP, Liverman CT, Kraak VI, editors. Preventing childhood obesity: health in the balance. Washington, DC: The National Academies Press; 2005.)

be a national public health priority [5]. More specific to younger children was the summary of the "Conference on Preventing Childhood Obesity," where it was remarked, "The prenatal period, infancy, and early childhood may be stages of particular vulnerability to obesity development because they are unique periods for cellular differentiation and development. This unique vulnerability might make it possible for actions taken at these stages to determine the future course of adiposity [6]." This statement has been magnified by the numerous studies demonstrating the association between rapid or accelerated infant weight gain and subsequent obesity [7–24], as well as hypertension [25–28], coronary heart disease [29,30], and type 2 diabetes mellitus [31,32]. Further, numerous studies have now shown that overweight infants and toddlers are at increased risk of staying overweight as they age [9,16,33–46]. It has been theorized that overnutrition in infancy adversely "programs" the components of the metabolic syndrome and the way energy is stored [47,48]. These relationships may be especially true for those born to overweight parents, as genetic and familial influences, combined with pregnancy weight gain, are strongly associated with obesity in offspring [19,34,35,49,50].

Whereas all of the concerns about infant growth and subsequent morbidity make a strong case for very early intervention, there is little evidence regarding what, if anything, works to prevent the development of obesity during the first years of life although the extant literature provides some suggestions regarding potentially promising approaches [5,51]. Early intervention and prevention hold great promise for interrupting the vicious cycle of obese children becoming obese adults who subsequently have obese offspring themselves. The following sections summarize numerous aspects of infant life that affect weight status, the way information on this subject should be communicated with parents, and interventions that can be suggested to families to prevent the development of obesity, based on the currently available evidence.

OBESITY PREVENTION DURING THE NEWBORN PERIOD AND EARLY INFANCY
Role of clinicians in addressing infant weight gain
Many parents, grandparents, and clinicians propagate the belief that "a chubby baby is a healthy baby" despite evidence even in the short term to the contrary [52–55], and substantial long-term evidence as described earlier. During infancy, growth charts are typically used by health care providers to ensure adequate and proportional growth with respect to weight, length, and head circumference, but information is usually communicated to parents without significant explanation so long as the child does not (a) raise concern for failure to thrive, or (b) demonstrate disproportionate or very excessive growth on 1 of the 3 measurements.

In addition, there is often a disconnect between health care provider definitions of overweight and obesity and parents' interpretation of these terms [53,56–65]. Many parents believe heavier infant weight and appearance indicates good infant health and higher levels of parenting competence, particularly parents from poor or minority backgrounds [57,65–70]. In contrast, parents often perceive their children as picky eaters even when their weight gain is progressing normally [71], and infants and children perceived as too small often are given developmentally inappropriate nutrition, including the early introduction of solids or table foods [68,70]. The association of food with love in some cultures may also contribute to higher infant weight [72].

Potential intervention
Given the childhood obesity epidemic and the evidence that early upward crossing of major percentile lines on the growth curve is associated with later obesity [7–11,13–15,73], clinicians must pay closer attention to patterns of growth during early childhood and the way parents interpret infant growth. Providers must better understand healthy infant growth patterns and communicate this information regularly and accurately to parents. In addition, they must be familiar with early interventions that can prevent unhealthy patterns of weight gain in infancy and corrective interventions when problems are identified (Table 1).

Early feeding mode
Epidemiologic and experimental evidence has consistently indicated that breastfeeding offers modest protection against obesity later in life compared

Table 1
Potential interventions to prevent or address obesity during infancy

Opportunity	Intervention
Early infancy	
Growth monitoring	Educate parents about growth charts, percentiles, and their meaning – Support of breastfeeding as the preferred source of infant nutrition – Plot breastfed infants on the WHO growth chart, particularly when there are weight gain concerns
Infant feeding mode	– Educate parents on satiety cues – For bottle-fed infants, emphasize to parents that the volume of formula consumed should be child, not parent driven
Sleep	Educate parents on methods to lengthen sleep duration and soothe at night without feeding as a first response to nocturnal crying
Parental regulation of distress	– Respond quickly to crying early in infancy, but use alternative methods to soothe than feeding – Use nonfood items as rewards later in infancy
Introduction of solid foods	– Delay introduction of complementary foods until at least age 4 months – Avoid placing cereal into a bottle; complementary foods should only be fed with a spoon – Use repeated exposure to healthy foods as a response to normal infant neophobia
Later infancy	
Parent feeding style	Avoid coercive or restrictive feeding styles
Transition to cow's milk	Use low-fat cow's milk
Sweet beverage consumption	– Do not give juice to children ≤6 months old – Limit daily consumption of 100% fruit juice to ≤6 ounces (170 g) per day – Give 100% juice only in a cup, never in a bottle – Do not allow children to easily transport juice so that they will not steadily consume it throughout the day – Completely avoid fruit drinks and soft drinks
Transitional feeding and table foods	– Emphasize healthy dietary choices that have high nutritional value and low energy density such as fresh fruits, cooked vegetables, cheese, yogurt, wholegrain breads and crackers, and cereals – Avoid foods with added salt or sugar
Physical activity and sedentary behaviors	– Choose physical activities that are interactive, stimulating, easy to do, and incorporated into daily routines – Avoid television watching for children younger than 2 years – Keep televisions out of bedroom

with formula feeding [74–80], and both exclusivity and duration of breastfeeding strengthen this association [75,77,78,80–83]. There are several reasons or mechanisms by which this protection may occur. First, breastfeeding promotes self-regulation of intake by the infant, and breastfed infants regulate the volume of feeds in response to the energy density of breast milk [84]. In contrast, formula feeding is a more parent-driven feeding activity, with the regulation of intake directed by the parents rather than the infant. Compared with nursing infants, bottle-fed infants are fed on a more regular schedule and the volume of feeds is very consistent, suggesting that parents are driving intake patterns [85]. Subsequent research has shown that common bottle feeding practices, such as "emptying the bottle" and serving larger volumes of formula at feedings, are associated with excess weight gain in the first 6 months of life [86].

The composition of breast milk may also contribute to the protective effects of breastfeeding. Human breast milk contains hundreds of components serving nutritive and nonnutritive functions within the infant [87], both of which may affect short- and long-term growth patterns of children [88]. Interspecies comparisons suggest that the high lactose and cholesterol content of human milk supports growth of the central nervous system, whereas the high protein and mineral content of other species' milk (eg, cow's milk) supports substantial and rapid gains in physical size [88,89]. Recent experimental research in humans suggest that the high levels of protein and minerals in formula may stimulate excess physical growth later in infancy, with persistent effects even at 2 years of age [90].

Other "bioactive" components of breast milk may have potential roles in the regulation of growth and development of the infant [91]. Human milk contains growth-regulating components such as leptin, ghrelin, insulinlike growth factor-1, and adiponectin [92–94], and blood leptin levels in breastfed infants are comparatively higher to formula-fed infants [92]. Subsequent research focused solely on breastfed infants has shown that maternal milk leptin levels are negatively associated with weight gain during early infancy and through 2 years of age [95,96].

The sum of this early feeding experience for breastfed and formula-fed infants produces clear growth differences by feeding mode that persists for at least the first 2 years after birth [97]. Limited research assessing body composition has shown that growth differences are likely due to increases in adiposity in formula-fed infants between 6 months and 24 months old [98]. These growth differences were viewed historically as a sign that breastfed infants were not thriving, and the widely used CDC 2000 growth reference has been criticized as inadequate for monitoring the growth of breastfed infants because it is based predominantly on data from formula-fed infants in the United States. The creation of the World Health Organization (WHO) International Growth Standards, based on an international sample of healthy breastfed infants, has helped to support the perception of breastfeed infants' growth as the "reference" growth pattern and formula-fed infants' growth as deviant from this reference [99–101]. Of note, when comparing how breastfed infants' growth trajectories track along the CDC versus the WHO charts across the first 2 years after birth, substantial differences in expected growth are apparent [101]. With this comparison, when using the WHO chart as the growth reference, a normal deceleration of growth for breastfed infants is easily apparent after age 2 months and a slower rate of growth is evident through the first year after birth. In contrast, when using the CDC chart as the growth reference, the average breastfed infant would cross below the 50th percentile at age 7 months and proceed further below the 50th percentile through the first year. Without reference to a growth chart for breastfed infants, some infants might come to attention for failure to thrive when in fact their growth is normal. Further highlighting this is the fact that at 12 months of age, the WHO median weight for age is 1.2 kg lower for females and 1.5 kg lower for males in comparison with CDC charts.

Potential intervention
The CDC Guide to Breastfeeding Interventions outlines evidence-based practices for promoting breastfeeding, and improving breastfeeding duration and exclusivity [102]. Optimal breastfeeding practices can be promoted through a variety of avenues, including the health care system, places of work/employment, the community, and broader society. Among the interventions that can improve breastfeeding rates are several changes that can be made within the health care system. Prenatal, intrapartum, and postpartum education to improve breastfeeding knowledge and skills is an integral part of the promotion of breastfeeding. In addition, access to professional support (eg, lactation consultants, nurses, physicians) when families experience problems is a critical component of a supportive health care system. Institutional changes within the hospital or clinical setting have been shown to improve breastfeeding initiation and duration rates. The changes may be discrete, such as not handing out formula promotion gift packs to families, or they may be comprehensive, such as becoming a designated Baby Friendly Hospital Initiative hospital [102].

For physicians who monitor the growth of infants, practice guidelines should emphasize the expected, natural, and health-promoting aspects of "slower" growth in breastfed infants during the second 6 months after birth and beyond. Physicians should reassure parents who may be concerned about their infant's performance on CDC growth charts that the growth patterns of breastfed infants are healthy. Plotting children on the appropriate WHO growth standard may provide both physicians and parents with needed reassurance.

For families choosing to formula feed their infant, parents should be given specific education aimed at reducing problematic bottle-feeding behaviors. For example, parents should be encouraged to feed their infants when they are hungry, rather than on a set schedule outside of the immediate newborn period. Parents should be instructed to be responsive to infant cues for satiety, rather than ensuring their infant finishes the bottle contents. Age-specific guidelines for how much formula should be dispensed at a feeding would help parents start the feed with an appropriate portion size for their infant. Finally, encouraging parents to discern whether an infant is hungry or needing alternative soothing may reduce overfeeding of the bottle-fed infant.

Sleep

Short sleep duration may have other health effects other than fatigue. There is some evidence that it may be a contributor to the development of obesity. During the past 40 years, sleep duration in the United States has decreased by 1 to 2 hours per day whereas the prevalence of obesity has markedly increased [103–105]. It is estimated that children, a group with a rapid increase in the prevalence of obesity, are currently sleeping 1 to 2 hours less than they require, and that approximately 15 million American children are affected by inadequate sleep [106,107].

The link between short sleep duration and childhood obesity was first shown by a study of French 5-year olds, in which investigators found a significant risk for overweight among children who slept less than 11 hours per day [108]. Since the publication of that study, several investigations have shown that short sleep duration during early childhood (age 3–5 years) is associated with overweight, obesity, and higher body fat during school age [9,11,74,109,110]. Most recently, Taveras and colleagues demonstrated that sleep duration of less than 12 hours during infancy is a risk factor for overweight and adiposity in preschool-aged children [111].

There are several mechanisms by which shorter sleep duration may lead to overweight even among the youngest of children. The first 2 months after birth represent a critical period in the development of sleep patterns, a period during which feeding and sleeping are inextricably linked with infants waking every 2 to 4 hours, typically to feed [112–115]. These first months are also central for the development of normal circadian rhythms [116]. As a result of these rhythms, infants have periods of arousal from sleep, and how parents handle the infant's night waking represents a source of variability in infants' developing nighttime sleep patterns [117,118].

To evaluate different parenting styles and the impact on sleep, St. James-Roberts evaluated a "proximal care" model of parenting infants characterized by prolonged holding, frequent breastfeeding, rapid response to infant frets and cries, and cosleeping with infants at night with other approaches to infant care that have less parent-infant contact per day [117]. He found that the proximal care group of infants had more frequent night waking and crying at age 12 weeks. In another investigation, infants whose parents were present when their child fell asleep were more likely to wake at night than infants whose parents were not present, suggesting that infants who were able to self-soothe in the absence of feeding were more likely to sleep through the night [119].

The early development of sleeping through the night and its association with subsequent weight status is based on several findings. First, children who are unable to achieve a sleep duration of 6 hours by age 5 months have a much greater risk of short sleep duration and sleep problems later in childhood [120,121]. Second, relative sleep duration for age compared with norms for age was shown to remain constant for approximately 90% of children in a recent longitudinal study of sleep in children [122].

Next, to understand a potential physiologic mechanism for a relationship between sleep and obesity, one might consider adult data that have demonstrated that sleep restriction results in a significant reduction in the anorexigenic hormone, leptin, and an increase in the appetite stimulating peptide, ghrelin [123]. Reduced leptin and increased ghrelin were associated with a significant increase in hunger and appetite. The relationship between short sleep duration, reduced leptin, and increased ghrelin was also found in another investigation with more than 1000 participants whereby the links were shown to exist independent of BMI [124]. Although limited data on this subject exist for infants and children, lower cord blood ghrelin levels have been linked to slower weight gain from age 0 to 3 months [125]. These findings suggest that efforts to increase sleep duration for children could result in lower ghrelin levels, which could limit rapid weight gain during infancy. The importance of research studying potential links between sleep and obesity in children is becoming apparent, and was emphasized in a recent editorial in the *Archives of Internal Medicine* [126]. There, Bass and Turek wrote, "It is now critical to determine the importance of a lack of sleep during the early formative years in putting our youth on a trajectory toward obesity and the metabolic syndrome—a trajectory that could be altered if sleep loss is indeed playing a role in this epidemic." In summary, the roots of short sleep duration can be found in infancy, and are linked to parenting practices surrounding sleeping and feeding with potential long-term consequences for weight status.

Two seemingly conflicting theories regarding the prevention of obesity intersect in the discussion of sleep. Whereas prolonged sleep duration may be protective for obesity, breastfeeding, which is also protective for obesity, is associated with shorter sleep segments, increased night waking, and reduced total daily sleep [121,127–130]. This shorter sleep duration can persist even after the child has been weaned [121,127]. Breastfed infants also may be more easily aroused from sleep than those that are bottle fed [131]. Further, more frequent night waking has been described as a source of distress for mothers and a cause for them changing from breastfeeding to formula feeding [121,132]. Clearly the relationship between sleep duration, breastfeeding, and weight status is complex, but interventions to promote longer sleep duration such as those now described could achieve objectives of breastfeeding promotion and obesity prevention.

Potential intervention

Because short sleep duration in infancy and childhood is linked to childhood obesity, interventions designed increase sleep duration during infancy may have long-term protective effects against obesity. Of note, some research suggests that sleep duration during infancy can be significantly lengthened with appropriate interventions, even for breastfed infants. An intervention developed by Pinilla and Birch was successful in increasing nocturnal sleep duration in breastfed infants, who were taught to sleep for at least 5 consecutive hours by age 8 weeks [133]. In this study, parents in the treatment group were given a simple set of instructions to gradually lengthen intervals between middle-of-the-night feedings by performing alternative caregiving behaviors before feeding (eg, reswaddling, diapering, rocking). By age 3 weeks, treatment infants showed significantly longer sleep episodes at night, and by 8 weeks 100% of treatment infants were sleeping a 5-hour duration overnight, compared with 23% of control infants. Of note, Infants made up for the reduced nocturnal milk consumption with a larger early morning feed. One of the interventions described in the study, swaddling, has been shown to calm infants, reduce arousals during sleep, improve sleep efficiency, and reduce spontaneous awakenings [134,135]. In addition, other pediatric practitioners have expanded on these techniques in an attempt to calm and soothe infants, and improve infant sleep through the addition of "white noise," gentle rocking, and nonnutritive sucking [136,137]. However, like the use of pacifiers, the techniques described in this study should not be attempted until breastfeeding success is well established.

Whereas those who advocate for breastfeeding "on demand" may initially be averse to attempts to lengthen sleep duration, it is important to recognize that there is no uniform definition of "on demand" and mothers may interpret "feeding on demand" in a highly variable fashion. Thus, teaching mothers sleep-lengthening techniques may potentially enhance their ability to distinguish hunger cues from other distress cues, improve feelings of parental competence, reduce formula use, and increase the duration of breastfeeding.

Parental regulation of distress, temperament, and self-regulation of emotion

The ability to regulate behavior and emotion are important developmental tasks [138]. Moreover, the *inability* to successfully regulate one's emotional state characterizes many childhood problem behaviors [139]. The self-regulation of emotion may also have important implications for other areas of development such as physical health, more specifically weight gain. There are several possible reasons why emotion regulation may be important in understanding and potentially preventing abnormal weight gain. First, infant difficultness, a temperamental quality characterized by fussiness and difficulty soothing, has been related to rapid weight gain [140] and later body composition [141] in childhood, whereas negative child emotionality has been linked to adult body mass [142]. Next, studies of emotion and eating in adults show emotions, particularly negative emotions, to be related to increased eating, prompting theorists to hypothesize that obese individuals eat to reduce discomfort [143]. Finally, there is increasing evidence that mental health problems such as depression and conduct disorder are strong predictors of adulthood obesity [144]. This link may be biologic, as several central nervous system processes responsible for feeding regulation also are involved in regulating emotion

[145]. Taken together, these data suggest that the ability to self-regulate emotion may be an important factor in preventing obesity.

Developmental theorists agree that the soothing environment provided by the parent serves not only to alleviate immediate distress but also facilitates the infant's development of self-regulation [138,146]. Soothing a distressed infant models emotion regulatory strategies and demonstrates the effectiveness of various behaviors for reducing distress. Previous research has shown parental sensitivity, or contingent responsiveness to infant cues, predict infant crying and behavior [147]. That is, parents exhibiting high sensitivity had infants who cried less both concurrently and longitudinally. Furthermore, whereas some researchers have examined the effect of certain soothing techniques on reducing infant distress or supporting concurrent infant regulation [148,149], only one study has demonstrated the carry-over effect of parental regulation to infant self-regulation. Jahromi and Stifter found that mothers who were most effective in soothing their infants at 2 months had infants who cried less with immunization injections 4 months later [148].

Unfortunately from an obesity prevention perspective, many parents use feeding as a method to soothe a distressed infant, and this practice may have negative consequences for weight gain [150]. Using food to reward or punish behavior in children has similarly been associated with binge eating and heavier weight status when those children become adults [151]. Thus, whereas parent regulation of distress is important to the development of the child's ability to self-regulate his or her emotion, the use of food to soothe or reward may contribute to unhealthy outcomes.

Potential intervention

As feeding in infancy is predominantly under the control of the parent, using food in circumstances unrelated to hunger and sustenance may lead to children's understanding that food has other 'rewardlike' qualities. Infants may learn to eat in response to cues other than hunger, such as the presence of food, or their own emotional distress. This compromised ability to self-regulate their food intake may put them at risk for overweight. Given this evidence and that parents report using food to soothe their children [67], parental regulation seems to be a critical variable in the development of children's overall self-regulation skills.

One simple strategy parents can employ is to use nonfood items to soothe during early infancy and nonfood rewards for good behaviors during later infancy. Alternative soothing strategies for young infants, as discussed earlier in relation to sleep, can be applied during the day as well. For older infants, praise or rewards with stickers, toys, book reading, singing songs, playing, or visits to special places may be good alternatives to rewarding good behaviors with food.

As for the core issue of improving parental regulation, the results of 2 studies suggest that the effect of improving parental sensitivity may be most important for the highly reactive infant. In one study, an intervention focused on mothers of irritable infants found that training mothers to respond contingently and appropriately to the fussing and crying of the infant improved maternal interactive behavior and infant self-soothing, exploration, and attachment [152]. In the second study, an intervention aiming to improve mother-infant attachment found the effect to be greatest for those infants who were highest in negative emotionality [153]. Taken together, these studies suggest that parents should (1) recognize that infant distress is a signal to act, (2) respond quickly as waiting does not reduce crying, and (3) use strategies such as rocking, presenting alternative activities, and providing a pacifier to reduce the crying and fussing. Not only does this ameliorate the infant's distress but, if applied consistently, will enhance the parent-child relationship, and demonstrate how the child might self-regulate his or her own emotions in the future. Promoting improved parental regulation of infant distress as well as less intense negative responses from the infant seems to be essential to the development of the child's ability to self-regulate. Furthermore, interventions that provide the parents with alternative strategies to using food to soothe may not only be practical and economical, but may directly prevent childhood obesity.

Introduction of solid foods

Timing of solid food introduction

The American Academy of Pediatrics (AAP) suggests that the introduction of solid foods should begin between 4 and 6 months because, in general, exclusive milk feeding is adequate to support growth until this time, and supplementary foods are not needed [154,155]. Others add that solids should not be introduced until an infant has good head and neck control and can sit with support [156]. Recent NHANES data suggest, however, that about 30% of breastfed infants and about 50% of formula-fed infants are consuming some infant cereal by 2 to 3 months [157]. Further, data from the Early Childhood Longitudinal Study showed that in a nationally representative cohort, children placed in child care before age 3 months were nearly twice as likely to receive introduction of solids before turning 4 months [158]. Also, many parents continue to add cereal to their infant's bottle, a practice not supported by the AAP because it can lead to excessive weight gain [159]. Related to the previous discussion about sleep and regulation of distress, one commonly attempted approach to improve infant sleep is to give infant cereal at bedtime, a practice that has not been shown to be effective at helping infants sleep despite the widespread belief that the early addition of solids promotes sleeping through the night [160]. Of note, the time when solids are first introduced may be related to increased caloric intake, rapid weight gain, and the subsequent development of overweight.

When the topic of the relationship between the timing of introduction of complementary foods and subsequent obesity has been evaluated in large, population-based studies, there has been minimal to little influence of this variable on the development of obesity [79,80]. However, several more focused studies have revealed important associations. Shukla and colleagues [161] found that overweight status at 13 weeks was related to the extra calories provided by solid foods early in life, and overweight status at age 13 weeks persisted through 1 year. Von Kries and colleagues [11] similarly showed a relationship between the introduction of solids before age 4 months and the risk of over-weight status between the age of 5 and 6 years. Others have further character-ized this relationship by showing the association between increased rate of weight gain in the first 6 to 12 months after birth and early introduction of solids, particularly for formula-fed infants [158,162–164]. The analysis of the Danish National Birth Cohort by Baker and colleagues revealed perhaps the most intriguing data on this subject. Their regression analyses showed that the relationship between maternal obesity and greater weight gain during the first year could be nearly eliminated by breastfeeding for more than 40 weeks and delaying the introduction of complementary foods until after age 20 weeks [165].

Method of solid food introduction and the use of repeated exposure
Across cultures, dietary diversity is vast, but all infants begin life consuming the same food: milk. However, as omnivores, they are prepared to learn to consume the diet of their culture. Infants "come equipped" to prefer sweet and salty tastes, to be "neophobic" and reject new foods when they are first offered (at least those that are not sweet or salty), and to learn to like foods of the adult diet of their culture and ethnicity, via various associative condi-tioning processes that involve the pairing of food with the aspects of the social contexts and physiologic consequences of eating [166]. Given this set of predis-positions, all normal infants will readily accept sweet and salty foods such as French fries and sweetened drinks. In contrast, many healthy foods such as pureed vegetables, infant cereals, meats, and dairy products, which are not high in sugar or salt, will be initially rejected by infants. These findings have revealed that infants typically need several opportunities to sample these new foods before intake will increase [167,168]. The liking for complex food flavors that are not dominated by sweet or salty tastes must be learned.

Potential intervention
In addition to delaying the introduction of complementary foods until age 4 to 6 months, parents should be instructed on the infant neophobic response to new foods. Parents often interpret the initial rejection of new foods as "she doesn't like it," and the food is not offered again. However, the infant's initial neophobic response is usually transient, and that infants', toddlers', and preschoolers' intake of new healthy foods will typically increase if the infant has repeated opportunities to taste them [167–170]. As few as 1 or 2 exposures [168] or as many as 5 or 10 exposures [169] may be needed, depending on the age of the child; and all foods will not be accepted by some children, despite repeated exposure. However, parents must be instructed that such repeated exposure is necessary if not sufficient for acceptance of new foods that are not very sweet or salty. Most of the healthy foods that are developmentally appropriate for infants and toddlers fall into this category, including most

vegetables, complex carbohydrates, and meat and dairy products. Although exceptions to these instructions are cases in which food aversions and dislikes develop when consumption is followed by nausea or vomiting, or when eating is coerced or unpleasant, parents need guidance on how to introduce new foods, to increase the likelihood that the child will learn to consume a variety of foods that will constitute a balanced diet promoting healthy weight gain.

In addition to repeated exposure to healthy foods, parents should be alerted to cues for fullness when feeding complementary foods. Pursed lips, closed mouth, spitting out food, turning of the head, and leaning back are examples of cues to stop feeding [156].

OBESITY PREVENTION DURING LATER INFANCY AND THE EARLY TODDLER YEARS
Parent feeding style
During the first years of life, infants and young children are learning an enormous amount about food and eating as they are being introduced to the adult diet of their culture. Growing children learn when to eat, what is food and what is not, how much to eat, and as a result of their experiences with food and eating, are developing food preferences and dislikes. The period from birth to 3 years is also a crucial one for the development of the controls of food intake, and the development of food preferences and eating behaviors [166]. There is evidence that early feeding practices are linked to patterns of food acceptance and the developing controls of food intake [166,171,172]. A feeding style using coercion is unlikely to be successful in the short term and can result in unhealthy weight status in the long term, as recent data suggest that maternal control of feeding during the first years after birth moderates infant weight gain [173,174]. Coercive feeding practices include tactics such as (1) pressuring children to finish their vegetables or (2) restricting their access to sweets and junk food, or using such foods as rewards [71]. In addition to promoting dislikes for healthy foods, and increased liking and wanting of restricted junk foods, coercive practices can also promote dysregulation of intake by promoting overeating, and learning to eat in response to the presence of food on the plate (as in "finish your vegetables") [175–177].

Potential intervention
When introducing solids, parents should be aware that new foods may be initially rejected, and should be advised to be patient, as learning to like new foods takes time. If parents offer new foods repeatedly, over a series of 5 or 10 days, many of these foods will eventually be accepted and even preferred [167–169]. However, pressuring or coercive feeding practices engender resistance and foster dislikes, and should be discouraged in favor of providing repeated experience in positive contexts. During the transition to table foods, parents can be effective positive models, promoting infant acceptance and liking for healthy foods by consuming healthy foods and avoiding "junk foods" at family meals. The use of positive feeding practices such as repeated exposure

and modeling are more likely to promote the establishment of healthy diets than the use of coercive feeding practices [178]. Parents should be advised to avoid pressure and restriction in feeding, and encouraged to put their efforts into promoting the liking and acceptance of table foods that are part of a healthy diet.

Transition from human milk or formula to cow's milk

Although consumption of human milk or infant formula may continue for over 1 year, most infants transition to cow's milk at age 1 year. As opposed to children 2 years or older, however, many do not recommend the use of nonfat or low-fat milk for children 12 to 23 months old [179–182]. This recommendation likely stems from concerns from years ago that infants consume a sufficient quantity of dietary fat and essential fatty acids for normal growth and development. However, as opposed to the evidence for infants younger than 12 months, the recommendation for 12- to 23-month-old infants is not evidence based [183].

The question of milk fat intake is important because the preference for high-fat foods develops early in life, and children still consume 20% to 25% of their calories from cow's milk between the ages of 1 and 2 years [184,185]. Further, a majority of preschool children drink whole milk, particularly those who are from minorities or low-income households [186,187].

Potential intervention

Reducing milk fat intake has been previously identified as a target for dietary fat reduction and obesity prevention in toddlers and preschool children [188–190], and reducing fat intake among infants and toddlers has been shown to be well tolerated without adverse effects on growth, nutrient intake, or development [191–193]. In contrast, high fat intake between 12 and 23 months of age has been associated with inhibition of the normal decrease in body fat between the ages of 2 and 5 years [194]. Given that contemporary diets for children older than 1 year typically contain a significant amount of dietary fat from nonmilk sources [195], the common advice to only use whole milk for children 12 to 23 months old is no longer necessary for infants who consume a well-balanced diet [186]. In fact, the 2008 AAP policy statement "Lipid Screening and Cardiovascular Health in Childhood" includes as its first recommendation the use of reduced fat milk for 12- to 23-month-old children [196]. Although studies of older children have suggested that consumption of dairy fat is not associated with weight gain [197], because each cup of whole milk contains 146 kcal compared with only 86 kcal per cup of nonfat milk [198], a change to low-fat or even nonfat milk could reduce energy consumption without adverse effects for infants.

Sweet beverage consumption

Over the past 3 decades, the percentage of daily calories obtained from soft drinks, fruit drinks, sweetened beverages, and fruit juice each have steadily increased among American children [199]. Among children 12 to 24 months old, 100% juice and sweetened beverages account for the second and third greatest source of dietary calories, respectively, exceeded only by milk [185]. Although data have in general not supported a link between consumption of 100% juice and obesity unless consumed in excess [200], there is a strong association between sweetened beverages and soft drinks with obesity [201]. Further, as suggested by Skinner and colleagues [202], because early life diet preferences predict later preferences, the development of beverage consumption patterns before age 2 years is important for long-term consumption.

Regarding infant and toddler consumption of juice, the AAP has recommended that juice (a) not be given to infants younger than 6 months, (b) only be given to infants that can drink from a cup and never given in a bottle, (c) not be given in a fashion that allows for a child to easily transport it with easy consumption throughout the day, and (d) not be given in quantities greater than 6 ounces (170 g) per day [203]. Data from the Feeding Infants and Toddlers Study (FITS), a national dietary survey, demonstrated that many infants consume fruit juice before 6 months of age, and exceed the recommended amount of juice later during infancy and the toddler years [202].

Unlike fruit juice, the AAP has no formal policy statement or recommendation regarding the consumption of other sweetened beverages and soft drinks prior to school entry, but the Institute of Medicine has recommended the avoidance of high-calorie, nutrient-poor beverages [5]. Of note, consumption of sweet drinks has been associated with obesity even among preschool children [204,205]. In addition, in FITS, sweetened drinks and soda also were being consumed at the expense of milk in this sample of infants and toddlers [203]. Further, several investigators have suggested that reducing intake of sweetened beverages is one of the most important and promising obesity prevention strategies [204–207].

Potential intervention
Given the current evidence, adherence to the AAP policy regarding fruit juice is appropriate. Further, because they have no nutritional benefit and are associated with obesity and other morbidities, the use of sweetened beverages, soft drinks, and fruit drinks should be totally discouraged for infants and toddlers. Given the alternatives of milk, water, and the now increasingly available low-calorie flavored water, there are sufficient options for parents to give their young children.

Transitional feeding and table foods
The transition from the exclusive milk diet of infancy to a modified adult diet is completed by age 3 years, and during this early period children already have begun acquiring food preferences and aversions [166]. Children are learning a great deal about when, what, and how much to eat. Unfortunately, recent data from FITS revealed that energy intakes among typical infants and toddlers exceed requirements by 20% to 30% [208]. Of note, in FITS this excess already was apparent in infants aged 4 to 6 months, in whom intake exceeded energy requirements by 10%, suggesting that patterns of intake promoting excessive

weight gain and obesity were being established at an early age. In addition to consuming too much energy, from an early age (4 to 24 months) children consume significant amounts of developmentally inappropriate foods, high in energy density and low in nutrients, while consuming too few of the foods that should form the basis of a healthy weaning diet [195]. The high energy density of foods offered appeared to be the same ones that contribute to energy intakes that were in excess of energy requirements in other age groups studied [208]. For example, in children 7 and 24 months old, 18% and 33%, respectively, consumed no servings of vegetables during a given 24-hour period. Twenty-three percent of 7-month-old and 33% of 24-month-old children did not consume any fruits. Further, parents reported that French fries were the third most common vegetable consumed by infants 9 to 11 months old, and by 15 to 18 months were the most common vegetable consumed. The diets of infants in this age group may, not surprisingly, be deficient of key nutrients [209].

Potential intervention

The FITS findings underscore the need to provide parents with anticipatory guidance regarding the transition to a modified adult diet. The Start Healthy Feeding Guidelines for Infants and Toddlers provides excellent guidance on the nutritional needs of children younger than 2 years [210]. As opposed to giving children French fries, parents should be encouraged to meet these nutritional requirements with fresh fruits, cooked vegetables, cheese, yogurt, wholegrain breads and crackers, and cereals [156,211,212]. All of these foods should not have added sugar or salt.

Physical activity and sedentary behaviors

There is substantial epidemiologic evidence that regular physical activity is essential for good physical and psychological health and disease prevention among children and adults. However, to date the recommendations for infant and toddler physical activity (from birth to age 5 years) have not been evidence based. Rather, the guidelines developed by the National Association for Sport and Physical Education [213] were adapted from evidence accumulated among older children and adolescents [214]. The recommendations for infants suggest that they should be: (1) interacting with caregivers in daily physical activities that promote movement and exploration of their environment, (2) engaging in activities that promote the development of movement skills and large muscle activities, and (3) placed in safe settings that facilitate physical activity and do not restrict physical activity for prolonged periods of time. These recommendations suggest that toddlers should: (1) accumulate at least 30 minutes of daily structured physical activity, (2) engage in at least 60 minutes and up to several hours a day of unstructured physical activity and should not be sedentary for more than 60 minutes at a time except when sleeping, and (3) develop movement skills that are building blocks for more complex movement behaviors [213]. Nonetheless, because physical activity and sedentary patterns, much like feeding and sleeping behaviors, become established in the early years, there is increasing support for promoting physical activity and reducing sedentary behaviors as soon as possible during the early infancy period [213,215].

Environmental risk factors associated with sedentary activities during the early infancy and toddler periods may predispose children to low levels of physical activity in later childhood. For example, restricting infants to car seats, swings, carriers, strollers, and small play spaces for long periods of time may limit motor development and delay physical activity such as crawling and walking [213,216]. Also, limited time for leisure activities and parent-child play, concern for neighborhood safety, and using television or computer games to occupy a child's attention may promote sedentary lifestyle during the first 3 years after birth [216,217]. Television viewing during the infancy and toddler years seems to be one particular sedentary practice that is an environmental risk factor for obesity development. It is reported that 82% of 1-year-old (11 average hours per week) and 96% of 2-year-old (15 average hours per week) children watch television or videos, and having a television in the bedroom elevates the risk of being overweight [218]. Also, Taveras and colleagues found that children who slept less than 12 hours per day and viewed 2 hours per day or more of television had an obesity probability at 3 years old of 17% [111].

Potential intervention
Although there is little debate that physical activity is important for obesity prevention, questions remain about how much and what types of physical activity during the infant and early toddler years is needed to prevent later obesity. In general, parents of infants should choose physical activities that are interactive, stimulating, easy to do, and incorporated into their daily routine, to reinforce the concept that physical activity is rewarding [213,215].

In addition, 2 existing programs offer possible blueprints for more extensive prevention efforts. The Infant Feeding Activity and Nutrition Trial is an early intervention to prevent childhood obesity that targets infants through age 18 months in Victoria, Australia. This program teaches parents about the development of positive diet and physical activity behaviors while reducing sedentary behaviors during infancy [219]. Parents in the program learn about age-appropriate physical activity behaviors, the risks associated with sedentary behaviors, and how parental modeling of physical activity and sedentary behaviors influences their child's behaviors.

The second program, Fighting Fit Tots, also aims to prevent obesity in the first years of life by promoting toddler physical activity and parent lifestyle education [220]. This program is currently being implemented in Lambeth, South London (United Kingdom) and consists of 11 weekly 2-hour sessions that include guided parent-child physical activity (eg, jumping, skipping, hopping, dancing, singing), snack (water and fruit), and parental education (eg, healthy lifestyle workshop) aimed at increasing physical activity behaviors, confidence, and decreasing BMI and waist circumference among children 18 to 30 months old.

Regarding sedentary behavior, one clear target for intervention is television viewing. Because most children watch television by age 2 years, educational efforts and interventions about limiting television/video viewing need to be implemented before this age to potentially impact overweight development. Of note, the AAP discourages television watching for children younger than 2 years, and suggests that televisions never be placed in children's bedrooms [221].

SUMMARY

Given the vast array of topics that are important to cover at infant health maintenance visits, extensive discussion about growth, growth charts, and healthy lifestyle may be challenging for providers. Nonetheless, obesity and its comorbidities threaten both individual patients and the health care system. To break the vicious cycle of obese children becoming obese adults who have obese offspring, preventing behaviors that lead to obesity must be implemented during the very earliest periods of life, the prenatal period and infancy. For pediatric care providers, there are numerous opportunities to intervene, and good communication with families about healthy growth and lifestyle are a promising beginning.

References

[1] Ogden CL, Carroll MD, Flegal KM. High body mass index for age among US children and adolescents, 2003–2006. JAMA 2008;299:2401–5.

[2] Ogden CL, Flegal KM, Carroll MD, et al. Prevalence and trends in overweight among US children and adolescents, 1999–2000. JAMA 2002;288:1728–32.

[3] Mei Z, Scanlon KS, Grummer-Strawn LM, et al. Increasing prevalence of overweight among US low-income preschool children: the Centers for Disease Control and Prevention pediatric nutrition surveillance, 1983 to 1995. Pediatrics 1998;101:E12.

[4] Kim J, Peterson KE, Scanlon KS, et al. Trends in overweight from 1980 through 2001 among preschool-aged children enrolled in a health maintenance organization. Obesity (Silver Spring) 2006;14:1107–12.

[5] Koplan JP, Liverman CT, Kraak VI, editors. Preventing childhood obesity: health in the balance. Washington, DC: The National Academies Press; 2005.

[6] Lederman SA, Akabas SR, Moore BJ. Editors' overview of the conference on preventing childhood obesity. Pediatrics 2004;114:1139–45.

[7] Eid EE. Follow-up study of physical growth of children who had excessive weight gain in first 6 months of life. Br Med J 1970;2:74–6.

[8] Ong KK, Ahmed ML, Emmett PM, et al. Association between postnatal catch-up growth and obesity in childhood: prospective cohort study. BMJ 2000;320:967–71.

[9] Reilly JJ, Armstrong J, Dorosty AR, et al. Early life risk factors for obesity in childhood: cohort study. BMJ 2005;330:1358–60.

[10] Stettler N, Zemel BS, Kumanyika S, et al. Infant weight gain and childhood overweight status in a multicenter, cohort study. Pediatrics 2002;109:194–9.

[11] von Kries R, Toschke AM, Wurmser H, et al. Reduced risk for overweight and obesity in 5- and 6-y-old children by duration of sleep—a cross-sectional study. Int J Obes Relat Metab Disord 2002;26:710–6.

[12] Cameron N, Pettifor J, De Wet T, et al. The relationship of rapid weight gain in infancy to obesity and skeletal maturity in childhood. Obes Res 2003;11:457–60.

[13] Mellbin T, Vuille JC. Physical development at 7 years of age in relation to velocity of weight gain in infancy with special reference to incidence of overweight. Br J Prev Soc Med 1973;27:225–35.

[14] Stettler N, Kumanyika SK, Katz SH, et al. Rapid weight gain during infancy and obesity in young adulthood in a cohort of African Americans. Am J Clin Nutr 2003;77:1374–8.

[15] Ekelund U, Ong K, Linne Y, et al. Upward weight percentile crossing in infancy and early childhood independently predicts fat mass in young adults: the Stockholm Weight Development Study (SWEDES). Am J Clin Nutr 2006;83:324–30.

[16] Monteiro PO, Victora CG, Barros FC, et al. Birth size, early childhood growth, and adolescent obesity in a Brazilian birth cohort. Int J Obes Relat Metab Disord 2003;27:1274–82.

[17] Wells JC, Hallal PC, Wright A, et al. Fetal, infant and childhood growth: relationships with body composition in Brazilian boys aged 9 years. Int J Obes (Lond) 2005;29:1192–8.

[18] Sachdev HS, Fall CH, Osmond C, et al. Anthropometric indicators of body composition in young adults: relation to size at birth and serial measurements of body mass index in childhood in the New Delhi birth cohort. Am J Clin Nutr 2005;82:456–66.

[19] Blair NJ, Thompson JM, Black PN, et al. Risk factors for obesity in 7-year-old European children: the Auckland Birthweight Collaborative Study. Arch Dis Child 2007;92:866–71.

[20] Dennison BA, Edmunds LS, Stratton HH, et al. Rapid infant weight gain predicts childhood overweight. Obesity (Silver Spring) 2006;14:491–9.

[21] Hui LL, Schooling CM, Leung SS, et al. Birth weight, infant growth, and childhood body mass index: Hong Kong's children of 1997 birth cohort. Arch Pediatr Adolesc Med 2008;162:212–8.

[22] Botton J, Heude B, Maccario J, et al. Postnatal weight and height growth velocities at different ages between birth and 5 y and body composition in adolescent boys and girls. Am J Clin Nutr 2008;87:1760–8.

[23] Yliharsila H, Kajantie E, Osmond C, et al. Body mass index during childhood and adult body composition in men and women aged 56–70 y. Am J Clin Nutr 2008;87:1769–75.

[24] Chomtho S, Wells JC, Williams JE, et al. Infant growth and later body composition: evidence from the 4-component model. Am J Clin Nutr 2008;87:1776–84.

[25] Singhal A, Cole TJ, Fewtrell M, et al. Is slower early growth beneficial for long-term cardiovascular health? Circulation 2004;109:1108–13.

[26] Huxley RR, Shiell AW, Law CM. The role of size at birth and postnatal catch-up growth in determining systolic blood pressure: a systematic review of the literature. J Hypertens 2000;18:815–31.

[27] Law CM, Shiell AW, Newsome CA, et al. Fetal, infant, and childhood growth and adult blood pressure: a longitudinal study from birth to 22 years of age. Circulation 2002;105:1088–92.

[28] Parker L, Lamont DW, Unwin N, et al. A lifecourse study of risk for hyperinsulinaemia, dyslipidaemia and obesity (the central metabolic syndrome) at age 49–51 years. Diabet Med 2003;20:406–15.

[29] Eriksson JG, Forsen T, Tuomilehto J, et al. Catch-up growth in childhood and death from coronary heart disease: longitudinal study. BMJ 1999;318:427–31.

[30] Barker DJ, Osmond C, Forsen TJ, et al. Trajectories of growth among children who have coronary events as adults. N Engl J Med 2005;353:1802–9.

[31] Forsen T, Eriksson J, Tuomilehto J, et al. The fetal and childhood growth of persons who develop type 2 diabetes. Ann Intern Med 2000;133:176–82.

[32] Bhargava SK, Sachdev HS, Fall CH, et al. Relation of serial changes in childhood body-mass index to impaired glucose tolerance in young adulthood. N Engl J Med 2004;350:865–75.

[33] Fisch RO, Bilek MK, Ulstrom R. Obesity and leanness at birth and their relationship to body habitus in later childhood. Pediatrics 1975;56:521–8.

[34] Charney E, Goodman HC, McBride M, et al. Childhood antecedents of adult obesity. Do chubby infants become obese adults? N Engl J Med 1976;295:6–9.

[35] Whitaker RC, Wright JA, Pepe MS, et al. Predicting obesity in young adulthood from child-hood and parental obesity. N Engl J Med 1997;337:869–73.

[36] Guo SS, Wu W, Chumlea WC, et al. Predicting overweight and obesity in adulthood from body mass index values in childhood and adolescence. Am J Clin Nutr 2002;76: 653–8.

[37] Mei Z, Grummer-Strawn LM, Scanlon KS. Does overweight in infancy persist through the preschool years? An analysis of CDC Pediatric Nutrition Surveillance System data. Soz Praventivmed 2003;48:161–7.

[38] Sayer AA, Syddall HE, Dennison EM, et al. Birth weight, weight at 1 y of age, and body composition in older men: findings from the Hertfordshire Cohort Study. Am J Clin Nutr 2004;80:199–203.

[39] Freedman DS, Khan LK, Serdula MK, et al. The relation of childhood BMI to adult adiposity: the Bogalusa heart study. Pediatrics 2005;115:22–7.

[40] Nader PR, O'Brien M, Houts R, et al. Identifying risk for obesity in early childhood. Pedi-atrics 2006;118:e594–601.

[41] Vogels N, Posthumus DL, Mariman EC, et al. Determinants of overweight in a cohort of Dutch children. Am J Clin Nutr 2006;84:717–24.

[42] Jouret B, Ahluwalia N, Cristini C, et al. Factors associated with overweight in preschool-age children in southwestern France. Am J Clin Nutr 2007;85:1643–9.

[43] Serdula MK, Ivery D, Coates RJ, et al. Do obese children become obese adults? A review of the literature. Prev Med 1993;22:167–77.

[44] Garn SM, LaVelle M. Two-decade follow-up of fatness in early childhood. Am J Dis Child 1985;139:181–5.

[45] Rolland-Cachera MF, Deheeger M, Guilloud-Bataille M, et al. Tracking the development of adiposity from one month of age to adulthood. Ann Hum Biol 1987;14:219–29.

[46] Muramatsu S, Sato Y, Miyao M, et al. A longitudinal study of obesity in Japan: relationship of body habitus between at birth and at age 17. Int J Obes 1990;14:39–45.

[47] Singhal A, Lucas A. Early origins of cardiovascular disease: is there a unifying hypothesis? Lancet 2004;363:1642–5.

[48] Gillman MW. The first months of life: a critical period for development of obesity. Am J Clin Nutr 2008;87:1587–9.

[49] Oken E, Taveras EM, Kleinman KP, et al. Gestational weight gain and child adiposity at age 3 years. Am J Obstet Gynecol 2007;196(322):e1–8.

[50] Whitaker RC. Predicting preschooler obesity at birth: the role of maternal obesity in early pregnancy. Pediatrics 2004;114:e29–36.

[51] Gillman MW, Rifas-Shiman SL, Kleinman K, et al. Developmental origins of childhood over-weight: potential public health impact. Obesity (Silver Spring) 2008;16:1651–6.

[52] Jaffe M, Kosakov C. The motor development of fat babies. Clin Pediatr (Phila) 1982;21: 619–21.

[53] Shibli R, Rubin L, Akons H, et al. Morbidity of overweight (> or =85th percentile) in the first 2 years of life. Pediatrics 2008;122:267–72.

[54] Wake M, Hardy P, Sawyer MG, et al. Comorbidities of overweight/obesity in Australian preschoolers: a cross-sectional population study. Arch Dis Child 2008;93:502–7.

[55] Taveras EM, Rifas-Shiman SL, Camargo CA Jr, et al. Higher adiposity in infancy associated with recurrent wheeze in a prospective cohort of children. J Allergy Clin Immunol 2008;121:1161–6, e3.

[56] Jain A, Sherman SN, Chamberlin LA, et al. Why don't low-income mothers worry about their preschoolers being overweight? Pediatrics 2001;107:1138–46.

[57] Sherry B, McDivitt J, Birch LL, et al. Attitudes, practices, and concerns about child feeding and child weight status among socioeconomically diverse white, Hispanic, and African-American mothers. J Am Diet Assoc 2004;104:215–21.

[58] Jackson J, Strauss CC, Lee AA, et al. Parents' accuracy in estimating child weight status. Addict Behav 1990;15:65–8.

[59] Baughcum AE, Chamberlin LA, Deeks CM, et al. Maternal perceptions of overweight preschool children. Pediatrics 2000;106:1380–6.

[60] Maynard LM, Galuska DA, Blanck HM, et al. Maternal perceptions of weight status of children. Pediatrics 2003;111:1226–31.

[61] Jeffery AN, Voss LD, Metcalf BS, et al. Parents' awareness of overweight in themselves and their children: cross sectional study within a cohort (EarlyBird 21). BMJ 2005;330:23–4.

[62] Carnell S, Edwards C, Croker H, et al. Parental perceptions of overweight in 3–5 y olds. Int J Obes (Lond) 2005;29:353–5.

[63] Eckstein KC, Mikhail LM, Ariza AJ, et al. Parents' perceptions of their child's weight and health. Pediatrics 2006;117:681–90.

[64] Campbell MW, Williams J, Hampton A, et al. Maternal concern and perceptions of overweight in Australian preschool-aged children. Med J Aust 2006;184:274–7.

[65] Reifsnider E, Flores-Vela AR, Beckman-Mendez D, et al. Perceptions of children's body sizes among mothers living on the Texas-Mexico border (La Frontera). Public Health Nurs 2006;23:488–95.

[66] Kramer MS, Barr RG, Leduc DG, et al. Maternal psychological determinants of infant obesity. Development and testing of two new instruments. J Chronic Dis 1983;36:329–35.

[67] Baughcum AE, Burklow KA, Deeks CM, et al. Maternal feeding practices and childhood obesity: a focus group study of low-income mothers. Arch Pediatr Adolesc Med 1998;152:1010–4.

[68] Bentley M, Gavin L, Black MM, et al. Infant feeding practices of low-income, African-American, adolescent mothers: an ecological, multigenerational perspective. Soc Sci Med 1999;49:1085–100.

[69] Contento IR, Basch C, Zybert P. Body image, weight, and food choices of Latina women and their young children. J Nutr Educ Behav 2003;35:236–48.

[70] Boyington JA, Johnson AA. Maternal perception of body size as a determinant of infant adiposity in an African-American community. J Natl Med Assoc 2004;96:351–62.

[71] Birch LL, Fisher JO. Development of eating behaviors among children and adolescents. Pediatrics 1998;101:539–49.

[72] Bruss MB, Morris J, Dannison L. Prevention of childhood obesity: sociocultural and familial factors. J Am Diet Assoc 2003;103:1042–5.

[73] Karaolis-Danckert N, Buyken AE, Bolzenius K, et al. Rapid growth among term children whose birth weight was appropriate for gestational age has a longer lasting effect on body fat percentage than on body mass index. Am J Clin Nutr 2006;84:1449–55.

[74] Lederman SA, Akabas SR, Moore BJ, et al. Summary of the presentations at the conference on preventing childhood obesity, 2003. Pediatrics 2004;114:1146–73.

[75] Owen CG, Martin RM, Whincup PH, et al. Effect of infant feeding on the risk of obesity across the life course: a quantitative review of published evidence. Pediatrics 2005;115:1367–77.

[76] Owen CG, Martin RM, Whincup PH, et al. The effect of breastfeeding on mean body mass index throughout life: a quantitative review of published and unpublished observational evidence. Am J Clin Nutr 2005;82:1298–307.

[77] Arenz S, Ruckerl R, Koletzko B, et al. Breast-feeding and childhood obesity—a systematic review. Int J Obes Relat Metab Disord 2004;28:1247–56.

[78] Dewey KG. Is breastfeeding protective against child obesity? J Hum Lact 2003;19:9–18.

[79] Hediger ML, Overpeck MD, Kuczmarski RJ, et al. Association between infant breastfeeding and overweight in young children. JAMA 2001;285:2453–60.

[80] Gillman MW, Rifas-Shiman SL, Camargo CA Jr, et al. Risk of overweight among adolescents who were breastfed as infants. JAMA 2001;285:2461–7.

[81] Bogen DL, Hanusa BH, Whitaker RC. The effect of breastfeeding with and without concurrent formula feeding on the risk of obesity at 4 years of age: a retrospective cohort study. Obes Res 2004;12:1527–35.

[82] von Kries R, Koletzko B, Sauerwald T, et al. Breast feeding and obesity: cross sectional study. BMJ 1999;319:147–50.

[83] Harder T, Bergmann R, Kallischnigg G, et al. Duration of breastfeeding and risk of overweight: a meta-analysis. Am J Epidemiol 2005;162:397–403.

[84] Dewey KG, Heinig MJ, Nommsen LA, et al. Maternal versus infant factors related to breast milk intake and residual milk volume: the DARLING study. Pediatrics 1991;87: 829–37.

[85] Wright P, Fawcett J, Crow R. The development of differences in the feeding behaviour of bottle and breast fed human infants from birth to two months. Behav Processes 1980;5: 1–20.

[86] Dewey KG, Nommsen-Rivers LA, Lonnerdal B. Plasma insulin and insulin-releasing amino acid (IRAA) concentrations are higher in formula fed than breastfed infants at 5 months of age [abstract]. Experimental Biology meeting, 2004.

[87] Jensen RG, editor. Handbook of milk composition. San Diego (CA): Academic Press; 1995.

[88] Hambraeus L. Proprietary milk versus human breast milk in infant feeding. A critical appraisal from the nutritional point of view. Pediatr Clin North Am 1977;24:17–36.

[89] Oftedal OT, Iverson SJ. Comparative analysis of nonhuman milks: phylogenetic variation in the gross composition of milks. In: Jensen RG, editor. Handbook of milk composition. San Diego (CA): Academic Press; 1995. p. 749–89.

[90] EU Childhood Obesity Programme. EU Childhood Obesity Programme press pack. Budapest, Hungary: Danone Institute; 2007.

[91] Read LC, Penttila IA, Howarth GS, et al. Role and function of growth factors in infant nutrition. In: Raiha NCR, Rubaltelli FF, editors. Infant formula: closer to the reference. Philadelphia: Vevey/Lippincott Williams & Wilkins; 2002. p. 185–95.

[92] Savino F, Fissore MF, Grassino EC, et al. Ghrelin, leptin and IGF-I levels in breast-fed and formula-fed infants in the first years of life. Acta Paediatr 2005;94:531–7.

[93] Elmlinger MW, Hochhaus F, Loui A, et al. Insulin-like growth factors and binding proteins in early milk from mothers of preterm and term infants. Horm Res 2007;68:124–31.

[94] Martin LJ, Woo JG, Geraghty SR, et al. Adiponectin is present in human milk and is associated with maternal factors. Am J Clin Nutr 2006;83:1106–11.

[95] Dundar NO, Anal O, Dundar B, et al. Longitudinal investigation of the relationship between breast milk leptin levels and growth in breast-fed infants. J Pediatr Endocrinol Metab 2005;18:181–7.

[96] Miralles O, Sanchez J, Palou A, et al. A physiological role of breast milk leptin in body weight control in developing infants. Obesity (Silver Spring) 2006;14:1371–7.

[97] Dewey KG. Growth characteristics of breast-fed compared to formula-fed infants. Biol Neonate 1998;74:94–105.

[98] Dewey KG, Heinig MJ, Nommsen LA, et al. Breast-fed infants are leaner than formula-fed infants at 1 y of age: the DARLING study. Am J Clin Nutr 1993;57:140–5.

[99] American Academy of Pediatrics policy statement. breastfeeding and the use of human milk. Pediatrics 2005;115:496–506.

[100] de Onis M, Garza C, Victora CG, et al. The WHO Multicentre Growth Reference Study: planning, study design, and methodology. Food Nutr Bull 2004;25:S15–26.

[101] de Onis M, Garza C, Onyango AW, et al. Comparison of the WHO child growth standards and the CDC 2000 growth charts. J Nutr 2007;137:144–8.

[102] Shealy K, Li R, Benton-Davis S, et al. The CDC guide to breastfeeding interventions. Atlanta: US Department of Health and Human Services, Centers for Disease Control and Prevention; 2005.

[103] National Sleep Foundation. "Sleep in America" poll. Washington, DC: National Sleep Foundation; 2000.

[104] National Sleep Foundation. "Sleep in America" poll. Washington, DC: National Sleep Foundation; 2001.

[105] National Sleep Foundation. "Sleep in America" poll. Washington, DC: National Sleep Foundation; 2002.
[106] National Sleep Foundation. "Sleep in America" poll. Washington, DC: National Sleep Foundation; 2004.
[107] Smaldone A, Honig JC, Byrne MW. Sleepless in America: inadequate sleep and relationships to health and well-being of our nation's children. Pediatrics 2007;119(Suppl 1): S29–37.
[108] Locard E, Mamelle N, Billette A, et al. Risk factors of obesity in a five year old population. Parental versus environmental factors. Int J Obes Relat Metab Disord 1992;16:721–9.
[109] Sekine M, Yamagami T, Hamanishi S, et al. Parental obesity, lifestyle factors and obesity in preschool children: results of the Toyama Birth Cohort study. J Epidemiol 2002;12:33–9.
[110] Agras WS, Hammer LD, McNicholas F, et al. Risk factors for childhood overweight: a prospective study from birth to 9.5 years. J Pediatr 2004;145:20–5.
[111] Taveras EM, Rifas-Shiman SL, Oken E, et al. Short sleep duration in infancy and risk of childhood overweight. Arch Pediatr Adolesc Med 2008;162:305–11.
[112] Moore T, Ucko LE. Night waking in early infancy. Arch Dis Child 1957;32:333–42.
[113] Parmelee AH, Wenner WH, Schulz HR. Infant sleep patterns: from birth to 16 weeks of age. J Pediatr 1964;65:576–82.
[114] Anders TF, Keener M. Developmental course of nighttime sleep-wake patterns in full-term and premature infants during the first year of life. I. Sleep 1985;8:173–92.
[115] James-Roberts IS, Conroy S, Hurry J. Links between infant crying and sleep-waking at six weeks of age. Early Hum Dev 1997;48:143–52.
[116] Glotzbach SF, Edgar DM, Boeddiker M, et al. Biological rhythmicity in normal infants during the first 3 months of life. Pediatrics 1994;94:482–8.
[117] St James-Roberts I, Alvarez M, Csipke E, et al. Infant crying and sleeping in London, Copenhagen and when parents adopt a "proximal" form of care. Pediatrics 2006;117:e1146–55.
[118] Anders TF. Night-waking in infants during the first year of life. Pediatrics 1979;63:860–4.
[119] Adair R, Bauchner H, Philipp B, et al. Night waking during infancy: role of parental presence at bedtime. Pediatrics 1991;87:500–4.
[120] Touchette E, Petit D, Paquet J, et al. Factors associated with fragmented sleep at night across early childhood. Arch Pediatr Adolesc Med 2005;159:242–9.
[121] Wolke D, Meyer R, Ohrt B, et al. Co-morbidity of crying and feeding problems with sleeping problems during infancy: concurrent and predictive associations. Early Dev Parenting 1995;4:191–208.
[122] Jenni OG, Molinari L, Caflisch JA, et al. Sleep duration from ages 1 to 10 years: variability and stability in comparison with growth. Pediatrics 2007;120:e769–76.
[123] Spiegel K, Tasali E, Penev P, et al. Brief communication: sleep curtailment in healthy young men is associated with decreased leptin levels, elevated ghrelin levels, and increased hunger and appetite. Ann Intern Med 2004;141:846–50.
[124] Taheri S, Lin L, Austin D, et al. Short sleep duration is associated with reduced leptin, elevated ghrelin, and increased body mass index. PLoS Med 2004;1:e62.
[125] James RJ, Drewett RF, Cheetham TD. Low cord ghrelin levels in term infants are associated with slow weight gain over the first 3 months of life. J Clin Endocrinol Metab 2004;89: 3847–50.
[126] Bass J, Turek FW. Sleepless in America: a pathway to obesity and the metabolic syndrome? Arch Intern Med 2005;165:15–6.
[127] Wright P, MacLeod HA, Cooper MJ. Waking at night: the effect of early feeding experience. Child Care Health Dev 1983;9:309–19.
[128] Elias MF, Nicolson NA, Bora C, et al. Sleep/wake patterns of breast-fed infants in the first 2 years of life. Pediatrics 1986;77:322–9.
[129] Eaton-Evans J, Dugdale AE. Sleep patterns of infants in the first year of life. Arch Dis Child 1988;63:647–9.

[130] Scher A, Tirosh E, Jaffe M, et al. Sleep patterns of infants and young children in Israel. Int J Behav Dev 1995;18:701–11.

[131] Horne RS, Parslow PM, Ferens D, et al. Comparison of evoked arousability in breast and formula fed infants. Arch Dis Child 2004;89:22–5.

[132] Ball HL. Breastfeeding, bed-sharing, and infant sleep. Birth 2003;30:181–8.

[133] Pinilla T, Birch LL. Help me make it through the night: behavioral entrainment of breast-fed infants' sleep patterns. Pediatrics 1993;91:436–44.

[134] Gerard CM, Harris KA, Thach BT. Spontaneous arousals in supine infants while swaddled and unswaddled during rapid eye movement and quiet sleep. Pediatrics 2002;110:e70.

[135] Franco P, Seret N, Van Hees JN, et al. Influence of swaddling on sleep and arousal characteristics of healthy infants. Pediatrics 2005;115:1307–11.

[136] Karp H. The happiest baby on the block. New York: Bantam Books; 2002.

[137] Karp H. The "fourth trimester": a framework and strategy for understanding and resolving colic. Contemp Pediatr 2004;21:94–116.

[138] Kopp CB. Regulation of distress and negative emotions: a developmental review. Dev Psychol 1989;25:343–54.

[139] Loeber R, Hay D. Key issues in the development of aggression and violence from childhood to early adulthood. Annu Rev Psychol 1997;48:371–410.

[140] Carey W, Hegvik R, McDevitt S. Temperamental factors associated with rapid weight gain and obesity in middle childhood. J Dev Behav Pediatr 1988;9:197–8.

[141] Wells JC, Stanley M, Laidlaw AS, et al. Investigation of the relationship between infant temperament and later body composition. Int J Obes Relat Metab Disord 1997;21:400–6.

[142] Pulkki-Raback L, Elovainio M, Kivimaki M, et al. Temperament in childhood predicts body mass in adulthood: the Cardiovascular Risk in Young Finns Study. Health Psychol 2005;24:307–15.

[143] Canetti L, Bachar E, Berry EM. Food and emotion. Behav Processes 2002;60:157–64.

[144] Pine DS, Cohen P, Brook J, et al. Psychiatric symptoms in adolescence as predictors of obesity in early adulthood: a longitudinal study. Am J Public Health 1997;87:1303–10.

[145] Kishi T, Elmquist JK. Body weight is regulated by the brain: a link between feeding and emotion. Mol Psychiatry 2005;10:132–46.

[146] Thompson RA. Emotion regulation: a theme in search of definition. Monogr Soc Res Child Dev 1994;59:25–52.

[147] Crockenberg S, Leerkes E. The family context of infant development. In: Zenah C, editor. Handbook of infant mental health. New York: Guilford; 1999. p. 60–90.

[148] Jahromi LB, Putnam SP, Stifter CA. Maternal regulation of infant reactivity from 2 to 6 months. Dev Psychol 2004;40:477–87.

[149] Crockenberg SC, Leerkes EM. Infant and maternal behaviors regulate infant reactivity to novelty at 6 months. Dev Psychol 2004;40:1123–32.

[150] Baughcum AE, Powers SW, Johnson SB, et al. Maternal feeding practices and beliefs and their relationships to overweight in early childhood. J Dev Behav Pediatr 2001;22:391–408.

[151] Puhl RM, Schwartz MB. If you are good you can have a cookie: how memories of childhood food rules link to adult eating behaviors. Eat Behav 2003;4:283–93.

[152] van den Boom D. Behavioral management of early infant crying in irritable babies. In: Barr RG, St James-Roberts I, Keefe MR, et al, editors. New evidence on unexplained infant crying: its origins, nature, and management. New Brunswick (NJ): Johnson & Johnson Pediatric Institute; 2001. p. 209–28.

[153] Velderman MK, Bakermans-Kranenburg MJ, Juffer F. van IMH. Effects of attachment-based interventions on maternal sensitivity and infant attachment: differential susceptibility of highly reactive infants. J Fam Psychol 2006;20:266–74.

[154] Chapter 6: Complementary feeding. In: Kleinman RE, editor. Pediatric nutrition handbook. Elk Grove (IL): American Academy of Pediatrics; 2004.

[155] Gartner LM, Morton J, Lawrence RA, et al. Breastfeeding and the use of human milk. Pediatrics 2005;115:496–506.
[156] Parents' survival guide to transitional feeding. The Institute of Pediatric Nutrition; 2003. Available at: http://abbottnutrition.com/home/breastfeeding/index.aspx?p=0.5.2_ForHealthCareProfessionals.
[157] US Department of Health and Human Services, National Center for Health Statistics. Third National Health and Nutrition Survey, 1988–1994, NHANES III. Examination data file: CD-ROM series 11 No 1A and No 2A. In: Hyattsville (MD): Public use data file documentation number 76200; July 1997 and April 1998, respectively.
[158] Kim J, Peterson KE. Association of infant child care with infant feeding practices and weight gain among US infants. Arch Pediatr Adolesc Med 2008;162:627–33.
[159] Shelov SP, Hannemann RE, editors. Caring for your baby and young child: birth to age 5. 4th edition. New York: Bantam Books; 2004.
[160] Macknin ML, Medendorp SV, Maier MC. Infant sleep and bedtime cereal. Am J Dis Child 1989;143:1066–8.
[161] Shukla A, Forsyth HA, Anderson CM, et al. Infantile overnutrition in the first year of life: a field study in Dudley, Worcestershire. Br Med J 1972;4:507–15.
[162] Ferris AG, Laus MJ, Hosmer DW, et al. The effect of diet on weight gain in infancy. Am J Clin Nutr 1980;33:2635–42.
[163] Kramer MS, Barr RG, Leduc DG, et al. Determinants of weight and adiposity in the first year of life. J Pediatr 1985;106:10–4.
[164] Ong KK, Emmett PM, Noble S, et al. Dietary energy intake at the age of 4 months predicts postnatal weight gain and childhood body mass index. Pediatrics 2006;117:e503–8.
[165] Baker JL, Michaelsen KF, Rasmussen KM, et al. Maternal prepregnant body mass index, duration of breastfeeding, and timing of complementary food introduction are associated with infant weight gain. Am J Clin Nutr 2004;80:1579–88.
[166] Birch LL. Development of food preferences. Annu Rev Nutr 1999;19:41–62.
[167] Sullivan SA, Birch LL. Infant dietary experience and acceptance of solid foods. Pediatrics 1994;93:271–7.
[168] Birch LL, Gunder L, Grimm-Thomas K, et al. Infants' consumption of a new food enhances acceptance of similar foods. Appetite 1998;30:283–95.
[169] Birch LL, Marlin DW. I don't like it; I never tried it: effects of exposure on two-year-old children's food preferences. Appetite 1982;3:353–60.
[170] Birch LL, McPhee L, Shoba BC, et al. What kind of exposure reduces children's food neophobia? Looking vs. tasting. Appetite 1987;9:171–8.
[171] Birch LL. Development of food acceptance patterns in the first years of life. Proc Nutr Soc 1998;57:617–24.
[172] Dietz WH, Franks AL, Marks JS. The obesity problem. N Engl J Med 1998;338:1157 [author reply 8].
[173] Farrow C, Blissett J. Does maternal control during feeding moderate early infant weight gain? Pediatrics 2006;118:e293–8.
[174] Farrow CV, Blissett J. Controlling feeding practices: cause or consequence of early child weight? Pediatrics 2008;121:e164–9.
[175] Birch LL, McPhee L, Shoba BC, et al. "Clean up your plate". Effects of child feeding practices on the conditioning of meal size. Learn Motiv 1987;18:301–17.
[176] Galloway AT, Fiorito L, Lee Y, et al. Parental pressure, dietary patterns, and weight status among girls who are "picky eaters". J Am Diet Assoc 2005;105:541–8.
[177] Galloway AT, Fiorito LM, Francis LA, et al. 'Finish your soup': counterproductive effects of pressuring children to eat on intake and affect. Appetite 2006;46:318–23.
[178] Ventura AK, Birch LL. Does parenting affect children's eating and weight status? Int J Behav Nutr Phys Act 2008;5:15.
[179] Gidding SS, Dennison BA, Birch LL, et al. Dietary recommendations for children and adolescents: a guide for practitioners. Pediatrics 2006;117:544–59.

[180] Green M, editor. Bright futures: guidelines for health supervision of infants, children, and adolescents. Arlington (VA): National Center for Education in Maternal and Child Health; 1994.

[181] Dietz WH, Stern L, editors. American Academy of Pediatrics: guide to your child's nutrition. New York: Villard; 1999.

[182] Kleinman RE, editor. Pediatric nutrition handbook. 5th edition. Elk Grove (IL): American Academy of Pediatrics; 2004.

[183] American Academy of Pediatrics. Committee on Nutrition. Cholesterol in childhood. Pediatrics 1998;101:141–7.

[184] Birch LL. Children's preferences for high-fat foods. Nutr Rev 1992;50:249–55.

[185] Fox MK, Reidy K, Novak T, et al. Sources of energy and nutrients in the diets of infants and toddlers. J Am Diet Assoc 2006;106:S28–42.

[186] Dennison BA, Erb TA, Jenkins PL. Predictors of dietary milk fat intake by preschool children. Prev Med 2001;33:536–42.

[187] Kranz S, Lin PJ, Wagstaff DA. Children's dairy intake in the United States: too little, too fat? J Pediatr 2007;151:642–6, 6 e1–e2.

[188] Basch CE, Shea S, Zybert P. Food sources, dietary behavior, and the saturated fat intake of Latino children. Am J Public Health 1992;82:810–5.

[189] Sigman-Grant M, Zimmerman S, Kris-Etherton PM. Dietary approaches for reducing fat intake of preschool-age children. Pediatrics 1993;91:955–60.

[190] Dixon LB, McKenzie J, Shannon BM, et al. The effect of changes in dietary fat on the food group and nutrient intake of 4- to 10-year-old children. Pediatrics 1997;100:863–72.

[191] Friedman G, Goldberg SJ. An evaluation of the safety of a low-saturated-fat, low-cholesterol diet beginning in infancy. Pediatrics 1976;58:655–7.

[192] Niinikoski H, Viikari J, Ronnemaa T, et al. Regulation of growth of 7- to 36-month-old children by energy and fat intake in the prospective, randomized STRIP baby trial. Pediatrics 1997;100:810–6.

[193] Lagstrom H, Seppanen R, Jokinen E, et al. Influence of dietary fat on the nutrient intake and growth of children from 1 to 5 y of age: the Special Turku Coronary Risk Factor Intervention Project. Am J Clin Nutr 1999;69:516–23.

[194] Karaolis-Danckert N, Gunther AL, Kroke A, et al. How early dietary factors modify the effect of rapid weight gain in infancy on subsequent body-composition development in term children whose birth weight was appropriate for gestational age. Am J Clin Nutr 2007;86:1700–8.

[195] Fox MK, Pac S, Devaney B, et al. Feeding Infants and Toddlers Study: what foods are infants and toddlers eating? J Am Diet Assoc 2004;104:s22–30.

[196] Daniels SR, Greer FR. Lipid screening and cardiovascular health in childhood. Pediatrics 2008;122:198–208.

[197] Berkey CS, Rockett HR, Willett WC, et al. Milk, dairy fat, dietary calcium, and weight gain: a longitudinal study of adolescents. Arch Pediatr Adolesc Med 2005;159:543–50.

[198] USDA National Nutrient Database for Standard Reference. Available at: http://www.nal.usda.gov/fnic/foodcomp/cgi-bin/nut_search_new.pl. Accessed February 7, 2008.

[199] Nielsen SJ, Popkin BM. Changes in beverage intake between 1977 and 2001. Am J Prev Med 2004;27:205–10.

[200] O'Connor TM, Yang SJ, Nicklas TA. Beverage intake among preschool children and its effect on weight status. Pediatrics 2006;118:e1010–8.

[201] American Dietetic Association. Childhood overweight evidence analysis project: factors associated with overweight. Available at: http://www.adaevidencelibrary.com/topic.cfm?cat=2792. Accessed February 15, 2007.

[202] Skinner JD, Ziegler P, Ponza M. Transitions in infants' and toddlers' beverage patterns. J Am Diet Assoc 2004;104:s45–50.

[203] American Academy of Pediatrics. The use and misuse of fruit juice in pediatrics. Pediatrics 2001;107:1210–3.

[204] Welsh JA, Cogswell ME, Rogers S, et al. Overweight among low-income preschool children associated with the consumption of sweet drinks: Missouri, 1999–2002. Pediatrics 2005;115:e223–9.

[205] Warner ML, Harley K, Bradman A, et al. Soda consumption and overweight status of 2-year-old Mexican-American children in California. Obesity (Silver Spring) 2006;14:1966–74.

[206] Murray R, Frankowski B, Taras H. Are soft drinks a scapegoat for childhood obesity? J Pediatr 2005;146:586–90.

[207] James J, Kerr D. Prevention of childhood obesity by reducing soft drinks. Int J Obes (Lond) 2005;29(Suppl 2):S54–7.

[208] Devaney B, Ziegler P, Pac S, et al. Nutrient intakes of infants and toddlers. J Am Diet Assoc 2004;104:s14–21.

[209] Picciano MF, Smiciklas-Wright H, Birch LL, et al. Nutritional guidance is needed during dietary transition in early childhood. Pediatrics 2000;106:109–14.

[210] Butte N, Cobb K, Dwyer J, et al. The Start healthy feeding guidelines for infants and toddlers. J Am Diet Assoc 2004;104:442–54.

[211] Ryan C, Dwyer J. The toddler's smorgasbord. Nutr Today 2003;38:164–9.

[212] McConahy KL, Picciano MF. How to grow a healthy toddler—12 to 24 months. Nutr Today 2003;38:156–63.

[213] National Association for Sport and Physical Education. Active start: a statement of physical activity guidelines for children birth to five years. New York: AAHPERD Publications; 2002.

[214] Corbin C, Pangrazi R, Beighle A, et al. Guidelines for appropriate physical activity for elementary school children 2003 update. A position statement. Council for Physical Education for Children (COPEC) of the National Association for Sport and Physical Education, an Association of the American Alliance for Health Physical Education and Recreation. New York: AAHPERD Publications; 2003.

[215] Gunner KB, Atkinson PM, Nichols J, et al. Health promotion strategies to encourage physical activity in infants, toddlers, and preschoolers. J Pediatr Health Care 2005;19:253–8.

[216] Dennison BA, Boyer PS. Risk evaluation in pediatric practice aids in prevention of childhood overweight. Pediatr Ann 2004;33:25–30.

[217] Neumark-Sztainer D. Childhood and adolescent obesity: an ecological perspective. Basic Pediatrics 2003;101:12–20.

[218] Dennison BA, Erb TA, Jenkins PL. Television viewing and television in bedroom associated with overweight risk among low-income preschool children. Pediatrics 2002;109:1028–35.

[219] Campbell K, Hesketh K, Crawford D, et al. The Infant Feeding Activity and Nutrition Trial (INFANT) an early intervention to prevent childhood obesity: cluster-randomised controlled trial. BMC Public Health 2008;8:103.

[220] Wolman J, Skelly E, Kolotourou M, et al. Tackling toddler obesity through a pilot community-based family intervention. Community Pract 2008;81:28–31.

[221] American Academy of Pediatrics. Children, adolescents, and television. Pediatrics 2001;107:423–6.

Advances in Pediatrics 56 (2009) 135–144

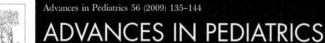

ADVANCES IN PEDIATRICS

ELSEVIER
MOSBY

Relationships Among Serum Iron, Inflammation, and Body Mass Index in Children

Ajay P. Sharma, MD[a], Ann Marie McKenna, MD, BSc[a], Nathalie Lepage, PhD[b], Ed Nieuwenhuys, BSc[c], Guido Filler, MD, PhD, FRCPC[a],*

[a]Department of Paediatrics, Children's Hospital at London Health Sciences Centre, University of Western Ontario, 800 Commissioners Road East, London, Ontario, Canada N6A 5W9
[b]Department of Pathology and Laboratory Medicine, Children's Hospital of Eastern Ontario, University of Ottawa, Ottawa, Ontario, Canada
[c]Sanquin Research-Academic Medical Center, Landsteiner Laboratory, Amsterdam, The Netherlands

O ver the last 3 decades, the National Health and Nutrition Examination Survey (NHANES) revealed a 3-fold increase in overweight prevalence, from 4% to 15%, among children and adolescents aged 6 to 19 years [1]. This trend continues in the most recent NHANES data [2]. Moreover, the National Longitudinal Survey of Youth demonstrated a marked increase in the degree of obesity among overweight children aged 4 to 12 years [3]. The increase in cardiovascular, renal, and endocrine disorders with childhood obesity is well recognized [4]. Some studies on adults [5–7] and children [8–11] also point to an association between obesity and low serum iron levels.

The underlying mechanisms to explain low serum iron levels with obesity are less well understood. The decrease in serum iron traditionally is considered to be a result of true iron deficiency, arising from a combination of lower iron intake because of an unbalanced diet [9], and higher iron requirement resulting from blood volume increase [10,12]. Alternatively, obesity has been reported to induce an inflammatory state [13–15], which can potentially aggravate iron sequestration into the reticuloendothelial system. Reduced iron bioavailability consequently may lower serum iron levels despite no real iron deficiency.

This work was supported by grants from Dade Behring GmbH, Marburg, Germany, and Dade Behring Inc., Canada.

*Corresponding author. Department of Paediatrics, Children's Hospital of Western Ontario, 800 Commissioners Road East, London, Ontario, Canada N6A 5W9. E-mail address: guido.filler@lhsc.on.ca (G. Filler).

0065-3101/09/$ – see front matter
doi:10.1016/j.yapd.2009.08.014

A recent study suggested that inflammation contributes to low serum iron levels in adult subjects [16]. This issue has not been evaluated in children. Based on the evidence that inflammatory process sets in during childhood [17], a similar role of inflammation in children is also possible, although younger age may alter the nature of this association [18]. If a contributory role of inflammation in lower serum iron levels with higher body mass index (BMI) is proven, weight reduction could potentially augment the response to iron therapy by decreasing inflammation. The detrimental effect of iron deficiency on physical and psychological growth in children makes this subject more relevant in the pediatric age group [19–21].

To evaluate the role of inflammation in the inverse relationship between BMI and serum iron levels, we (the authors of this article) studied the relationship among BMI, inflammation, and serum iron levels in apparently healthy children.

METHODS

From March 2005 to March 2006, 220 otherwise healthy children, scheduled for elective surgeries such as hernia repair, circumcision, hypospadiasis repair, tympanostomy, strabismus repair, hardware removal, and minor orthopedic or dental interventions, were recruited from the operative lists at the Children's Hospital of Eastern Ontario (CHEO). Exclusion criteria included an associated acute medical illness, a weight change of more than 10 body weight percentiles over the preceding 3 months, medication use that could affect body weight, or refused consent. Patients aged 2 years or younger were also excluded due to the lack of reference data for BMI z-score calculation. A study nurse approached the selected patients at the preoperative anesthesia assessment visit. Written informed consent was obtained from the parents for limited anthropometric data and also for blood sampling at the time of vascular access being secured for surgery. The Institutional Review Board gave full approval for the study.

All included patients had their age, gender, ethnicity, weight, and height recorded, and blood collected to assess hematological, iron, and inflammatory profiles. The hematological parameters included hemoglobin (Hb), mean corpuscular volume (MCV), mean corpuscular hemoglobin (MCH), mean corpuscular hemoglobin concentration (MCHC), and red blood cell distribution width (RDW). The iron profile included serum iron, soluble transferrin receptor (sTfR), and ferritin levels. Inflammatory status was assessed by serum C-reactive protein (CRP).

Weight and height were recorded in hospital gowns, fasting, on the same digital scale and stadiometer. The equipment was calibrated before each subject's measurement. BMI was calculated from the ratio of weight (kg) and the square of the height (m). As BMI is age- and gender-dependent, we calculated BMI z scores.

For the z score calculation, we used the reference intervals from the most recent NHANES III database compiled by the National Center for Health Statistics (NCHS, USA) [22]. These NCHS-CDC growth charts provide the

L, M, and S parameters needed to generate exact percentiles and z scores. The LMS parameters are the power in the Box-Cox transformation (L), the median (M), and the generalized coefficient of variation (S). To obtain a z score or percentile (X), we used the equation from the same Web site. The equation reads: $X = M(1+LSZ)^{**}(1/L)$; where L, M, and S are the values from the appropriate table corresponding to the age in months of the child (** indicates an exponent, such that $M(1+LSZ)^{**}(1/L)$ means raising $(1+LSZ)$ to the $(1/L)$th power and then multiplying the M; $\exp(X)$ is the exponentiation function, e to the power X).

The children with BMI z scores >1.95 (2 standard deviations) constituted the high BMI group, whereas rest of the children comprised the normal BMI group.

Serum iron was measured by dry slide technology (Vitros 250, Ortho Clinical, Rochester, NY) with coefficient of variation (CV) of 2.15% at the level of 12.0 mmol/L, 1.97% at 27.65 mmol/L, and 2.47% at 41.81 mmol/L. Serum ferritin was measured by immunonephelometry (Dade Behring BN Prospec, Marburg, Germany), with CV of 5.64% at the level of 96.41 μg/L, 5.39% at 105.64 μg/L, and 3.44% at 148.24 μg/L. sTfR was measured by immunonephelometry (Dade Behring BN Prospec), with CV of 4.67% at the level of 0.90 mg/L, 2.37% at 1.21 mg/L, and 9.57% at 1.76 mg/L. Hb was measured on CellDyn 3200 (Abbott), with CV of 1.05% at the level of 161.29 g/L, 0.73% at 120.24 g/L, and 0.95% at 79.07 g/L. CRP was measured by immunonephelometry (Dade Behring BN Prospec) with CV of 4.02% at the level of 12.79 mg/L and 4.48% at 50.87 mg/L.

Due to the age dependency of Hb, Hb z scores were calculated from the measured Hb concentration for the age groups ranging from 2 to 6, 6 to 12, and 12 to 18 years. As there were no gender differences observed in the Hb values except in children aged 12 to 18 years, data were pooled for both genders and were analyzed separately only for boys and girls aged 12 to 18 years. z Scores for ferritin levels were also calculated.

STATISTICAL ANALYSIS

Statistical analysis was performed with the GraphPad Prism version 4.02 for Windows (GraphPad Software, San Diego, CA). The Fisher exact test was used to compare frequencies between the normal and the high BMI groups. Contiguous data were analyzed for normal distribution with the D'Agostini Pearson omnibus test [23]. Simple descriptive tests were employed using appropriate parametric tests for normally distributed parameters and nonparametric tests otherwise. Log transformations were done as indicated. For multivariate regression analysis, only the variables significant in the univariate regression models were entered as the independent variables, with serum iron as the dependent variable. A P value of <0.05 was considered statistically significant.

RESULTS

From the initial 220 subjects, 41 patients were not included in the study due to different exclusion criteria. Finally, 179 constituted the study sample, 75 (42%)

of whom were girls. In the study cohort, 22 (12%) boys and 21 (11%) girls were older than 12 years. Fifty-eight children (31%) were younger than 5 years, 60 (34%) were aged 5 to 10 years, and 61 (35%) were older than 10 years. The majority, 159 (89%), were Caucasians, whereas Asians, Africans, and others constituted 12 (6%), 3 (2%), and 5 (3%) of the study sample, respectively.

The characteristics of the high BMI group (n = 30) were compared with the normal BMI group (n = 149). As shown in Table 1, the difference in the BMI z scores between the 2 groups was statistically significant ($P<.001$). The high BMI group had significantly lower serum iron levels ($P = .01$) (Fig. 1), and markedly higher CRP ($P = .008$) and sTfR levels ($P = .03$). The 2 groups had no significant difference in age, gender, and ferritin z scores.

Regression coefficients of age, BMI z score, ferritin z score, sTfR, and CRP with serum iron as the dependent variable are shown in Table 2. In the normal BMI group, serum iron did not correlate with sTfR and ferritin z score; however, it correlated significantly with both BMI z score ($\beta = -0.24$; confidence interval (CI) -3.47, -0.57; $P = .007$) and CRP ($\beta = -0.36$; CI -0.22, -0.08; $P = .001$) (Fig. 2). In the high BMI group, serum iron exhibited significant correlation with BMI z score ($\beta = -0.50$; CI -4.76, -0.80; $P = .009$), CRP ($\beta = -0.73$; CI -0.51, -0.23; $P<.001$) (Fig. 3), and sTfR ($\beta = -0.46$; CI -17.02, -1.93; $P = .01$). Evident from these results is that the association between serum iron, CRP, and BMI z score was stronger in the high BMI group.

On adjusted regression analysis, only CRP retained a statistically significant association with serum iron in both groups (normal BMI group: $\beta = -0.29$; CI -1.70, -0.40; $P = .004$; high BMI group: $\beta = -0.60$; CI -0.45, -0.12; $P = .001$).

On separate correlation analyses in the whole group, serum iron had significant association with other hematological parameters including Hb z score

Table 1		
Characteristics of the normal and high body mass index groups		
	Normal BMI Group (n=149)	High BMI Group (n=30)
Age (years)	8.07 (7.25, 8.89)	8.75 (6.86, 10.64)
Females (%)	64 (43%)	11 (37%)
BMI z score	0.24 (0.10, 0.37)	3.28 (2.99, 3.85)[a]
Ferritin z score	0.39 (−1.93, 1.14)	−0.03 (−2.13, 1.26)
sTfR (mg/L)	1.70 (1.64, −1.76)	1.83 (1.67, 1.92)[a]
CRP (mg/L)	0.75 (0.47, 1.03)	2.20 (0.27, 4.13)[a]
Iron (mmol/L)	14.98 (13.86, 16.09)	11.66 (9.25, 14.07)[a]

Data expressed as % for gender and mean (95% confidence interval) for rest of the variables.
BMI, body mass index; CRP, C-reactive protein; high BMI group, BMI z score >1.95 (2 standard deviations); sTfR, soluble transferrin receptors.
[a]P value <0.05.

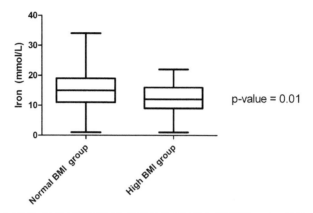

Fig. 1. Serum iron levels in the high body mass index (BMI) and normal BMI groups. The high BMI group comprised children with BMI z score >1.95 (2 standard deviations). The normal BMI group comprised children with BMI z score ≤1.95.

($r = 0.15$; $P = .02$), MCV ($r = 0.21$; $P = .002$), MCH ($r = 0.26$; $P = .000$), MCHC ($r = 0.18$; $P = .01$), and RDW ($r = -0.22$; $P = .002$).

DISCUSSION

The recognized inverse relationship between serum iron levels and obesity [5–7,9–11] has been traditionally attributed to true iron deficiency, resulting from dietary iron inadequacy, and increased iron demand with higher BMI. Based on the observations suggesting a proinflammatory potential of obesity [13,14], we suspected a contribution of functional iron deficiency, resulting from inflammation, in the iron-obesity relationship.

Low serum iron level in our high BMI group was consistent with the observations from previous studies [5–7,9–11]. A stronger correlation coefficient between BMI z score and serum iron levels in both BMI groups again supported this association.

To evaluate the role of inflammation in the BMI-iron relationship, we compared serum CRP levels between the 2 BMI groups. Serum CRP was significantly higher in the high BMI group. On further analysis, CRP had a strong inverse association with serum iron in both groups on unadjusted regression analysis. The association remained significant after adjusting for age, BMI z score, ferritin z score, and sTfR. In relative terms, the CRP-serum iron relationship was stronger in the high BMI group than in the normal BMI group. The positive association between BMI and CRP, and the inverse relationship between CRP and serum iron, suggest a contribution of inflammation in the BMI-iron relationship.

The role of inflammation in the BMI-iron relationship has not been previously evaluated in healthy children. Yanoff and colleagues [16] explored this

Table 2

Regression analysis in the normal and high body mass index groups with serum iron as the dependent variable

	Normal BMI group		High BMI group	
	Unadjusted β (95% CI)	Adjusted β (95% CI)	Unadjusted β (95% CI)	Adjusted β (95% CI)
Age (years)	0.17 (−0.00, 0.46)	—	0.07 (−0.47, 0.68)	—
BMI z score	−0.24[a] (−3.47, −0.57)	−0.17 (−2.86, 0.02)	−0.50[a] (−4.76, −0.80)	−0.08 (−2.91, 1.94)
Ferritin z score	0.06 (−0.69, 1.39)	—	0.30 (−1.67, 0.27)	—
sTFR (mg/L)	−0.13 (−5.72, 0.89)	—	−0.46[a] (−17.02, −1.93)	−0.19 (−11.94, 4.21)
Log CRP (mg/L)	−0.36[a] (−0.22, −0.08)	−0.29[a] (−1.70, −0.40)	−0.73[a] (−0.51, −0.23)	−0.60[a] (−0.45, −0.12)

β, regression coefficient; BMI, body mass index; CI, confidence interval; CRP, C-reactive protein; high BMI group, BMI z score >1.95 (2 standard deviations); sTFR, soluble transferrin receptors.

[a]P value <0.05.

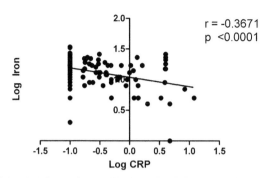

Fig. 2. Relationship between C-reactive protein (CRP) and serum iron levels on regression analysis in the normal BMI group. The normal BMI group comprised children with BMI z score ≤1.95 (2 standard deviations).

question in healthy adults, and reported a similar relationship between serum iron levels and inflammation in obese subjects. Similar to our observations, serum iron in the adult subjects showed a stronger association with CRP than with sTfR [16]. In addition, Yanoff and colleagues analyzed dietary iron intake in their study sample, and reported no relationship between iron intake and serum iron levels. For the first time, our results suggest a similar contribution of inflammation to the lower iron levels with an increase in the BMI in children. Kopp and colleagues [24] showed a decrease in the inflammatory markers in obese adults with weight reduction following gastroplasty. Whether weight reduction can improve the response to iron therapy with a decrease in the inflammatory state in children with high BMI needs to be evaluated.

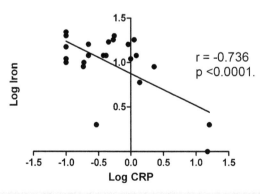

Fig. 3. Relationship between CRP and serum iron levels on regression analysis in the high BMI group. The high BMI group comprised children with BMI z score >1.95 (2 standard deviations).

We speculated the possible mechanisms to link obesity and low serum iron levels through inflammation. Obesity has been shown to be a proinflammatory state [13,14]. Adipose tissue enhances the expression of inflammatory cytokines, including tumor necrosis factor-α, interleukin (IL)-6, and IL-18 [12,13]. Inflammation has been proposed to lower serum iron levels through a combination of functional iron deficiency, by reticuloendothelial iron sequestration, and true iron deficiency through reduced intestinal iron absorption [22,23]. Inflammation has recently been shown to increase the expression of an iron-regulating protein, hepcidin, on adipose tissue [25,26]. Hepcidin could be the potential connecting link between inflammation and serum iron, as its elevation decreases macrophagic iron release [26] and reduces enterocytic iron absorption [27]. Future studies on the relationship of hepcidin and inflammation in context with BMI and serum iron will be helpful in establishing the proposed hypothesis.

On comparing the conventional markers of true iron deficiency, the high BMI group exhibited higher serum sTfR levels, but serum ferritin levels did not significantly differ between the groups. Serum iron showed a positive association with sTfR on unadjusted regression analysis; however, unlike with CRP, sTfR-serum iron association did not reach a statistically significant level after adjusting for other variables.

Our observation is novel but it needs to be looked at in the context of the limitations of the study. Due to the cross-sectional study design, a cause-and-effect relationship among the studied variables cannot be established. A Caucasian predominance limits the applicability of our observations to children from other ethnicities. We did not obtain menstrual history in the adolescent girls. A relatively small proportion of the girls (11%) who were older than 12 years, and the possibility of no menstruation in a few of those, should minimize a confounding effect from menstrual blood loss, although this additional information would have potentially strengthened our observation. The proportion of children with defined obesity was relatively smaller in our study sample. Despite this limitation, the observed relationship among BMI, inflammation, and serum iron raises the possibility of a continuous nature of the association even below the conventional cutoffs used to define obesity. Although an unrelated infection or inflammation could affect the CRP measurement, the exclusion of subjects with acute medical issues decreases the likelihood of such a confounding effect. Elevation of CRP with increase in BMI is consistent with the recent observations suggesting obesity as a low-grade inflammatory state, resulting from chronic activation of the innate immune system [28,29]. Serum CRP level has also been found to be associated with other markers of inflammation, such as serum adiponectin and IL-6 levels, in obesity [24].

While interpreting ferritin and sTfR for assessing iron deficiency, it should be noted that ferritin is a positive acute-phase reactant, and sTfR increases with accelerated erythropoiesis. A selection of otherwise healthy subjects decreases the likelihood of a significant acute-phase ferritin increase. Although the subjects were not formally screened for hemoglobinopathies, no previous history of hemolytic anemia, as well as an inverse relationship between serum sTfR and serum ferritin in the enrolled children, suggest against a significant impact from undiagnosed hemolysis on our results. A better association between serum iron and sTfR, rather than with serum ferritin, was consistent with a higher sensitivity of sTfR in predicting marrow iron, although its age dependency and lower specificity to predict marrow iron limit the utility of sTfR as a stand-alone test to diagnose iron deficiency [30–34]. It seems less likely that the limitations of sTfR for the diagnosis of iron deficiency should have influenced our primary observation on the possible role of inflammation in the BMI-iron relationship.

We conclude that inflammation is associated with lower serum iron levels in children with high BMI. This observation may have a clinical implication, as weight reduction can potentially improve response to iron therapy with a decrease in inflammatory state in children with high BMI. Longitudinal studies with larger study samples are needed to confirm this association.

Acknowledgments

The authors are grateful to Dr. Abeer Yasin, PhD, for help with the statistical analysis.

References

[1] Ogden CL, Flegal KM, Carroll MD, et al. Prevalence and trends in overweight among US children and adolescents, 1999–2000. JAMA 2002;288(14):1728–32.

[2] Ogden CL, Carroll MD, Flegal KM. High body mass index for age among US children and adolescents, 2003–2006. JAMA 2008;299(20):2401–5.

[3] Strauss RS, Pollack HA. Epidemic increase in childhood overweight, 1986–1998. JAMA 2001;286(22):2845–8.

[4] Ball GD, McCargar LJ. Childhood obesity in Canada: a review of prevalence estimates and risk factors for cardiovascular diseases and type 2 diabetes. Can J Appl Physiol 2003;28(1):117–40.

[5] Micozzi MS, Albanes D, Stevens RG. Relation of body size and composition to clinical biochemical and hematologic indices in US men and women. Am J Clin Nutr 1989;50(6):1276–81.

[6] Whitfield JB, Treloar S, Zhu G, et al. Relative importance of female-specific and non-female-specific effects on variation in iron stores between women. Br J Haematol 2003;120(5):860–6.

[7] Lecube A, Carrera A, Losada E, et al. Iron deficiency in obese postmenopausal women. Obesity (Silver Spring) 2006;14(10):1724–30.

[8] Wenzel BJ, Stults HB, Mayer J. Hypoferraemia in obese adolescents. Lancet 1962;2:327–8.

[9] Seltzer CC, Mayer J. Serum iron and iron-binding capacity in adolescents. II. comparison of obese and nonobese subjects. Am J Clin Nutr 1963;13:354–61.

[10] Pinhas-Hamiel O, Newfield RS, Koren I, et al. Greater prevalence of iron deficiency in overweight and obese children and adolescents. Int J Obes Relat Metab Disord 2003;27(3):416–8.

[11] Nead KG, Halterman JS, Kaczorowski JM, et al. Overweight children and adolescents: a risk group for iron deficiency. Pediatrics 2004;114(1):104–8.

[12] Failla ML, Kennedy ML, Chen ML. Iron metabolism in genetically obese (ob/ob) mice. J Nutr 1988;118(1):46–51.

[13] Greenberg AS, Obin MS. Obesity and the role of adipose tissue in inflammation and metabolism. Am J Clin Nutr 2006;83(2):461S–5S.

[14] Weiss R, Dziura J, Burgert TS, et al. Obesity and the metabolic syndrome in children and adolescents. N Engl J Med 2004;350(23):2362–74.

[15] Visser M, Bouter LM, McQuillan GM, et al. Low-grade systemic inflammation in overweight children. Pediatrics 2001;107(1):E13.

[16] Yanoff LB, Menzie CM, Denkinger B, et al. Inflammation and iron deficiency in the hypoferremia of obesity. Int J Obes (Lond) 2007;31(9):1412–9.

[17] Osganian SK, Stampfer MJ, Spiegelman D, et al. Distribution of and factors associated with serum homocysteine levels in children: Child and Adolescent Trial for Cardiovascular Health. JAMA 1999;281(13):1189–96.

[18] Warnberg J, Marcos A. Low-grade inflammation and the metabolic syndrome in children and adolescents. Curr Opin Lipidol 2008;19(1):11–5.

[19] Lozoff B, Jimenez E, Hagen J, et al. Poorer behavioral and developmental outcome more than 10 years after treatment for iron deficiency in infancy. Pediatrics 2000;105(4):E51.

[20] Grantham-McGregor S, Ani C. A review of studies on the effect of iron deficiency on cognitive development in children. J Nutr 2001;131(2S–2):649S–66S [discussion: 666S–8S].

[21] Looker AC, Dallman PR, Carroll MD, et al. Prevalence of iron deficiency in the United States. JAMA 1997;277(12):973–6.

[22] Available at:http://www.cdc.gov/nchs/about/major/nhanes/growthcharts/zscore/zscore. htm. National Center for Health Statistics—2000 CDC growth charts: United States. In; 1999–2002. Accessed June 2, 2008.

[23] Oztuna D, Elhan AH, Tuccar E. Investigation of four different normality tests in terms of type 1 error rate and power under different distributions. Turk J Med Sci 2006;36(3):171–6.

[24] Kopp HP, Krzyzanowska K, Mohlig M, et al. Effects of marked weight loss on plasma levels of adiponectin, markers of chronic subclinical inflammation and insulin resistance in morbidly obese women. Int J Obes (Lond) 2005;29(7):766–71.

[25] Bekri S, Gual P, Anty R, et al. Increased adipose tissue expression of hepcidin in severe obesity is independent from diabetes and NASH. Gastroenterology 2006;131(3): 788–96.

[26] Nemeth E, Rivera S, Gabayan V, et al. IL-6 mediates hypoferremia of inflammation by inducing the synthesis of the iron regulatory hormone hepcidin. J Clin Invest 2004;113(9):1271–6.

[27] Laftah AH, Ramesh B, Simpson RJ, et al. Effect of hepcidin on intestinal iron absorption in mice. Blood 2004;103(10):3940–4.

[28] Bastard JP, Maachi M, Lagathu C, et al. Recent advances in the relationship between obesity, inflammation, and insulin resistance. Eur Cytokine Netw 2006;17(1):4–12.

[29] Heilbronn LK, Campbell LV. Adipose tissue macrophages, low grade inflammation and insulin resistance in human obesity. Curr Pharm Des 2008;14(12):1225–30.

[30] Means RT Jr, Allen J, Sears DA, et al. Serum soluble transferrin receptor and the prediction of marrow aspirate iron results in a heterogeneous group of patients. Clin Lab Haematol 1999;21(3):161–7.

[31] Mast AE, Blinder MA, Gronowski AM, et al. Clinical utility of the soluble transferrin receptor and comparison with serum ferritin in several populations. Clin Chem 1998;44(1):45–51.

[32] Punnonen K, Irjala K, Rajamaki A. Serum transferrin receptor and its ratio to serum ferritin in the diagnosis of iron deficiency. Blood 1997;89(3):1052–7.

[33] Ritchie B, McNeil Y, Brewster DR. Soluble transferrin receptor in Aboriginal children with a high prevalence of iron deficiency and infection. Trop Med Int Health 2004;9(1):96–105.

[34] Danise P, Maconi M, Morelli G, et al. Reference limits and behaviour of serum transferrin receptor in children 6–10 years of age. Int J Lab Hematol 2008;30(4):306–11.

Advances in Pediatrics 56 (2009) 145–164

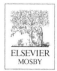

ADVANCES IN PEDIATRICS

The Gender Medicine Team: "It Takes a Village"

Marni E. Axelrad, PhD[a],*, Jonathan S. Berg, MD[b],
Leslie Ayensu Coker, MD[c],
Jennifer Dietrich, MD, MSc, FACOG[c], Lisa Adcock, MD[d],
Shannon L. French, MD[e], Sheila Gunn, MD[e],
B. Lee Ligon, PhD[f], Laurence B. McCullough, PhD[g],
V. Reid Sutton, MD[b], Lefkothea P. Karaviti, MD, PhD[e]

[a]Pediatric Service, Texas Children's Hospital, Houston, TX 77030, USA
[b]Department of Molecular and Human Genetics, Baylor College of Medicine, Texas Children's Hospital, Houston, TX 77030, USA
[c]Department of Obstetrics and Gynecology, Baylor College of Medicine, Texas Children's Hospital, Houston, TX 77030, USA
[d]Neonatology Section, Pediatrics, Baylor College of Medicine, Houston, TX 77030, USA
[e]Pediatrics-Endocrinology and Metabolism, Baylor College of Medicine, Houston, TX 77030, USA
[f]Department of Pediatrics, Baylor College of Medicine, Houston, TX 77030, USA
[g]Center for Medical Ethics and Health Policy, Baylor College of Medicine, Houston, TX 77030, USA

According to the Intersex Initiative, an organization based in North America, approximately 1 in 2000 children (ie, approximately 5 children per day in the United States alone) is born with a visible intersex condition [1], herein called disorders of sex differentiation (DSDs). As the Intersex Society of North America (ISNA) has suggested that the term intersex disorder or condition not be used, and more appropriate nomenclature be adopted [2] the authors have chosen to use the term disorders of sex differentiation rather than some of the other terms that have been suggested (those suggesting that all conditions are "disordered") because it better designates the continuum of sex variations that occur that are not necessarily a biopsychosocial pathologic condition.

The traditional approach to defining sex and gender according to an absolute sexual dimorphism of "male" or "female," once believed to be a natural

No potential, perceived, or real conflict of interest, especially any financial arrangement with a company whose product is discussed in the manuscript, exists. Genentech and Ross Pharmaceuticals contributed an educational grant to the Baylor College of Medicine Continuing Medical Education (CME) Gender Medicine course. No products were discussed during the CME course/this paper.

*Corresponding author. E-mail address: meaxelra@texaschildrenshospital.org (M.E. Axelrad).

0065-3101/09/$ – see front matter
doi:10.1016/j.yapd.2009.08.001

conceptualization, has been shown by developmental biology to be inadequate [3]. Nonetheless, societal norms, which often have political and legal ramifications, require that all infants be designated as "male" or "female." Traditionally, the responsibility for determining the sex of a child born with a DSD has fallen primarily or exclusively on physicians, and often surgery has been performed accordingly to align external genitalia with the chosen sex of rearing.

In the past several decades, the medical community and organizations for individuals with DSDs have called for a more comprehensive approach to meet the multifaceted needs of these individuals [4,5]. Most recently, the need for a multidisciplinary team approach for management of DSDs has been articulated [2,6]. This article describes a multidisciplinary team approach that has been in use for several years at Baylor College of Medicine (BCM) and Texas Children's Hospital (TCH), Houston, Texas. Our clinical practice model was presented in a Continuing Medical Education (CME) conference in October 2005, the first CME course on DSDs, and at the meeting of the Endocrine Society in June 2006. It is more comprehensive than those suggested by other groups [2,6] in that it includes legal and ethical experts and parents, in the decision-making process (Fig. 1).

MANAGEMENT OF DISORDERS OF SEX DIFFERENTIATION
Historical approaches to the management of disorders of sex differentiation
The management of DSDs has evolved as advances in the understanding of these conditions and in surgical techniques, and societal norms and biases,[7], have been incorporated. Before the 1950s, a child born with a DSD was not surgically altered [8]. However, in the 1950s, major changes in management approaches occurred as a result of psychologist John Money's highly publicized theory concerning the factors that determine gender identity [9]. For approximately the next half-century, the standard approach to treating individuals

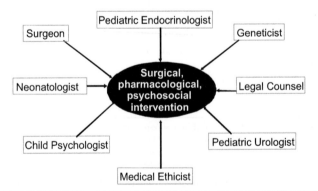

Fig. 1. The various members of our multidisciplinary team. Our paradigm includes a medical ethicist, legal counsel, and extensive parental education. Each member is involved in the decision-making process, which includes involvement of the parents.

with DSDs, the "optimal gender policy," rested on Money's notion that gender identity is not irrevocably fixed at birth and that children adapt to the social, psychological, and other environmental factors encountered in life and develop their psychosocial and gender identities accordingly, with no biologic constraints [10]. Decisions regarding sex assignment, typically made by the urologist, were driven largely by anatomic considerations, the primary importance being placed on optimizing the appearance and functional capabilities of the external genitalia and then rearing the child in the "assigned" sex.

This approach gained widespread attention in 1973 when the popular press reported on an "experiment" conducted by Money on identical male twins, 1 of whom had his penis accidentally ablated while undergoing circumcision. The child's testes were removed, his genitalia were reconstructed to appear female, and the parents were told to rear the child as a girl [11,12]. The case made headlines, and with the doctors' report that the child and the parents had successfully adapted to the alteration, the concept that masculine and feminine behavior can be altered without biologic constraints appeared to be confirmed [8]. Subsequently, however, Diamond and Sigmundson reported the long-term effects on the child, who expressed at the age of 14 his belief that he was a boy and began the process of remasculinization [11]. Since then, detrimental outcomes in other patients have been well documented. In 1998, Milton Diamond, speaking before the Section of Urology of the American Academy of Pediatrics (AAP), endorsed the position of the ISNA and called for a moratorium on all reconstructive genital surgery on newborns with ambiguous genitalia [4,13].

The fallacy in Money's theory, namely that there are no biologic constraints on sex and gender, has now been well documented and widely recognized [4,14,15]. Scientific advances have revealed that gender is not defined merely by external genitalia or environmental factors, although these factors are important, and that numerous other biologic factors are involved [16,17]. Therefore, more extensive biopsychosocial considerations must be taken into account when making gender assignments [18,19]. To meet these biopsychosocial needs, the authors propose the implementation of a more extensive multidisciplinary team.

Complexities of the sex assignment decision-making: two case studies

Several of our cases help to illustrate the variety of clinical and psychosocial complexities involved in making sex assignment or sex of rearing decisions and the need to apply an ethical framework that involves a team of specialists and the parents (Table 1). The cases summarized demonstrate the types of challenges the team has had to address and manage responsibly. These cases illustrate our clinical practice standards and the team's approach to helping families and children be more comfortable with DSDs.

Case 1 (transition from pink to blue)
A family with a 1-month-old child who had ambiguous genitalia and had been given a female sex assignment at birth was referred to the Gender Medicine

Table 1
A composite of components in sex assignment decisions

Chromosomal Sex	Male/Female
Molecular sex	Male/female
Brain sex	Male/female
Hormonal sex	Male/female
Appearance of the external genitalia	Male/female
Ability to achieve orgasm	Male/female
Internal genitalia	Male/female
Sex of rearing	Male/female
Reproductive sex	Male/female
Religious beliefs	Male/female
Overall impression	Male/female

Research has shown that sex is determined by a composite of components that must be considered when making a sex assignment or decision for sex of rearing. The authors have developed a matrix that codes the parents' responses of how they perceive the different sex components and how they respond before and after they receive education by our team.

Team. The subsequent evaluation and laboratory work included input from the team geneticist and indicated components consistent with a predominant male sex assignment. The components involved in the sex assignment process were the presence of male chromosomes, and lack of uterus, ovaries, or vaginal opening.

These factors supported a male sex assignment. After extensive consultation with the team ethicist, focusing on the concordance of the components of sexual differentiation, the findings were discussed with the family. The endocrinologist presented the results of the evaluation, including laboratory work, to the family in the presence of the psychologist. The psychologist discussed with the family the implications of changing the child's sex assignment, including feelings of guilt and grief they would likely experience, and how to explain the change to siblings, other family members, and friends. The family immediately chose to change the child's sex assignment to male. The parents expressed their full understanding that they arrived at their decision themselves after receiving education and support from medical professionals and that they have no guarantee that the child will have a male gender identity. The team psychologist established the groundwork for long-term follow-up care. Although it will not be known for some time whether this decision will be accepted by the patient, our model provided education for the parents within an ethical framework.

Case 2

A 3-day-old infant with ambiguous genitalia and presumed congenital adrenal hyperplasia (CAH) was given a female sex assignment at birth and was transferred to TCH for further work-up. Prenatal diagnosis based on the obstetrician's readings of the prenatal ultrasound was consistent with female sex. The parents prepared a pink nursery and chose a feminine name for their baby. However, the genetics consultation at TCH revealed 46,XY. Pelvic and abdominal ultrasound revealed persistence of Müllerian ducts and undescended testes. Sex assignment was established as male after several sessions with the team and input from the urologists about the male sex assignment, including functionality and surgical possibility of removal of the persistent Müllerian duct structures. The parents, with the team's help, participated in the process by evaluating anticipated surgical procedures and expressing their desire to have components not concordant with male sex assignment removed. They concluded that additional surgery at that particular juncture would not contribute to the male sex assignment.

Each of these cases illustrates the dynamics that influence the decision-making process. Obviously these decisions have far-reaching implications for the patient and the family. The authors concur with those physicians and other individuals who advocate making a sex assignment that is determined by concordance of the various components with input from the family. The authors have developed an expansive multidisciplinary model designed to respond to the complexity and particular biopsychosocial needs of each case.

REASSESSMENT OF MANAGEMENT STRATEGIES
Determinants of sexual development and gender identity

The process of sexual development involves a complex interplay between genetic and hormonal factors, reviewed extensively elsewhere [20–22]. Sex determination is the process by which the bipotential embryonic gonads commit to developing into either ovaries or testes, largely under genetic control. Subsequently, a cascade of genetic and hormonal events drives the process of sex differentiation, in which internal genitalia arise through regression or maturation of the Müllerian ducts (which form the cervix, uterus, and fallopian tubes in typical females) or Wolffian ducts (which form the epididymis, vas deferens, and seminiferous tubules in typical males). Later, under the influence of androgens, the external genitalia develop from the indifferent genital tubercle (which forms the phallus or clitoris), fold (which forms the urethra), and swelling (which forms the labia majora or scrotum). However, individuals in whom chromosomal or genetic definitions of sex may not match the phenotypic sex challenge dichotomous concepts of sex and demonstrate the need for concepts that take into consideration qualitative variations in chromosome complement, genital morphology, and hormonal activity.

Individuals with gender identity disorders (in whom cognitive and psychological measures of gender may be at odds with the genetic or phenotypic sex of the individual) also pose challenges to traditional approaches. Early theories suggested that gender identity is malleable early on and is not established until the child is 3 years old, but more recent studies indicate that such identity may not be fixed in childhood and instead is an evolving process that is not complete until after the individual undergoes pubertal development [23]. Various factors, including androgens and hormones, and environmental and sociocultural influences, seem to be involved in the process, and contribute to the formation of gender identity [24–28]. The urge to engage in sexual activity also seems to be hormonally influenced if not mediated, instead of being produced solely by social cues [29]. The process by which the brain is sexually differentiated and in which the individual develops gender-stereotyped behavior, gender identity, and sexual preference is less well understood [30].

Traditionally, sexual differentiation of the brain was not a consideration in gender assignment, primarily because nothing was known about it, and the general tendency was to accept Money's conclusion that "psychologically, sexuality is undifferentiated at birth and that it becomes differentiated as masculine or feminine in the course of various experiences of growing up."[31] Subsequent studies have indicated otherwise [32–34]. Studies in knockout mouse models suggest that estrogen receptors α and β have effects on the brain that determine female-typical and male-typical behaviors [35]. Recent studies indicate that certain structural differences in the brain seem to be related to gender identity and sexual orientation [36]. Furthermore, Gorski asserts that brain sex is a function of circulating androgens [37]. Research has shown that the brains of men and women do not respond to various stimuli in the same manner and that women have numerous cortical regions showing increased concentrations of gray matter [38], and increased T1 signal intensity and decreased fractional anisotropy in the corpus callosum [39], compared with men. Functional magnetic resonance imaging (fMRI) has shown that women exhibit greater signal intensity changes in middle, inferior, and orbital prefrontal cortices than do men when performing auditory verbal working memory tasks [40], and male and female brains differ considerably in architecture and activity [38,41]. Animal studies support a role for postnatal androgens in brain/behavior development, leading some researchers to suggest that gender assignment in infants with DSDs should be made in light of the possibility that postnatal testicular hormones at ages 1 to 6 months may affect gender identity [42,43]. Given the current neuro-anatomic data, results of studies on the patient's brain will likely play a greater role in making more reliable sex assignment decisions in the future when these data are better understood.

Reconsiderations of treatment decisions

In addition to numerous cases reported in the scientific literature, the actions of DSD activist groups began to question the standard protocol for treating individuals with DSDs in the 1990s. In 1996, 26 activists formed the first public demonstration by individuals with DSDs in modern history to protest against the AAP's support of what the activists termed "intersex genital mutilation."[44] More recently, ISNA has published on its Web site a call for a shift in the paradigm for treatment of DSDs [45].

There is a need to establish a basis for evidence-based medicine regarding sex assignment and treatment options to avoid making premature decisions leading to irreversible interventions before a reliable diagnosis has been established [46]. It can no longer be assumed that a child born with a DSD will grow into the sex and gender that is determined at birth based on the "optimal" approach [47]. A broader spectrum of considerations must be incorporated into our management model. Social, psychological, religious, legal, and ethical concerns must be addressed in addition to the medical issues. With the call for a shift in the treatment paradigm from the "concealment-centered model" to the "patient-centered model,"[44,45] physicians now must consider the role parents and patients should play in the decision-making process and provide them with the education required to make informed decisions [17,48,49].

A MULTIDISCIPLINARY APPROACH TO TREATING PATIENTS WITH DISORDERS OF SEX DIFFERENTIATION

Structure and composition of the multidisciplinary team

ISNA [2] and other groups [6,50] have identified the need for a multidisciplinary team approach to treating children with DSDs. In their Treatment Guidelines, the authors of the ISNA Clinical Guidelines describe the important role the team can play in creating a climate of commitment to the health and welfare of children born with DSDs, and to their families [2]. Their paradigm calls for, in alphabetical order: child psychologist/psychiatrist, geneticist, gynecologist, nurse specialist, pediatric endocrinologist, pediatric urologist, and social worker, and "others as needed." In the past several years, the authors have formed a multidisciplinary team of experts similar to that prescribed by the ISNA [2] and others [6,50], with the difference being that our team includes a medical ethicist, legal counsel, and extensive parental involvement. The authors have concentrated efforts on identifying how the various clinical, social, psychological, ethical, and legal factors affect the well-being of the patients and their families. The roles and responsibilities of the team leader (TL) and the different members of the team are described.

Team leader

One individual on the team, in our case an endocrinologist, serves as the formal head of the team. The TL assembles the team and oversees the efforts of its members. In addition to coordinating the efforts of the team as a whole and in individual cases, the TL is the point-of-contact person for the family of the child born with the DSD and explains to the family their options and how the team is prepared to assist them. The TL also helps educate the family with regard to the evidence in favor of one sex assignment versus another.

Endocrinologist

Because many DSDs result from a primary endocrine abnormality, the endocrinologist is typically involved in the initial evaluation. For example, female virilization, previously termed female pseudohermaphroditism (see later discussion on nomenclature), may be caused by CAH, maternal exposure to androgens, aromatase deficiency, or teratogenic conditions [51–54]. Male undervirilization, previously termed male pseudohermaphroditism, may result from androgen resistance, Leydig cell unresponsiveness, testosterone biosynthetic defects, 5α-reductase deficiency, or defects in anti-Müllerian hormones. These conditions might lead to cryptorchidism, anorchia, hypospadias, or teratogenic conditions [55–58]. Chromosome analysis and fluorescence in situ hybridization (FISH) are a necessary part of the initial evaluation of the infant born with a DSD and can establish the first branch of the decision-making tree (eg, whether the patient is an undervirilized male or a virilized female with possible CAH).

Geneticist

Chromosomal complement plays an important role in sex determination; however, chromosomes do not fully define sex. As indicated earlier, sexual differentiation requires complex interactions of many genes, some of which are dose sensitive. Numerous genes, including *SF1*, *WT1*, *SRY*, *SOX9*, and *DAX1*, when altered can lead to gonadal dysgenesis and/or discordance between the phenotype of internal and/or external genitalia with the chromosomal sex. If a common cause of ambiguous genitalia is not identified on initial evaluation, further specialized genetic testing may be needed. Some DSDs can include systemic manifestations such as skeletal dysplasia, renal abnormalities, adrenal failure, or other abnormalities that require evaluation by a genetic specialist.

Urologist

The pediatric urologist is a critical member of the multidisciplinary team and should be involved throughout the evaluation and management process. Patients with DSDs are usually identified on the initial genitourinary examination. Genital abnormalities are liable to have significant consequences for sexual and reproductive function. In addition, because developments of the genital and urinary systems are tightly integrated, urinary tract function is often profoundly affected in these patients. The urologist should be involved early after birth to help guide diagnostic evaluation and to frame the decision-making process for any surgical interventions.

The decision to perform gender reassignment surgery has become more complex in recent years. Historically, the consensus was that ambiguous genitalia, left uncorrected, would cause the patient unnecessary psychological distress. Hence, an immediate decision was made concerning the child's sex, and surgery was performed accordingly. Today, however, genital surgery is 1 of the most controversial decisions in managing patients with DSDs [59]. Many researchers and advocate groups question the earlier approach and advocate postponing surgery until the patient can be involved in making the decision [60,61]. Numerous arguments have been posited to delay feminizing genital surgery in young children. One such argument is that many patients require further surgery in adolescence [62]; another is that ablative surgery, such as clitoroplasty and clitorectomy, may impair later sexual function [63,64]. Some activist groups also argue strongly against performing surgery, charging that cosmetic genital surgery on infants with DSDs violates their human rights and subordinates the value of sexual pleasure or notions of heterosexual normality [65], whereas others have challenged their position [66].

These issues must be taken into account and discussed with the family when deciding on the timing and approach to reconstructive genitoplasty. The urologist plays a significant role in explaining to the parents the implications of performing surgery early on and in waiting, in describing the types of surgical interventions available, and in addressing the ethical concerns regarding surgical alteration of the child's genitals. As parents play a greater role in the decision-making process, the treatment paradigm is being redefined [67].

Neonatologist
The neonatologist is often responsible for informing the parents of their child's condition at birth. The announcement must be made judiciously, using appropriate terminology and emotional tone, both of which can have lasting effects on how the parents conceptualize their child's genital development and, in turn, how they relate to their child [68]. ISNA has published scripts that can be used to explain to the parents what needs to be done immediately, what decisions can be made at a later date, and what matters will need to be addressed in the future, and ways to answer common questions (available on-line at www.isna.org).

Psychologist
The birth of a child with a DSD often evokes emotional and psychological reactions from the parents and other family members, including parental guilt, fear, anger, anxiety, and a desire to have an immediate resolution to the situation. The psychologist plays a critical role in helping parents understand their child's condition and relate to the child in a positive manner, dispel feelings of guilt and/ or anger, and gain an understanding of the child's long-term psychological needs. Of practical concern to parents is how to explain the child's condition to siblings, other family members, and friends. The psychologist often will need to explain different scenarios to the parents to help them grasp the psychosocial challenges that they and their child may face, depending on their decisions regarding sex assignment and surgical intervention, and counsel them on how to recognize and cope with immediate challenges. Subsequently, as the child grows and begins to recognize that other children have a different physical appearance, the intervention of the psychologist is needed again, especially if psychopathology develops [28]. As the child matures, the psychologist has the opportunity to help the child develop a stable gender identity and to assist the parents in supporting this identity. The various factors that contribute to the development of gender identity are beyond the scope of this article, but the importance of the psychologist cannot be overemphasized. Frequently, the family will need the intervention of a psychologist who can help the child, other family members, and other adults involved in a child's care (daycare or school) cope with issues of sexual identity and behavior, and self-image and social interactions. The psychologist's role in the life of a child born with a DSD is a long-term one, with consultation as needed throughout the individual's life.

Ethicist
The birth of an infant with a DSD presents immediate ethical concerns, including ensuring the provision of adequate information to the parents regarding their child's condition and the options available for treatment [69].

The ethicist's role is to help structure clinical ethical judgments and decision-making about diagnostic and treatment plans and discussions with the parents and eventually with the child.

The consensus ethical framework for the informed consent process in clinical practice generally [70], and pediatrics in particular [71], should guide the process of informing parents about their newborn with a DSD and of making decisions about the clinical management of the infant's condition. The physician is obligated to provide information about the patient's diagnosis, the medically reasonable alternatives for the clinical management of the diagnosis, and the biopsychosocial benefits and risks of each alternative. Medically reasonable means that the best available evidence supports a prognostic judgment that an intervention will result in clinical benefit for the patient [72]. When the best available evidence supports the clinical judgment that there is only 1 effective treatment of the patient's condition or that 1 among 2 or more alternatives is clinically superior, the physician is justified in making a recommendation for that intervention [73]. When there is uncertainty about which of 2 or more alternatives is clinically superior, there is a considerable role for parental autonomy. Parents are ethically obligated to authorize treatment that is life-saving [70].

When discussing sex assignment, physicians should be clear that the decision concerns sex of rearing. The physician should explain that a child's ultimate gender identity, as a biopsychosocial phenomenon, develops under the influence of biologic sex, including genomic, hormonal, brain, and gonadal sex, and psychosocial factors. When the components of biologic sex are highly in concordance and when the best available evidence indicates satisfaction with ultimate gender, a reliable prognosis of ultimate gender and psychosocial well-being can be made and the appropriate sex of rearing can be assigned with considerable confidence [74]. In such circumstances, physicians are ethically justified in strongly recommending the appropriate sex assignment. However, when the biologic components of sex are in discordance, prognosis becomes more uncertain and strong recommendations should not be made. The alternatives should be considered carefully, and the parents should be assisted in making a decision about the sex of rearing, with the caveat that the ultimate gender the child chooses may be different (eg, in cases of 5α-reductase deficiency in children who are raised as girls).

The surgical management of DSDs also poses ethical challenges. The physician should explain that surgery, by itself, cannot assign a sex of rearing, much less determine the ultimate gender. A chance to cut should not be understood or presented as a chance to cure, which represents a change in surgical thinking. Surgical management should be considered only after reliable prognostic judgment is formed about the child's DSD. When that prognostic judgment is highly reliable, surgery to correct dysfunction (eg, hypospadias) is justified. In such cases, surgery to align anatomy with assigned sex of rearing may be justified, but only when it has an acceptable biopsychosocial risk/benefit ratio, especially concerning preservation of sexual sensitivity and function. As prognostic judgment becomes more uncertain, irreversible surgery for disorders in which ultimate gender is likely to be different from sex of rearing should not be recommended, especially when surgery can be postponed safely until the child becomes old enough to participate in the pediatric assent process [70].

Legal counselor

The numerous debates that have occurred in the treatment of children born with DSDs have involved primarily physicians, psychiatrists, ethicists, sociologists, historians, and DSD activists. Very little attention has been paid to the legal implications [8]. Yet, the legal contexts should be of utmost concern, especially considering that a person's sex affects such legal documents as birth certificate, passport, and driver's license and has implications for marriage, military service, and pension rights, liability under sex crime statutes, insurance actuarial tables, prison assignment, athletics, and a host of other matters [8,75]. Other legal and ethical issues that arise during the course of treating the child may become primary considerations when explaining conditions to older patients who have chromosomal conditions that were not identified or explained during early childhood and yet affect the definition of their gender [73,76,77].

Recent court decisions have exposed the arbitrary nature of sex as it is defined by the legislative and judicial systems. Legal institutions have used various factors to establish legal sex, including exclusively chromosomes, surgical and hormonal modifications, or even Merriam-Webster Dictionary's definition of male and female [8]. Some decisions threaten to deprive individuals with DSDs of basic civil rights [78,79], whereas others protect the rights of transsexuals (the legal term) not to be required to conform to a particular gender role in the workplace [80,81]. The Defense of Marriage Act (DOMA), intended to prevent same-sex marriages, may inadvertently deprive individuals with DSDs of their rights, if "male" or "female" sex is defined simplistically by chromosome complement or the outward phenotypic appearance (as has been the ruling in some court cases) [8].

Although many of the far-reaching legislative decisions lie outside the realm of our immediate influence, these issues highlight the difficulty of making a clear definition of sex that does not infringe on the rights of some individuals, which could extend to practical concerns such as health insurance, restroom facility use, roommate assignments in college residence halls, housing in penitentiaries, and state and federal discrimination statutes. Because of the ramifications of sex assignment on one's legal status, input from legal counsel may be needed throughout the course of the patient's life.

Other

A nurse coordinator also plays an important role in helping the parents and patients cope and in educating them. Assistance from a social worker who understands the complex issues surrounding DSDs can be of great value in navigating the paperwork (such as birth certificate, application for insurance, and so forth.) that invariably accompanies a birth, and in obtaining resources for patients with special needs later in life. Assistance may also be obtained from some of the activists groups, which provide information on coping with these issues.

A paradigm for sex assignment: team procedures with parental involvement and informed decision-making

Our procedure for treating an infant born with a DSD begins immediately on identification of the DSD in the neonatal intensive care unit (NICU) (Fig. 2).

Initial team procedure

The endocrine team, composed of an endocrine fellow and endocrinologist, is notified, and endocrine, genetic, and urologic work-ups are initiated. During this time, the neonatologist and the TL inform the family about what is known and not known at this early stage in the evaluation of the child's DSD, the tests being performed, and the possible options that will be available once a complete diagnosis is established. Of utmost importance is to engage the family in a positive manner regarding their child's condition and to offer reassurance, answer questions, and begin to educate them so that they can start the process of

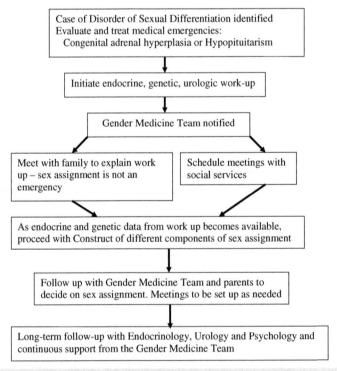

Fig. 2. The procedure followed by the multidisciplinary team once a child with a DSD is identified in the NICU.

making an informed decision. The psychologist also meets with the parents to address their concerns, to discuss the resources available to aid their understanding and ability to cope, and to lay the groundwork for educating them regarding the psychosocial implications of their child's condition. At this time, practical concerns regarding how to dress the child, what to call the child, and how to share the information with others are addressed.

The TL then contacts the other team members, and a team conference is scheduled to discuss the results of the laboratory work-up and diagnostic and treatment options. The endocrinologist and geneticist analyze the results to determine the diagnosis, the urologist examines the child and makes suggestions for types and timing of surgical procedures, the psychologist presents information regarding the family's level of understanding, and the medical ethicist reviews the information and the options regarding treatment and surgery. The team identifies and addresses the ethical issues, especially whether one sex assignment should be strongly recommended to the parents. The goal is to assign sex with parental understanding of the bases, limits, and uncertainties of the proposed sex assignment. Legal counsel is consulted as necessary with regard to the child's condition. As we become more informed regarding the implications of "brain sex," or the effects of hormones on the brain with regard to gender-related behavior and sexual drive and identity, the neurologist most likely will play a greater role in the decision-making process.

Parental involvement
Parental involvement in the decision-making process for sex assignment or sex of rearing is a major component of our approach. Parents are provided with all of the diagnostic data and a significant amount of time is spent explaining the meaning of the data. Parents are given the opportunity to ask the opinion of each respective specialist concerning the most appropriate sex assignment before making a decision. The psychologist participates in these discussions to ensure that the parents understand the information presented to them. In addition to presenting information, the team members frequently encourage the parents to voice questions or concerns, engage them in dialog, and have them review the information. It is made clear to the parents that sex assignment or sex of rearing in these cases encompasses the most likely gender role, sexual function, reproductive function, and partner preference based on the biologic data. We always stress the uncertainty about such sex assignments and explain that sexual orientation cannot be predicted for any child with perfect accuracy by either the family or physician.

In cases in which the sex is not clear, families may opt to delay performing definitive genital surgery. In these instances, acceptance of a temporary, indeterminate genital phenotype provides adequate time for decision-making.

Education matrix
One of the critical responsibilities of the team is to provide the parents with adequate education regarding their child's diagnosis [82,83]. The authors

have developed a matrix to assess the value and efficacy of the educational process (Table 1). The matrix codes the parents' responses to a series of questions that they answer before and after receiving education from the team. Their answers have demonstrated that education helps to redefine the parents' perception of the situation. The authors also believe that the education empowers the parents by involving them in the decision-making process, and helps parents understand that in some situations surgical intervention is not indicated immediately. By providing a matrix for decision-making, we help parents decide on a sex assignment based on all of the available information, with the understanding that the determination may not be certain until the child has matured and assumed a gender role and indicated a partner preference.

Efficacy of the team approach with parental involvement
Advantages. Our approach, which includes ethical and legal considerations, provides education for the families, and engages the parents in the decision-making process, has numerous advantages. For instance, an immediate sex assignment by the treating physicians is avoided, thus gaining time to ensure that an adequate diagnostic evaluation is made, and parents have the opportunity to understand and in turn provide accurate information about the baby's condition to other family members and to make informed decisions regarding the child's sex of rearing. Numerous other advantages have been outlined earlier.

Caveats. Despite its many advantages, this process may be difficult for the patient, family, and society. The frustration that parents may experience in having to cope with the uncertainties of DSDs and their clinical, psychological, and social management requires understanding, encouragement, and support. The authors recognize that, in the short term, our approach may be more stressful for some parents and families than the older model in which the physician authoritatively determined the child's sex; however, that approach did a disservice to many patients and families in the long run, as noted earlier. In our model, sex assignment is made as soon as possible (always in the first few months of life but not necessarily before discharge from the hospital) and is delayed only long enough to permit establishing an adequate initial diagnostic evaluation of the likely cause of the ambiguous genitalia. Obviously, a delay in making a determination will present some challenges for the families, including the difficulty of explaining the situation to other family members and friends. These are areas in which the psychologist plays an integral role in assisting the family.

Risk/benefit. Our primary concern is with the long-term effects on the infant, for whom a delay of a couple of months seems to have advantages over making an immediate decision, especially if the decision is made for the sole purpose of providing comfort for the family. In our experience, educating the parents on ways to present the child's condition has proven to be productive so far.

Certainly, in less than ideal situations, as these cases are, one must keep in mind that no decision is perfect.

Financial reimbursement

One of the questions that has been posed is whether this model survive financially. At our institutions (BCM/TCH), each service (discipline) charges separately for the individual medical, psychological, or laboratory services provided, although the team members meet in conference with the parents to discuss the child's DSD and to provide education. The team also meets in conference to discuss follow-up of the patients. The institutions currently provide the ethicist and legal counsel, and patients are not charged for these services. The financial arrangements and responsibilities are explained to the parents in the first conference. In the formation of a multidisciplinary treatment team, each institution will need to work out its own financial arrangements.

A REVISED NOMENCLATURE ADOPTED BY THE GENDER MEDICINE TEAM

From a medical practice standpoint, implementation of this multidisciplinary model requires the commitment of numerous specialists and intense discussions with family members. In addition, identifying and explaining DSDs will require adoption of nomenclature for the various phenotypes that is more practical and less pejorative in connotation [2,84,85]. These terms will affect the child and family socially and psychologically, especially when the child enters school or engages in gender-based social activities. As proposed by Dreger and colleagues [84], the terms pseudohermaphrodite and hermaphrodite should be abandoned as they fail to connote accurately the biologic basis of certain disorders and may lead to confusion among patients, families, physicians, and others in society. Defining the conditions by their specific causes is preferable and more explanatory. Dreger and colleagues also suggest using an umbrella term to encompass all of these conditions. Among the possibilities for this term would be "Disorders of Sexual Development" or "Developmental Disorders of the Reproductive System [84]." A nomenclature that better defines the various DSDs and that eliminates certain stigma associated with the traditional terminology clearly needs to be adopted by the medical profession.

SUMMARY

Scientific advances and changing medical practice have demonstrated that we must redefine how sex assignment determinations are made in cases of ambiguous genitalia or other DSDs. These decisions require the multidisciplinary input of pediatric endocrinologists, geneticists, urologists, and psychologists. Legal and ethical standards are evolving and need to be better defined, requiring the expertise of an ethicist and legal counsel. Various considerations should be identified if we are to ensure that adequate protection is afforded to patients, their families, physicians, institutions, and, ultimately, society.

As legal and ethical concerns of DSDs become more the domain of the courts and as evidence regarding the genetic, endocrine, and psychosocial influences on DSDs continue to evolve, those of us who treat individuals with DSDs, gender identity disorders, and related matters must keep informed of the advances being made and must initiate plans and programs that will facilitate maximizing the available resources for optimal treatment options. Parents must be supported in a more proactive role, which requires education by the treatment team to allow the parents to make informed decisions regarding the management of their child's condition. The multidisciplinary team model with a matrix for educating parents such as described herein and in operation at Texas Children's Hospital in Houston, Texas, offers a means of providing integrated care to patients who present with DSDs.

Our model differs from others in that it is the first to explicitly implement a multidisciplinary framework, including not only members of various medical disciplines and psychology but also an ethicist, within which to make a sex assignment decision and this decision is carefully considered within a legal context. The authors do not consider sex assignment to be either a social or a surgical emergency, but a complex biopsychosocial set of decisions that require adequate time to identify diagnostic and treatment options, and to provide education and support to parents and involved extended family members. The authors consider the surgical component an important one that should be considered in the context of the laboratory data, psychosocial concerns, and legal and ethical implications.

In addition, the authors concur that the nomenclature used for DSDs needs to be updated to better define these conditions according to current scientific evidence, and we recommend that comprehensive practice guidelines for the management of DSDs be developed. Finally, increased social awareness and acceptance of DSDs is needed, and the legal definition of sex must be redefined to take into account the existence of individuals in whom incongruity may exist among various determinates of gender. The authors are committed to these goals.

Acknowledgments
The authors thank the Continuing Medical Education office of Baylor College of Medicine for their involvement in sponsoring a conference in October 2005 that led to the development of this paper and that benefited practicing pediatricians; the Learning Support Center for Child Psychology for providing assistance to families of children born with DSDs and for their involvement in launching the program; and Dr. Barbara Anderson for helping the model of the multidisciplinary team approach to materialize. Special thanks also to Dr. Morey Haymond and Dr. Dennis Bier for their support and assistance in the development of the multidisciplinary model and in the formation of the Baylor College of Medicine Gender Medicine Team, and to Dr. Judith Z. Feigin for her encouragement and support of the team.

References

[1] Intersex FAQ (frequently asked questions). Intersex Initiative. Available at: http://www. intersexinitiative.org/articles/intersex-faq.html. Accessed July 19, 2005. See also Minto CL, et al. The effect of clitoral surgery on clinical outcome in individuals who have intersex conditions with ambiguous genitalia: a cross sectional study. Lancet 2003;361(9365):1252.

[2] Consortium on the Management of Disorders of Sex Development. Clinical guidelines for the management of disorders of sex development in childhood. Intersex Society of North America, 2006. Available at: http://www.isna.org. Accessed April 15, 2008.

[3] Blackless M, Charuvastra A, Derryck A, et al. How sexually dimorphic are we? Review and synthesis. Am J Hum Biol 2000;12:151–66.

[4] Diamond M. Pediatric management of ambiguous and traumatized genitalia. J Urol 1999;162:1021–8.

[5] Diamond M, Sigmuundson HK. Management of intersexuality: guidelines for dealing with persons with ambiguous genitalia. Arch Pediatr Adolesc Med 1997;151:1046–50.

[6] Hughes IA, Houk C, Ahmed SF, et al. Consensus statement on management of intersex disorders. Available at: http://adc.bmjjournals.com. Accessed April 19, 2006, 10.1136/adc.2006/098319, also Arch Dis Child 2006; 91: 554–63.

[7] Kuhnle U, Krahl W. Impact of culture on sex assignment and gender development in intersex patients. Perspect Biol Med 2002;45:85–103.

[8] Greenberg J. Legal aspects of gender assignment. Endocrinologist 2003;13:277–86.

[9] Money J, Hampson JG, Hampson JL, et al. Imprinting and the establishment of gender role. Arch Neurol Psychiatry 1957;77:333–6.

[10] Money J. Hermaphroditism: recommendations concerning case management. J Clin Endocrinol Metab 1956;4:547–56.

[11] Diamond M, Sigmundson HK. Sex reassignment at birth: long-term review and clinical implications. Arch Pediatr Adolesc Med 1997;151:298–304.

[12] Calapinto J. As nature made him. New York: Harper Collins; 2000.

[13] Diamond DA, Burns JP, Mitchell Clamb K, et al. Sex assignment for newborns with ambiguous genitalia and exposure to fetal testosterone: attitudes and practices of pediatric urologists. J Pediatr 2006;148:445–9.

[14] Grumbach M, Conte F. Disorders of sex differentiation. In: Wilson JD, Foster DW, Kronenberg HM, et al, editors. Williams textbook of endocrinology. Philadelphia: WB Saunders; 1998. p. 1303–425.

[15] Berenbaum S, Sandberg D. Sex determination, differentiation, and identity. N Engl J Med 2004;350:2204–6.

[16] Al-Mutair A, Iqbal MA, Sakati N, et al. Cytogenetics and etiology of ambiguous genitalia in 120 pediatric patients. Ann Saudi Med 2004;24:368–72.

[17] Brown J, Warne G. Practical management of the intersex infant. J Pediatr Endocrinol Metab 2005;18:3–23.

[18] Thyen U, Richter-Appelt H, Wiesemann C, et al. Deciding on gender in children with intersex conditions: considerations and controversies. Treat Endocrinol 2005;4:1–8.

[19] Lee PA, Houk CP. Surgical, medical and psychological dilemmas of sex reassignment: report of a 46, XY patient assigned female at birth. J Pediatr Endocrinol Metab 2006;19: 111–4.

[20] Jordan BK, Vilain E. Sry and the genetics of sex determination. Adv Exp Med Biol 2002;511:1–3.

[21] Cotinot C, Pailhoux E, Jaubert F, et al. Molecular genetics of sex determination. Semin Reprod Med 2002;20:157–67.

[22] Houck CP, Lee PA. Intersex states, diagnosis and management. Endocrin Clin North Am 2005;34:791–810.

[23] Wisniewski AB, Migeon CJ. Gender identity/role differentiation in adolescents affected by syndromes of abnormal sex differentiation. Adolesc Med 2002;13:119–28, vii.

[24] Zucker KJ. Gender identity development and issues. Child Adolesc Psychiatr Clin N Am 2005;24:551–68.

[25] A Campo J, Nijman H, Merckelbach H, et al. Psychiatric comorbidity of gender identity disorders: a survey among Dutch psychiatrists. Am J Psychiatry 2003;160: 1332–6.

[26] Rich er-Appelt H, Discher C, Gedrose B. Gender identity and recalled gender related childhood play-behaviour in adult individuals with different forms of intersexuality. Anthropol Anz 2005;63:241–56.

[27] Giordano G, Giusti M. Hormones and psychosexual differentiation. Minerva Endocrinol 1995;20:165–93.

[28] Slijper FM, Drop SL, Molenaar JC, et al. Long-term psychological evaluation of intersex children. Arch Sex Behav 1998;27:125–44.

[29] Bancroft J. The endocrinology of sexual arousal. J Endocrinol 2005;186:411–27.

[30] Vega-Matuszczyk J, Larsson K. Sexual preference and feminine and masculine sexual behavior of male rats prenatally exposed to antiandrogen or antiestrogen. Horm Behav 1995;29:191–206.

[31] Money J, Hampson JG, Hampson JL. An examination of some basic sexual concepts: the evidence of human hermaphroditism. Bull Johns Hopkins Hosp 1955;97:301–19.

[32] Phoenix CH, Goy RW, Gerall AA, et al. Organizing action of prenatally administered testosterone propionate on the tissues mediating mating behavior in the female guinea pig. Endocrinology 1959;65:369–82.

[33] Ehrhardt AA, Epstein R, Money J. Fetal androgens and female gender identity in the early treated adrenogenital syndrome. Johns Hopkins Med J 1968;122:160–7.

[34] Imperato-McGinley J, Peterson RE, Gautier T, et al. Androgens and the evolution of male-gender identity among male pseudohermaphrodites with 5alpha-reductase deficiency. N Engl J Med 1979;300:1233–7.

[35] Kudwa AE, Michopoulos V, Gatewood JD, et al. Roles of estrogen receptors alpha and beta in differentiation of mouse sexual behavior. Neuroscience 2006;138:921–8.

[36] Swaab DF. Sexual differentiation of the human brain: relevance for gender identity, transsexualism and sexual orientation. Gynecol Endocrinol 2004;19:301–12.

[37] Gorski RA. Hypothalamic imprinting by gonadal steroid hormones. Adv Exp Med Biol 2002;511:57–70.

[38] Luders E, Narr KL, Thompson PM, et al. Mapping cortical gray matter in the young adult brain: effects of gender. Neuroimage 2005;26:493–501.

[39] Shin YW, Kim DJ, Ha TH, et al. Sex differences in the human corpus callosum: diffusion tensor imaging study. Neuroreport 2005;16:795–8.

[40] Goldstein JM, Jerram M, Poldarack R, et al. Sex differences in prefrontal cortical brain activity during fMRI of auditory verbal working memory. Neuropsychology 2005;19:509–19.

[41] Neubauer AC, Grabner RH, Fink A, et al. Intelligence and neural efficiency: further evidence of the influence of task content and sex on the brain-IQ relationship. Brain Res Cogn Brain Res 2005;25:217–25.

[42] Hrabovszky Z, Hutson JM. Androgen imprinting of the brain in animal models and humans with intersex disorders: review and recommendations. J Urol 2002;168:2142–8.

[43] Hines M. Abnormal sexual development and psychosexual issues. Bailliers Clin Endocrinol Metab 1998;12:173–89.

[44] Kitzinger C. The myth of the two biological sexes. Psychologist 2004;17:451–4.

[45] Dreger A. Shifting the paradigm of intersex treatment. Intersex Society o North America. Available at: http://www.isna.org.

[46] Hiort O, Thyen U, Holterhus PM. The basis of gender assignment in disorders of somatosexual differentiation. Horm Res 2005;64(Suppl 2):18–22.

[47] Minto CL, Liao KL, Conway GS, et al. Sexual function in women with complete androgen insensitivity syndrome. Fertil Steril 2003;80:157–64.

[48] Migeon CJ, Wisniewski AB, Gearhart JP, et al. Ambiguous genitalia with perineoscrotal hypospadias in 46, XY individuals: long-term medical, surgical, and psychosexual outcome. Pediatrics 2002;110:e31.

[49] Lee PA. A perspective on the approach to the intersex child born with genital ambiguity. J Pediatr Endocrinol Metab 2004;17:133–40.

[50] Lee PA, Houk CP, Ahmed SF, et al. Consensus statement on management of intersex disorders. Pediatrics 2006;118:488–500.

[51] Sultan C, Paris F, Jeandel C, et al. Ambiguous genitalia in the newborn. Semin Reprod Med 2002;20:181–8.

[52] Anhalt H, Neely EK, Hintz RL. Ambiguous genitalia. Pediatr Rev 1996;17:213–20.

[53] Ozkinay F, Yenigun A, Kantar M, et al. Two siblings with fetal hydantoin syndrome. Turk J Pediatr 1998;40:273–8.

[54] Kuhnle U, Bullinger M, Schwarz HP. The quality of life in adult female patients with congenital adrenal hyperplasia: a comprehensive study of the impact of genital malformations and chronic disease on female patients' life. Eur J Pediatr 1995;154:708–16.

[55] McPhaul MJ. Androgen receptor mutations and androgen insensitivity. Mol Cell Endocrinol 2002;198:61–7.

[56] Paris F, Jeandel C, Servant N, et al. Increased serum estrogenic bioactivity in three male newborns with ambiguous genitalia: a potential consequence of prenatal exposure to environmental endocrine disruptors. Environ Res 2006;100:39–43.

[57] Rajfer J, Walsh PC. The incidence of intersexuality in patients with hypospadias and cryptorchidism. J Urol 1976;116:769–70.

[58] Kaefer M, Diamond D, Hendren WH, et al. The incidence of intersexuality in children with cryptorchidism and hypospadias: stratification based on gonadal palpability and meatal position. J Urol 1999;162:1003–6.

[59] Creighton S. Managing intersex. Editorial. BMJ 2001;323:1264–5.

[60] Crouch NS, Creighton SM. Minimal surgical intervention in the management of intersex conditions. J Pediatr Endocrinol Metab 2004;17:1591–6.

[61] Kipnis K, Diamond M. Pediatric ethics and the surgical assignment of sex. J Clin Ethics 1998;9:398–410.

[62] Alizai NK, Thomas DF, Lilford RJ, et al. Feminizing genitoplasty for congenital adrenal hyperplasia: what happens at puberty? J Urol 1999;161:1588–91.

[63] Creighton SM, Minto CL, Steele SJ. Objective cosmetic and anatomical outcomes at adolescence of feminizing surgery for ambiguous genitalia done in childhood. Lancet 2001;358:124–5.

[64] Crouch NS, Minto CL, Laio LM, et al. Genital sensation after feminizing genitoplasty for congenital adrenal hyperplasia: a pilot study. BJU Int 2004;93:135–8.

[65] Chase C. Intersexual rights. Science (July/August) 1993;3.

[66] Eugster EA. Reality vs. recommendations in the care of infants with intersex conditions. Arch Pediatr Adolesc Med 2004;158:428–9.

[67] Nelson CP, Gearhart JP. Current views on evaluation, management, and gender assignment of the intersex infant. Nat Clin Pract Urol 2004;1:38–43.

[68] Committee on Genetics. American Academy of Pediatrics: evaluation of the newborn with developmental anomalies of the external genitalia. Pediatrics 2000;106:138–42.

[69] Daaboul J, Frader J. Ethics and the management of the patient with intersex: a middle way. J Pediatr Endocrinol Metab 2001;14:1575–83.

[70] Faden RR, Beauchamp TL. A history and theory of informed consent. New York: Oxford UP; 1986.

[71] Committee on Bioethics. American Academy of Pediatrics. Informed consent, parental permission, and assent in pediatric practice. Pediatrics 1995;95:314–7.

[72] Brett AS, McCullough LB. When patients request specific interventions: defining the limits of the physician's obligation. N Engl J Med 1986;315:1347–51.

[73] Whitney SN, McGuire AL, McCullough LB. A typology of shared decision making, informed consent, and simple consent. Ann Intern Med 2004;140:54–9.

[74] McCullough LB. A framework for the ethically justified clinical management of intersex conditions. Adv Exp Med Biol 2002;511:149–65 [discussion: 165–73].

[75] Franke K. Legal aspects of gender assignment. Columbia University School of Law. Available at: http://www2.law.clumbia.edu/faculty_franke/Gubbio%20Recent.pdf.

[76] Kirtane J. Ethics in intersex disorders. Issues Med Ethics 2000;8:47–8.

[77] Maharaj NR, Dhai A, Wiersma R, et al. Intersex conditions in children and adolescents: surgical, ethical, and legal considerations. J Pediatr Adolesc Gynecol 2005;18:399–402.

[78] Littleton v Prange, 9 S.W. 3d 223 (4th Cir 1999).

[79] In the Supreme Court of the State of Kansas, No. 85,030, In the Matter of the Estate of Marshall G. Gardiner, Deceased.

[80] Smith v City of Salem, Ohio, 369 F.3d 912 (6th Cir. 2004).

[81] Barnes v City of Cincinnati, 401 F.3d 729 (6th Cir. 2005).

[82] Lee PA, Money J. Communicating with parents of the newborn with intersex: transcript of an interview. J Pediatr Endocrinol Metab 2004;17:925–30.

[83] Myers C, Lee PA. Division of Neonatal Medicine and Pediatric Endocrinology, Department of Pediatrics, Penn State College of Medicine. Communicating with parents with full disclosure: a case of cloacal extrophy with genital ambiguity. J Pediatr Endocrinol Metab 2004;17:273–9.

[84] Dreger AD, Chase C, Sousa A, et al. Changing the nomenclature/taxonomy for intersex: a scientific and clinical rationale. J Pediatr Endocrinol Metab 2005;18:735–8.

[85] Houk CP, Hughes IA, Ahmed SF, et al. Writing Committee for the International Intersex Consensus Conference Participants. Summary of the consensus statement on intersex disorders and their management. Pediatrics 2006;118:753–7.

Advances in Pediatrics 56 (2009) 165–186

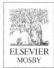

ELSEVIER
MOSBY

Fragile X: A Family of Disorders

Weerasak Chonchaiya, MD[a,b], Andrea Schneider, PhD[a,c],
Randi J. Hagerman, MD[a,d],*

[a]Medical Investigation of Neurodevelopmental Disorders (M.I.N.D.) Institute, University of California Davis Medical Center, 2825 50th street, Sacramento, CA 95817, USA
[b]Division of Growth and Development, Department of Pediatrics, Faculty of Medicine, Chulalongkorn University, 1873 Rama IV. Road, Pathumwan, Bangkok 10330, Thailand
[c]Department of Psychiatry and Behavioral Sciences, University of California Davis Health System, 2230 Stockton Blvd., Sacramento, CA 95817, USA
[d]Department of Pediatrics, University of California Davis Health System, 2315 Stockton Blvd., Sacramento, CA 95817, USA

I f you have seen a child with fragile X syndrome (FXS), you probably know that it is the most common inherited cause of intellectual disabilities (ID) and the most common single genetic cause of autism [1]. However, what you may not know is that there is a broad spectrum of involvement throughout the generations in a single family that includes medical and psychiatric involvement in those with the premutation and in those with the full mutation. In the carrier mother, who usually has a normal intelligence quotient (IQ), there is an increased risk for primary ovarian insufficiency [2] depression and anxiety [3,4], and late onset neurologic problems including hypothyroidism, fibromyalgia, neuropathy, and the fragile X-associated tremor ataxia syndrome [5] (FXTAS). In the grandparent who is the carrier, particularly the grandfather, there is a high risk for FXTAS and dementia [6]. There is often involvement in extended family members at all levels in the generations so a detailed family history that reviews many of the disorders that are associated with the premutation (55–200 CGG repeats on the front end of the FMR1 gene) and the full mutation (>200 repeats) is important.

You may have ordered a fragile X DNA test on a child with autism, found the premutation and believed that this was not a cause of his

This work was supported by the following National Institute of Child Health and Human Development grants HD036071, HD02274, National Institute of Dental & Craniofacial Research grant DE019583, National Institute on Aging grant AG032115, National Institute of Neurological Disorders and Stroke grant NS062412, National Institute on Drug Abuse TL1DA024854, and 90DD0596 from the Health and Human Services Administration on Developmental Disabilities.

*Correspondence author. Medical Investigation of Neurodevelopmental Disorders (M.I.N.D.) Institute, University of California Davis Medical Center, 2825 50th street, Sacramento, CA 95817, USA. E-mail address: randi.hagerman@ucdmc.ucdavis.edu (R.J. Hagerman).

0065-3101/09/$ – see front matter
doi:10.1016/j.yapd.2009.08.008

problems, because it was not a full mutation. We now know that some individuals with the premutation can have developmental problems [7] and this is related to an RNA gain-of-function secondary to elevated mRNA in those with the premutation. Chen and colleagues [8] have shown that premutation neuronal cell cultures demonstrate changes in branching and synaptic size compared with controls. Although those with the premutation usually have a normal IQ and are successful in life, developmental problems including attention deficit/hyperactivity disorder (ADHD), executive function deficits, memory problems, and autism spectrum disorders (ASD) can be seen, particularly in boys [7,9]. In individuals who have ID with the premutation, there is often a deficit of fragile X mental retardation protein (FMRP), the protein produced by the fragile X gene, and this is most commonly seen in the upper end of the premutation range in humans and in the premutation mouse model (120–200 CGG repeats) [10,11]. This review focuses on the latest research in FXS and in premutation involvement and their treatment.

EPIDEMIOLOGY
The premutation is common in the general population with a prevalence of 1 in 130 to 260 females and 1 in 250 to 810 males [12]. There is variability in the prevalence figures depending on where the study was done and the ethnic or racial background of the patients. The study recently reported by Cronister and colleagues [13], has shown that the premutation is less common in those of Chinese background and more common in the middle east, particularly Israel, as reported by others [14]. The allele frequency of the full mutation is approximately 1 in 2500 [12] although the affected prevalence has been shown to be 1 in 3600 [15] because some individuals with the full mutation do not have significant ID, particularly females.

To test for the premutation or the full mutation, a fragile X DNA test (also called the *FMR1* DNA test) is ordered. This is done in almost all university molecular laboratories and in commercial laboratories at a cost ranging from $200 to $500. It is usually covered by insurance companies or Medicaid. The DNA test includes a polymerase chain reaction and a Southern blot so that the number of CGG repeats and the presence of abnormal methylation, which typically occurs only in the full mutation, are reported. With complete methylation there is little or no *FMR1* mRNA in the full mutation leading to a deficit of FMRP (Fig. 1). In the premutation there is no methylation and the level of *FMR1* mRNA is increased. The premutation mRNA also contains the expanded CGG repeats although they are not translated. In the high end of the premutation this can lead to a mild block in translation so that a mild deficiency of FMRP can occur. If the FMRP level is significantly decreased the child with the premutation can have many features of FXS, such as prominent ears, hand flapping, connective tissue problems or poor eye contact. This can be confusing to the clinician because most individuals with FXS have the full mutation, although, on occasion FXS can be caused by the premutation with a significant FMRP deficit.

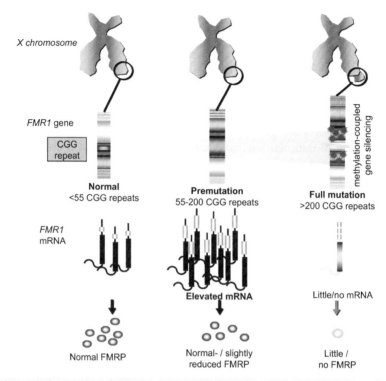

Fig. 1. The function of *FMR1* gene and the relationship among CGG repeat numbers, mRNA level, and FMRP production in normal, premutation and full mutation individuals.

PHENOTYPE OF FXS

Most physicians typically may not suspect FXS unless there are typical dysmorphic features or a family history of ID. However, approximately 30% of families with FXS do not have a family history of ID and about 30% of children with FXS do not have obvious physical features of this disorder. On examination there is a broad spectrum of morphologic, cognitive, behavioral, and psychological features, even though FXS is a single gene disorder. This variability is related to the differences in individual genetic background, environmental influences, and variations in the *FMR1* gene including the degree of mosaicism (both size and methylation mosaicism), *FMR1* mRNA levels, FMRP levels, and activation ratio (fraction of normal *FMR1* alleles that are active in females). An example of an environmental influence is the surgical pinning procedure that some families carry out to treat the prominent ears seen in most children with FXS. The most significant molecular variable is the level of FMRP. In those with the full mutation or mosaicism, FMRP levels correlate with the IQ and many physical features typical of fragile X including ear prominence. FMRP correlates with the level of involvement of premutation carriers as previously mentioned [1,7,16]. The phenotypic findings in those with the full mutation are presented in the following section.

PHYSICAL FEATURES

Most young individuals with FXS have changes in their connective tissue including prominent ears, hyperextensible finger joints, soft skin, and flat feet [17], related to changes in the elastin fibers of connective tissue [18]. Pectus excavatum, mitral valve prolapse, strabismus, long face, prominent chin, and enlargement of testicular size have also been documented in individuals with FXS [17]. Macroorchidism usually begins to present after the age of 8 years and the maximal size of the testicles (about 2 or 3 times normal) is seen in mid-adolescence [19].

COGNITIVE FEATURES

Most children with FXS will not be diagnosed until they are almost 3 years of age. Often the first diagnosis of children with FXS is autism because the behavioral features of poor eye contact, hand flapping, and social deficits are the most prominent features [17,20]. Because all individuals with autism or ASD are routinely screened for FXS, the cause of their autism will be readily apparent with *FMR1* DNA testing. Approximately 30% of boys with FXS will also have autism and an additional 20 to 30% will have pervasive developmental disorder not otherwise specified (PDDNOS) as described later [21]. Recently, decreased fine motor scores have been reported in 1- to 6-year-old children with FXS, particularly with autism and FXS together [22]. In addition, cognitive, language, and adaptive skills are lower in those with FXS plus autism compared with autism alone [23–25].

Parents typically notice that their children are not talking by the time they are 13 to 18 months [26]. They are brought to see primary physicians or pediatricians and are diagnosed with a developmental delay at an average age of 21 months [26]. Unusual sensory-motor development, such as object play skills (eg, spinning) and unusual motor patterns (eg, repetitive movements of the legs, unusual posture) at 9–12 months of age may be helpful to recognize FXS in early infancy. The lag time between the initial parental concerns and the diagnosis of developmental delay can be addressed through standardized developmental screening tests at the 9-, 18-, and 24- or 30-month well child visits to detect developmental disorders early [27]. The developmental trajectory in fragile X is slow (about 50% of normal in boys) and IQ decline may be seen in late childhood and adolescence, although mental age continues to increase even though the rate is slower than normal [28].

Approximately 85% of males and 25% to 30% of females with the full mutation have an IQ less than 70 (ID) [1,16]. The severity of IDs is related to FMRP deficiency [16,29]. Some individuals with only a mild decrease in FMRP level may present with a normal or borderline IQ with or without learning disabilities (LD). LD with a normal or borderline IQ is a typical presentation in females with FXS. Mathematics skill is the main area of academic underachievement in the girls and high-functioning boys with FXS [1,30]. Other cognitive impairments involve many domains including executive function, visual memory, visuospatial processing abilities, visual motor coordination, auditory short-term memory, processing of sequential information, sustained attention, and working memory [30–33]. Fortunately, children seem to have relative strengths in verbal-based skills, general knowledge, and activity of daily living skills [30,31]. Academic acquisition is not predicted by FMRP level or nonverbal IQ, but the level of maternal education and presence of autistic behaviors do predict academic strengths in children with FXS [30].

FMRP regulates several proteins important for synaptic plasticity [34]. FMRP typically inhibits the translation of proteins at the synapse, so in the absence of FMRP there is up-regulation of several proteins including proteins in the metabotropic glutamate receptor 5 pathway (mGluR5) leading to long-term depression (LTD) or weakening of synaptic connections [35]. Recently, cognitive deficits in memory have been found in the *Drosophila* model of FXS related to up-regulation of staufen and argonaute1 proteins [36]. These cognitive problems were reversed by treatment with puromycin which blocks protein production. Antagonists of the mGluR5 system have also reversed the cognitive deficits in animal models of FXS including the knock out mouse and *Drosophila* [37,38].

Epilepsy occurs in approximately 10% to 40% of individuals with FXS [39,40]. The seizures are usually generalized or partial complex seizures and they may occur at night [40,41]. Seizures are about 3 times as common in those with FXS plus autism compared with FXS without autism [41]. Seizures may be related to dysfunction in the mGluR5 pathway and in the γ-aminobutyric acid A (GABA$_A$) pathway. Dysfunction in the GABA system has been found in the KO mouse model of FXS and there seems to be down-regulation of the GABA pathways particularly the GABA$_A$ pathway [42]. Steve Warren's group has found that supplementation with medication that enhances the GABA system rescues the *Drosophila* model with FXS from death [43]. In addition, use of mGluR5 antagonists reverses the seizure phenotype in the KO mouse model of fragile X [44].

BEHAVIOR AND PSYCHOLOGIC FEATURES

Behavior and psychologic characteristics of FXS include shyness, social avoidance, anxiety, autistic behaviors (poor eye contact, perseverative behaviors or speech, sensory hypersensitivity, stereotypic or repetitive motor behaviors such as hand flapping and hand biting), distractibility, hyperactivity, inattention, impulsivity, tactile defensiveness, self-injurious behavior, aggression, mood instability, irritability, and inflexibility [17,24,45,46]. Females typically have milder behavioral and cognitive problems than those observed in males because they have some FMRP production from their normal X chromosome. Nonetheless, they are likely to develop emotional problems and maladaptive behaviors, including depression, social anxiety, and withdrawal [31]. Although most individuals with FXS are shy at first they do become friendly with time; those with FXS plus autism typically remain aloof [47].

The reason why children with FXS are more likely to have anxiety may be a result of their enhanced sympathetic response to stimuli and their inability to accommodate or habituate over time to stimuli. This autonomic dysregulation is likely related to the mGluR5 up-regulation and the GABA down-regulation previously described. Individuals with FXS also have enhanced cortisol release after stressful stimuli [48]. This hyperarousal to stimuli can lead to tantrum behavior and even aggression that often requires medical treatment as described later [49]. Dysregulation of the autonomic nervous system is more common in those with FXS plus autism [50].

In a family study there was a strong interaction between the behavior of the child with FXS and the adaptation of the mother [51]. The degree of the child's behavior problems had a strong effect on the mothers' stress level in addition to her depressive symptoms, anxiety, anger, and quality of life [51]. Because the mother also has the fragile X mutation, typically the premutation, which puts her at risk for anxiety and depression [3], it is important to recognize the problems that she is experiencing and recommend treatment if needed.

Once a proband is diagnosed, the evaluation of the whole family tree should take place with a genetic counselor. Many other individuals will have additional involvement from the premutation (described later) and the full mutation. A spectrum of psychiatric, endocrine, medical, and neurologic problems will be found related to these mutations [5,6,52,53]. The authors routinely recommend testing of family members who are at risk for either the premutation or full mutation involvement because of the many treatment options that may reduce the burden of disease over time [49,54]. For instance, identification of a carrier helps surveillance for hypertension and hypothyroidism, which are increased in carriers [5] and early treatment of these conditions decreases the medical complications of these problems. Early treatment of depression may influence the cognitive decline that occurs in older carriers related to FXTAS [54]. Early identification of those affected with FXS leads to early conventional treatments and targeted treatments described later.

RELATIONSHIP BETWEEN FXS AND AUTISM

There is a close relationship between FXS and autism. Two to 7% of children with autism have a mutation in *FMR1* [1]. The prevalence of autism in individuals with FXS has been reported to range from 15% to 35%, although when the Autism Diagnostic Observation Schedule (ADOS) is used, it is approximately 30% [21,24,25] with an additional 20% to 30% with PDDNOS [21]. Even those without ASD have several autistic-like features, such as poor eye contact, hand flapping, perseverative and repetitive behaviors, language, and self-talk [17,24,25].

There is an increased prevalence of autism in individuals with FXS likely because FMRP regulates the translation of several proteins known to be associated with autism, such as neuroligins, neurorexins, SHANK protein, PTEN,

CYFIP, PSD95, and many more [1,20,34,55]. The lack of FMRP interferes with synaptic plasticity, leads to dysconnectivity in the central nervous system (CNS), and causes dysregulation of GABA and glutamate systems, all of which are associated with other forms of autism [20]. Why autism occurs in some individuals with FXS and not others is not known. There are predictive factors including severity of IDs [24–56], degree of FMRP deficiency [57], increased age [57], presence of seizures or additional genetic disorders [41], poor adaptive social skills [24,56] and more behavioral problems [56], that are associated with increased autism or ASD in FXS. However, FMRP level was not related to the presence or severity of autism when the IQ was controlled suggesting that factors in addition to fragile X lead to the presence of autism [58].

Cognition, adaptive behavior, language, and social interaction are more severely impaired in those with FXS and autism compared with FXS alone as described earlier [24,25,47,56,57]. Language deficits in fragile X individuals with ASD are likely to involve more severe receptive deficits, including verbal reasoning, recognition of emotions, and labeling of emotions [23,45] than those with FXS alone. Social affective impairment in the child with FXS with ASD makes it challenging for them to learn language effectively. The language learning processes require more investigation to understand why language outcomes are variable in FXS with or without autism. Restricted, repetitive, and stereotyped behaviors are not the important clue for the autism diagnosis in individuals with IDs including FXS [24]. To diagnose autism in children with FXS, an assessment of communication deficits, social withdrawal behaviors, impairment in complex social interactions, and adaptive social skills is needed because these pivotal deficits are highly associated with autism [24,45,56]. High levels of social withdrawal characterized as avoidance in multiple social settings and low interest in others can be seen in individuals with autism and FXS [47]. Autistic behaviors in FXS may change and vary day to day, or even related to the time of day or emotional reactivity to events. Therefore a comprehensive evaluation involving different aspects of the assessment with different clinicians may be necessary to reach consensus on the diagnosis of autism. Such a diagnosis is essential to help children receive the appropriate intensive interventions needed for autism, although such interventions are also beneficial in those without autism who have FXS [21].

There are several neuroanatomic and neurobiologic similarities between FXS and idiopathic autism; particularly their common phenotypes including macrocephaly, which represents rapidly increased brain growth during the early childhood period [59]. A *PTEN* mutation has been reported in approximately 18% of those with idiopathic autism with extreme macrocephaly [60]. In FXS, PTEN activity is down-regulated (S. Zupan, personal communication, FRAXA Conference, Maine 2008) [34]. which is likely why children with FXS, especially those with FXS plus autism, have a larger head [59].

Several genetic conditions, such as Down syndrome [29], and Prader-Willi phenotype (PWP) of FXS [61] and medical conditions affecting the CNS, such as brain trauma, cerebral palsy, recurrent seizures, when added to FXS increase the risk for autism [41]. On the other hand, individuals with FXS and ASD may be more vulnerable to more medical problems affecting the CNS compared with the individual with FXS alone (38.6% vs 18.2%) [41]. For instance, seizures occur in about 28% of children with FXS and ASD, but occur in only 12% in those with FXS without ASD [41]. Neuronal excitability and susceptibility to develop seizures from underlying CNS conditions may be associated with emerging autism in FXS. On the other hand, abnormal electrical discharges from epilepsy possibly disrupt brain connectivity and lead to autism in those with FXS [20,41]. Nevertheless, it is important to search for seizures or abnormal spike-wave discharges in those with FXS and autism because anticonvulsant medication, such as valproate may be helpful for the seizures and for the autism [41,49].

ASD occurs in approximately 70% of those FXS with the PWP, suggesting a role for the second genetic hit in leading to autism [29,61]. The PWP in FXS does not have a 15q deletion or uniparental disomy like Prader-Willi syndrome. In the PWP of FXS, individuals have severe hyperphagia emerging in the first 3 to 8 years of life, lack of satiation after a meal, obesity, and hypogenitalia or delayed puberty. Recently, it was reported that the expression level of cytoplasmic *FMR1* interacting protein (CYFIP1), normally coded within the Prader-Willi syndrome region (15q region between break point 1 and 2), was lower in individuals with PWP and FXS than those with FXS but without PWP and typically developing individuals [61]. CYFIP interacts with Rac1, which has GTPase activity, and is essential in synaptic function and neuronal migration [61]. Lowered CYFIP expression may have an additional effect on synaptic plasticity and may predispose individuals with PWP and FXS to develop more autism. Recently, Buxbaum and colleagues [62] reported that deletion of CYFIP in mice causes autism. Why CYFIP is down-regulated in a small subgroup of patients with FXS who have the PWP is not known. FMRP regulates CYFIP translation and the absence of FMRP typically leads to elevation of CYFIP levels in FXS without the PWP compared with controls without FXS [61].

There is remarkable overlap between neurobiologic mechanisms leading to several known forms of autism and FXS with autism. In summary, the *FMR1* gene can regulate the expression of other genes and affect synaptic formation and plasticity [34,63]. Therefore, if FMRP is decreased or absent, there is significant dysregulation of various pathways/proteins that disrupt brain development pervasively leading to developmental delays, particularly autism. Disruption in critical networks occur in the absence of FMRP including up-regulation of the mGluR5 pathway [35], up-regulation of the mTOR pathway [34], down-regulation of the PTEN pathway, down-regulation of the $GABA_A$ receptors [42], down-regulation of the dopamine pathway [64], dysregulation of neuroligin 3, 4 and SHANK3 [34]. The authors assess dysregulation in GABA and mGluR5 systems with an electrophysiologic method including pre-pulse inhibition (PPI). In individuals with FXS and/or ASD, who have problems of frontal gating or sensory information processing, PPI is typically decreased [65]. This measure can also be used in the quantitation of brain improvements with the use of targeted treatments, such as mGluR5 antagonists in FXS explained later.

NEUROBIOLOGIC ADVANCES

FMR1 is involved in the control of protein synthesis, and recent studies have found that FMRP shuttles from nucleus to cytoplasm as an mRNP particle [34]. FMRP has been shown to be an mRNA-binding protein, which regulates synaptic and cytoskeleton-associated proteins. Formerly believed to be just a general repressor of translation, FMRP is now considered to be restricted to specific messages. Most importantly the mGluR signaling pathway is regulated by FMRP [35]. Besides the mGluR mechanism, other pathways have been identified for FMRP interaction (Fig. 2).

Dendritic spines are small membranous extensions on a neuronal dendrite in the brain. The spines serve as synaptic storage sites, support the electric signal transmission, and increase the number of possible contacts between neurons. On their surface, the dendritic spines express glutamate receptors (GluR), for example, the α-amino-3-hydroxy-5-methyl-4-isoxazolepropionic acid (AMPA) receptor and the N-methyl-D-aspartate (NMDA) receptor. A broad variety of proteins (eg, kinases) mediate the signaling from the GluRs. Cognitive function, motivation, learning, and memory are based on spine plasticity. Especially the long-term memory formation is mediated in part by the growth of new or existing dendritic spines to reinforce a particular neural pathway. Enhancing the ability of the presynaptic cell to activate the postsynaptic cell strengthens the connection between 2 neurons. After the formation of numerous dendritic spines during fetal cortical neurogenesis, the dendritic spines need to mature or they are pruned. Immature spines can be identified through their malformations (eg, long "necks" or lack of "heads"). Those immature spines show a significant impairment in signal transduction. Several studies show abnormalities in the spine formation in FXS, which can be directly correlated to the cognitive impairment. A neurophysiologic study by Wilson and Cox [66] in 2007 demonstrated a clear attenuation in the cortical long-term potentiation (LTP) in slices from FMRP-KO mice compared with the wildtype. The investigators suggest the decrease in LTP is caused by a diminished mGluR5-mediated activity in the neocortex. This leads to an enhanced LTD through the absence of FMRP inhibition of protein translation, implicating a complex interaction between FMRP and mGluRs. The changes in synaptic plasticity occur differently in various brain areas. LTD is associated with a reduction in the number of postsynaptic AMPA type GluRs that mediate excitatory activity in brain and shuttle between postsynaptic membrane and beneath in cytoplasm, regulating synaptic excitability [63].

FXS is associated with protein synthesis–dependent lengthening/thinning of dendritic spines. The synapses on thin dendritic spines have smaller postsynaptic density, fewer AMPA receptors, and a reduced number of synaptic vesicles docking at the presynaptic active zone [67]. The lengthening of dendritic

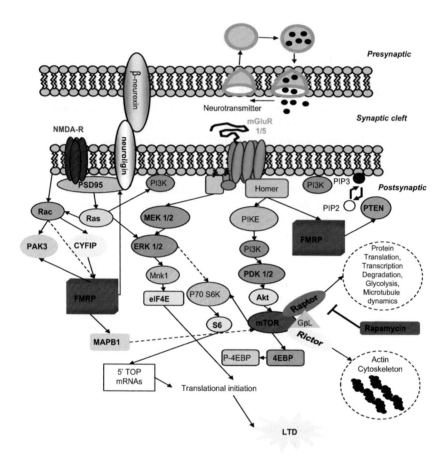

Fig. 2. Cascade of reactions leading to LTD and interactions with FMRP. The dotted lines are hypothetical and the T-shaped line is an inhibitory effect. 5′ TOP mRNAs, 5′ terminal oligo pyrimidine mRNAs that code for proteins important for translation; Akt, protein kinase B (PKB); CYFIP, cytoplasmic interacting FMR1 protein; elF4E, E74-like factor 4, expressed, translation initiation factor, cap-binding; ERK, extracellular signal-regulated kinases, synonym for mitogen-activated protein kinase (MAPK); FMRP, fragile X mental retardation protein; Homer, scaffolding protein; MAPB1, microtubule-associated protein 1B; MEK, mitogen-activated protein kinase (MAPK); mGluR, metabotropic glutamate receptors; Mnk, MAP kinase integrating kinase; mTOR, mammalian target of rapamycin/FK506 binding protein 12-rapamycin associated protein 1 (FRAP1); NMDA-R, ionotropic N-methyl-D-aspartic acid receptor; P-4EBP, phosphorylated emopamil binding protein (sterol isomerase); P70 S6K, p70 ribosomal S6 protein kinase; PAK3, P21 (CDKN1A)-activated kinase 3; PDK, 3-phosphoinositide-dependent protein kinase; PI3K, class I phosphoinositide 3-kinases; PIKE, PI 3-kinase enhancer, GTPase, enhances PI 3-kinase (PI3K) activity; PIP, prolactin-induced protein; PSD95, postsynaptic density protein; PTEN, phosphatase and tensin homolog; Rac/Ras, small guanosine triphosphatases (intracellular molecular switches).

spines suggests an interaction of FMRP with the Rac1 pathway and this is through CYFIP1 [61]. Rac1 has been shown to regulate actin dynamics, and dendritic spines are actin-rich structures.

A study by Nakamoto and colleagues [68] in 2007 on cultured hippocampal neurons demonstrated a hypersensitive AMPA receptor internalization with FMRP deficiency correlated to the excess mGluR signaling, pointing to the cellular defect in FXS that causes learning and memory deficits. The investigators used mGluR antagonists to reverse this pattern and "rescue" the excessive signaling in FXS cells. This study was based on the mGluR hypothesis of FXS, postulated by Bear and colleagues [35] in 2004. Bear and colleagues postulate that the loss of FMRP in FXS leads to an excessive expression of mRNA near synapses, making it impossible to regulate protein synthesis adequately, thus increasing LTD caused by receptor loss (Fig. 3).

Glutamate is the most common excitatory neurotransmitter in the mammalian brain. A major function is the stimulation of local protein synthesis at synapses required for synaptic function and inducing of LTD [38]. In the FMR1 knockout mouse, the mGluR-dependent activity is increased, leading to increased LTD (mGluR-LTD) [35]. In Bear's mGluR theory, the heterogeneous FXS phenotypes are caused by mGluR misregulation [35]. LTP and LTD are synaptically triggered and lead to long-lasting changes in synaptic strength. Cognitive functioning is dependent on synaptic plasticity, and impairment leads to learning and memory deficits. In neonates, LTP leads to retaining nascent synapses, and LTD activity–guided synapse elimination, providing the base for postnatal learning and memory storage. LTD is triggered by mGluR activation, which requires rapid translation of mRNA in postsynaptic dendrites. The lack of appropriate FMRP levels leads to exaggerated mGluR5 activation [35].

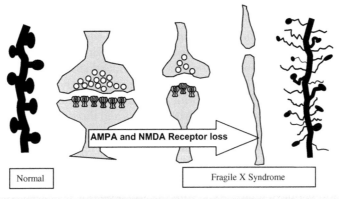

Fig. 3. Reduction of synaptic strength in the dendritic tree in FXS compared with normal individuals. (*Modified from* Bear MF, Huber KM, Warren ST. The mGluR theory of fragile X mental retardation. Trends Neurosci 2004;27(7):370–77.)

FMRP is widely expressed in the brain, and mGluR-dependent protein synthesis is exaggerated in absence of FMRP in various brain areas, particularly the hippocampus [35]. If LTD is associated with changes in synaptic receptors for glutamate, then FXS is treatable with drugs interacting with GluR receptors. One example for a GluR-interacting substance is 2-methyl-6-(phenylethynyl)-pyridine (MPEP), a potent and specific, noncompetitive antagonist of mGluR receptors. As postulated, several animal studies showed a beneficial effect of MPEP. The substance rescued behavioral abnormalities in the *FMR1* KO mouse [44], and the courtship and mushroom body defects in the *Drosophila* d*fmr1* mutants [69].

During human development, the synaptic connections in the brain undergo drastic changes, from thin, long, dendritic spines with small synapses to short, mushroom-shaped, dendritic spines with bigger synapses [70]. In FXS, the dendritic spines in the brain seem immature, and could lead to the conclusion that little or no pruning happened as a result of the neurochemical imbalance of FMRP and mGluR mechanisms. Pruning of synaptic connections is essential for the fine-tuning of neural networks and does happen but to a reduced degree in FXS with an absence of FMRP. The larger number of immature dendritic spines and weak synaptic connections could lead to cortical hyperexcitability.

In summary, the neurobiologic base of FXS is a disruption of interrelated neuronal signaling pathways involved in learning and memory.

NEUROIMAGING IN FXS

There have been numerous neuroimaging findings in FXS depending on the population studied and the techniques used. Individuals with FXS have reduced activation in the right ventrolateral prefrontal cortex, which is an area of the brain important for executive function, compared with both autistic and typically developing subjects. Hoeft and colleagues [71] hypothesized that the lateral prefrontal cortex abnormality, together with larger caudate volumes (which is associated with lowered FMRP level), may play a role in hyperactivity, frontostriatal dysfunction, and the response inhibition deficit seen in FXS (part of the executive function involved in sustained attention, target detection, and rule maintenance). Normally, the striatum has a main function in motivation and cognitive abilities; therefore individuals with FXS, who typically have frontostriatal dysfunction, may exhibit hyperactivity, stereotypic and repetitive motor behaviors. Girls with FXS have reduced basal forebrain and hippocampal activation related to FMRP deficits and these problems are important for attention and memory encoding. Enlarged hippocampal volumes bilaterally have been reported in children with FXS. This brain area is vital to memory processing, emotional and stress regulation [71,72].

Autism and FXS have some similar neuroimaging findings. For instance both disorders have a large cerebrum but the posterior cerebellar vermis, an area involved in sensory perception, cognition and motor function; is smaller or abnormal when compared with controls [20,72]. This reduced volume of the posterior cerebellar vermis accompanied by a large caudate nucleus may be associated with decreased FMRP, severe autistic behaviors, profound cognitive deficits, and aberrant behaviors [72]. Both FXS and autism individuals have similar decreased activation patterns in the fusiform gyrus that is correlated with deficits in gaze fixation to human faces [73]. However, the FXS group had greater activation than the autism and control groups in brain regions including the left hippocampus, the right insula, the left postcentral gyrus, and the left superior temporal gyrus, involved in fear, processing of emotional faces and complex auditory stimuli [73]. Amygdala dysfunction, a potential area underlying social deficits, has been described in fMRI amygdala activation studies to social cognition tasks in ASD and adult males with the premutation [74].

A lack of normal recruitment of the neural network involved in visual memory tasks to solve more difficult math problems or perform executive function tasks has been demonstrated on fMRI in FXS [75]. Furthermore, parietal lobe dysfunction is also associated with dorsal stream processing deficits that were investigated through biologic motion processing tasks and may be involved in visual motor deficits in both FXS and individuals with autism [1,32].

Other brain abnormalities in FXS include a larger hypothalamus. This structure is likely involved in the abnormal stress response with enhanced cortisol release, sleep disturbances, and abnormal melatonin release seen in FXS [71,76]. There is also a smaller insula and medial prefrontal cortex (involved in aberrant activation during gaze processing, hyperarousal, and cognitive and social features in FXS) and a smaller right superior temporal gyrus involved in cognitive deficits in FXS [20,71]. The complexity of the morphometric changes in the brain related to the deficiency or absence of FMRP is profound and related to the great number of pathways that are dysregulated with the absence of this protein [71].

NEUROPHYSIOLOGIC STUDIES IN FXS

Only a few electroencephalography (EEG) studies in FXS have been published so far. Among common findings are seizures, abnormally large somatosensory evoked potentials, and the occurrence of interictal paroxysmal EEG activity in prepubertal subjects with FXS. There are similarities between EEG findings in FXS and benign childhood epilepsy with centrotemporal spikes [40]. Additional abnormal EEG findings in FXS have been described [39], including an increase in slow waves, diffuse spike-wave, and focal spike-wave discharges, particularly in the temporal and central regions. A comparison of findings in single-photon emission computed tomography (SPECT) and EEG show a distinct overlap in the results, with a cerebral dysfunction in FXS, with slow-wave paroxysms and cerebral perfusion abnormality with focal deficits seen in frontal regions in females with FXS [77].

Another approach to evaluate perception and cognitive processes in the brain are event-related potentials (ERPs). The brain activity at a fixed time frame, dependent on the occurrence of a sensory or a cognitive stimulus (eg, the presentation of a tone or a picture) is measured with an EEG and averaged. The specific pattern of the amplitudes and latencies of the ERPs provides an insight into the underlying information processing in the brain. For example, an auditory ERP assesses the stimulus processing in auditory afferent pathways and corresponding cortical areas. The N1/N100 is the first prominent negativity in the auditory evoked potentials, generated by at least 3 sources in the temporal and frontal lobes [78].

In children with FXS, an augmentation of the auditory N1 has been shown [79], and abnormal P300 in auditory evoked potentials in adults with FXS [80]. During development, a maturation of auditory stimulus processing occurs in FXS, with an increased responsiveness to auditory stimuli [79]. Compared with a healthy control group, the FXS group showed a more frontal N1 scalp distribution, implicating immature processing. The increased global field power shows reduced inhibition and increased excitability. The FXS group did not show N1 habituation, which is considered to be a nonspecific arousal as part of the orienting reaction; the habituation is an indicator of the refractory properties of neurons in auditory cortex.

A magnetoelectroencephalography study on auditory evoked magnetic fields showed a higher amplitude for the N100m auditory evoked field component, and less lateralized N100m anterior-posterior dipole locations [81]. The investigators concluded that there is a more widespread activation of neurons that are activated by acoustic stimuli, consistent with the increased stimulus intensity experience in FXS. FMRP is considered to play a role in cortical hyperexcitability and abnormal synaptic transmission; the neuropathologic bases for the hyperexcitability are the enhanced dendritic connections and immature pruning in FXS.

Another research approach to show sensorimotor processing deficits in FXS is the prepulse inhibition of acoustic startle reflex (PPI), a behavioral model of basic sensorimotor processing. The sensorimotor gating abnormalities in FXS, a heightened sensitivity to sensory stimulation and sensory defensiveness are caused by the abnormalities in maturation of synaptic connections in sensory circuits [82]. Compared with other mental disorders, the deficit in PPI in FXS is even greater than in schizophrenia [83]. PPI has been established as a reliable measure in FXS that will be useful in medication trials [65].

Studies have shown hyperarousal and hyperreactive responses to sensory stimulation [50,84]. The electrodermal responses show an increased sensory sensitivity in FXS, and the magnitude of responses correlate negatively with FMRP expression [84].

The neurophysiologic approaches to cognition, arousal, and inhibition provide a useful base for outcome measures in future medication trials of FXS. Sensory processing and an improvement in cognitive functioning cannot be sufficiently assessed with broader neuropsychologic tests, and especially the EEG and ERP paradigms will provide a better method to look at even subtle changes in the improvement of information processing, indicating a change in the underlying deficit in dendritic spine morphology in FXS.

PREMUTATION INVOLVEMENT

Involvement in those with a premutation (55–200 CGG repeats) has a different molecular pathogenesis than those with the full mutation. In the premutation the elevated levels of FMR1 mRNA lead to toxicity in the cell, particularly the neuron [85]. The elevated mRNA causes dysregulation of several proteins including lamin A/C, myelin basic protein (MBP), and heat shock proteins leading to early cell death [86]. Although most individuals with the premutation do not suffer from significant medical, psychiatric, or cognitive problems related to this toxicity, others do, and the findings of primary ovarian insufficiency (POI) and the FXTAS are believed to be related to this RNA toxicity (see Fig. 1) [2,85].

Approximately 40% of older males with the premutation will eventually develop FXTAS and the features of this disorder include an intention tremor, ataxia, parkinsonism, neuropathy, cognitive deficits, particularly executive function deficits with eventual cognitive decline to dementia in some and autonomic dysfunction including hypertension, impotence, and eventual bladder and bowel incontinence [5,52,87,88]. Although some patients with FXTAS have a rapid decline over 5 or 6 years, others are stable for 1 or 2 decades. More rapid decline typically occurs when the features of FXTAS are combined with another disorder, such as multiple sclerosis (MS) [89], Alzheimer disease, [90] or Parkinson disease [91]. In female carriers, FXTAS occurs in approximately 8% [5] but it is usually not associated with cognitive decline, although cases of dementia have been reported.

The neuroanatomic hallmark of FXTAS is intranuclear eosinophilic inclusions in neurons and astrocytes throughout the brain but with highest numbers in the hippocampus and limbic system [91]. These inclusions can also occur outside the CNS and they have been found in Leydig and myotubular cells of the testicles [92] and in peripheral nerve ganglia throughout the body [93]. These inclusions contain the excess mRNA and several proteins including lamin A/C and MBP that are dysregulated by the elevated mRNA [86]. Although the inclusions themselves are probably not pathognomonic they are a marker for the RNA toxicity that is occurring in these cells.

It is important to recognize that other medical and psychiatric problems can occur in some carriers that are not necessarily part of POI and FXTAS but may also be related to the mRNA toxicity. Neuropathy is common in older carriers and can occur without other symptoms of FXTAS [5,87,94]. Hypertension is seen in most older carriers and may be secondary to the autonomic dysfunction related to RNA toxicity [5]. In a study of female carrier with and without FXTAS, hypothyroidism was seen in 50% and fibromyalgia was seen in more than 40% of those with FXTAS [5]. This suggests that autoimmune problems are more common in female carriers. The elevated mRNA in carriers up-regulates α B crystallin and heat shock proteins and perhaps this stimulates autoimmune activity. MS occurs in 2 to 3% of female carriers and this may be related to the α B crystallin up-regulation, because this is an important antigen in MS [5,89]. FXTAS has been reported in 1 woman with the premutation who had a long history of MS so both conditions can occur together [89].

Psychopathology that is more common in those with the premutation include anxiety, depression, and obsessive compulsive behavior [3,4]. Although not all individuals with the premutation have significant psychopathology, these problems are clinically significant for 25 to 40% of carriers. There is now emerging evidence that premutation involvement has a neurodevelopmental component in some children, especially boys, causing a higher incidence of ADHD, shyness, and social deficits including autism spectrum disorder [7,9,46]. Cell cultures of premutation neurons have also demonstrated abnormalities in dendritic branching and synaptic size compared with controls [8]. Further study of unselected premutation babies identified in the newborn period through screening will clarify what percentage of carriers will have neurodevelopmental problems and the benefit of early intervention. The new blood spot screening test for the premutation developed by Tassone and colleagues [95] will facilitate newborn screening studies that are now taking place at 4 centers in the United States.

TARGETED TREATMENTS

There are several currently available medications that are helpful in the treatment of various symptoms in children with FXS. Stimulants are usually beneficial for the 70 to 90% of boys and 30 to 40% of girls with FXS who have ADHD [49,96]. Research by Wang and colleagues [64] regarding dopamine dysregulation in the absence of FMRP in brain tissue demonstrates normalization of dopamine function with the use of a stimulant, so, in a sense, stimulants are a targeted treatment of FXS. Clonidine or guanfacine can also be used for treatment of ADHD and they have an overall calming effect for the hyperarousal [49]. In Italy, where stimulants are not used, L-acetylcarnitine has been used for ADHD in children with FXS with some efficacy [97]. Selective serotonin reuptake inhibitors (SSRIs) have been successful in the treatment of anxiety in children and adults with FXS [49]. Perhaps the most successful conventional medication in the treatment of FXS is aripiprazole (Abilify), an atypical antipsychotic which helps to stabilize mood, decrease anxiety, and improve attention [49]. However, many children with FXS can become more agitated or hyperaroused at high doses so a low dose is essential at the start (eg, aripiprazole 1 mg at bedtime in mid-childhood and 0.5 mg for children <5 years) [49]. For adolescents and adults, a dose of just 5 mg at bedtime is usually adequate for a clinical effect.

The use of targeted treatments is an exciting area of research and it holds the promise of reversing the epilepsy, behavioral problems, and cognitive deficits in FXS because these changes have been demonstrated in animal models with the use of mGluR5 antagonists (Fig. 4) as previously described. The initial clinical trial of fenobam, the first mGluR5 antagonist used in patients with FXS, was a single dose study in 12 adults that demonstrated no significant adverse effects, and there were favorable behavioral changes in most patients including calming

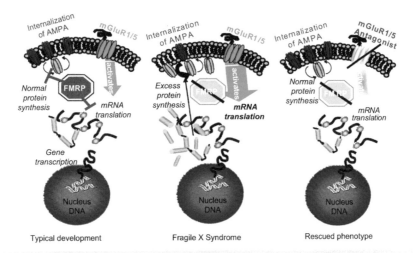

Fig. 4. mGluR1/5 pathways in normal individuals and in those with FXS after the use of an mGluR5 antagonist.

of the hyperactivity and anxiety [98]. In addition, significant improvement of the PPI deficit was seen in 50% of patients with FXS treated with fenobam. Within the next year there will be several trials of mGluR5 antagonists performed in multiple centers in the United States that are part of the Fragile X Clinical and Research Consortium set up by the National Fragile X Foundation (www.fragileX.org).

Another targeted treatment that may be helpful for children and adults with FXS is minocycline. In a study of newborn KO fragile X mice, a 1-month treatment with minocycline normalized synaptic connections by lowering matrix metalloproteinase 9 (MMP9), which is up-regulated without FMRP [99]. This exciting development has led to clinical instances of minocycline treatment of individuals with FXS and about two-thirds of families have noticed subtle but positive improvements in language, attention, and/or behavior. An open trial has been initiated in Canada recently and future controlled trials are needed. Minocycline can cause graying of the teeth in children who are younger than 7 years if their permanent teeth are not in place. Minocycline can also cause graying of other tissue with long-term use, and it can also cause enhanced sun sensitivity in most individuals and pseudotumor cerebri in rare instances. Further study of the neurobiology of FXS will likely lead to other targeted treatments and the combination of these treatments with educational endeavors to rehabilitate the cognitive deficits hold the promise of reversing the ID and behavioral problems in children and adults with FXS.

SUMMARY

There is a broad spectrum of clinical involvement throughout the generations in families affected by the fragile X mutations, both the full mutation and the premutation. A careful family history, assessment, and genetic counseling should lead to better treatments in all individuals affected by the many manifestations of these mutations. Individuals with ID, autism, ASD, neurologic problems of tremor, ataxia, neuropathy, and cognitive decline in addition to those with early menopause, infertility, and POI should be tested for the fragile X mutation. New targeted treatments give hope of reversing the ID and behavioral problems in children and adults with FXS. This review focuses on the latest research in both FXS and in premutation involvement and their treatment.

References

[1] Hagerman RJ, Rivera SM, Hagerman PJ. The fragile X family of disorders: a model for autism and targeted treatments. Curr Pediatr Rev 2008;4(1):40–52.

[2] Wittenberger MD, Hagerman RJ, Sherman SL, et al. The FMR1 premutation and reproduction. Fertil Steril 2007;87(3):456–65.

[3] Roberts JE, Bailey DB Jr, Mankowski J, et al. Mood and anxiety disorders in females with the FMR1 premutation. Am J Med Genet B Neuropsychiatr Genet 2009;150B(1):130–9.

[4] Hessl D, Tassone F, Loesch DZ, et al. Abnormal elevation of FMR1 mRNA is associated with psychological symptoms in individuals with the fragile X premutation. Am J Med Genet B Neuropsychiatr Genet 2005;139(1):115–21.

[5] Coffey SM, Cook K, Tartaglia N, et al. Expanded clinical phenotype of women with the FMR1 premutation. Am J Med Genet A 2008;146(8):1009–16.

[6] Bourgeois J, Coffey S, Rivera S, et al. Fragile X premutation disorders expanding the psychiatric perspective. J Clin Psychiatry 2009;70(6):852–62.

[7] Farzin F, Perry H, Hessl D, et al. Autism spectrum disorders and attention-deficit/hyperactivity disorder in boys with the fragile X premutation. J Dev Behav Pediatr 2006;27(2 Suppl):S137–44.

[8] Chen Y. Abnormal growth and synaptic architecture in hippocampal neurons cultured from a mouse model of FXTAS. Paper presented at: 11th International Fragile X Conference, July 23–27, 2008; St. Louis, MO.

[9] Aziz M, Stathopulu E, Callias M, et al. Clinical features of boys with fragile X premutations and intermediate alleles. Am J Med Genet 2003;121B(1):119–27.

[10] Brouwer JR, Severijnen E, de Jong FH, et al. Altered hypothalamus-pituitary-adrenal gland axis regulation in the expanded CGG-repeat mouse model for fragile X-associated tremor/ataxia syndrome. Psychoneuroendocrinology 2008;33(6):863–73.

[11] Tassone F, Hagerman RJ, Taylor AK, et al. Elevated levels of FMR1 mRNA in carrier males: a new mechanism of involvement in the fragile-X syndrome. Am J Hum Genet 2000;66(1): 6–15.

[12] Hagerman PJ. The fragile X prevalence paradox. J Med Genet 2008;45(8):498–9.

[13] Cronister A, Bhatt S, Wang Y, et al. Fragile X allele frequency comparisons among different ethnicities. Paper presented at: 58th Annual Meeting of the American Society of Human Genetics, November 11–15, 2008; Philadelphia.

[14] Toledano-Alhadef H, Basel-Vanagaite L, Magal N, et al. Fragile-X carrier screening and the prevalence of premutation and full-mutation carriers in Israel. Am J Hum Genet 2001;69: 351–60.

[15] Crawford DC, Meadows KL, Newman JL, et al. Prevalence of the fragile X syndrome in African-Americans. Am J Med Genet 2002;110(3):226–33.

[16] Loesch DZ, Huggins RM, Hagerman RJ. Phenotypic variation and FMRP levels in fragile X. Ment Retard Dev Disabil Res Rev 2004;10(1):31–41.

[17] Hagerman RJ. Physical and behavioral phenotype. In: Hagerman RJ, Hagerman PJ, editors. Fragile X syndrome: diagnosis, treatment and research. 3rd edition. Baltimore (MD): The Johns Hopkins University Press; 2002. p. 3–109.

[18] Hagerman RJ. Medical follow-up and pharmacotherapy. In: Hagerman RJ, Hagerman PJ, editors. Fragile X syndrome: diagnosis, treatment and research. 3rd edition. Baltimore (MD): The Johns Hopkins University Press; 2002. p. 287–338.

[19] Lachiewicz AM, Dawson DV. Do young boys with fragile X syndrome have macroorchidism? Pediatrics 1994;93(6 Pt 1):992–5.

[20] Belmonte MK, Bourgeron T. Fragile X syndrome and autism at the intersection of genetic and neural networks. Nat Neurosci 2006;9(10):1221–5.

[21] Harris SW, Hessl D, Goodlin-Jones B, et al. Autism profiles of males with fragile X syndrome. Am J Ment Retard 2008;113(6):427–38.

[22] Zingerevich C, Greiss-Hess L, Lemons-Chitwood K, et al. Motor abilities of children diagnosed with fragile X syndrome with and without autism. J Intellect Disabil Res 2009;53(1):11–8.

[23] Lewis P, Abbeduto L, Murphy M, et al. Cognitive, language and social-cognitive skills of individuals with fragile X syndrome with and without autism. J Intellect Disabil Res 2006;50(Pt 7):532–45.

[24] Kaufmann WE, Cortell R, Kau AS, et al. Autism spectrum disorder in fragile X syndrome: communication, social interaction, and specific behaviors. Am J Med Genet 2004;129(3):225–34.

[25] Rogers SJ, Wehner EA, Hagerman RJ. The behavioral phenotype in fragile X: symptoms of autism in very young children with fragile X syndrome, idiopathic autism, and other developmental disorders. J Dev Behav Pediatr 2001;22(6):409–17.

[26] Bailey DB Jr, Skinner D, Sparkman KL. Discovering fragile X syndrome: family experiences and perceptions. Pediatrics 2003;111(2):407–16.

[27] Council on Children With Disabilities, Section on Developmental Behavioral Pediatrics, Bright Futures Steering Committee, et al. Identifying infants and young children with developmental disorders in the medical home: an algorithm for developmental surveillance and screening. Pediatrics 2006;118(1):405–20.

[28] Skinner M, Hooper S, Hatton DD, et al. Mapping nonverbal IQ in young boys with fragile X syndrome. Am J Med Genet A 2005;132(1):25–32.

[29] Hagerman RJ. Lessons from fragile X regarding neurobiology, autism, and neurodegeneration. J Dev Behav Pediatr 2006;27(1):63–74.

[30] Roberts JE, Schaaf JM, Skinner M, et al. Academic skills of boys with fragile X syndrome: profiles and predictors. Am J Ment Retard 2005;110(2):107–20.

[31] Reiss AL, Hall SS. Fragile X syndrome: assessment and treatment implications. Child Adolesc Psychiatr Clin N Am 2007;16(3):663–75.

[32] Farzin F, Whitney D, Hagerman RJ, et al. Contrast detection in infants with fragile X syndrome. Vision Res 2008;48(13):1471–8.

[33] Cornish KM, Turk J, Hagerman R. The fragile X continuum: new advances and perspectives. J Intellect Disabil Res 2008;52(Pt 6):469–82.

[34] Bassell GJ, Warren ST. Fragile X syndrome: loss of local mRNA regulation alters synaptic development and function. Neuron 2008;60(2):201–14.

[35] Bear MF, Huber KM, Warren ST. The mGluR theory of fragile X mental retardation. Trends Neurosci 2004;27(7):370–7.

[36] Bolduc FV, Bell K, Cox H, et al. Excess protein synthesis in *Drosophila* fragile X mutants impairs long-term memory. Nat Neurosci 2008;11(10):1143–5.

[37] de Vrij FM, Levenga J, van der Linde HC, et al. Rescue of behavioral phenotype and neuronal protrusion morphology in Fmr1 KO mice. Neurobiol Dis 2008;31(1):127–32.

[38] Dolen G, Bear MF. Role for metabotropic glutamate receptor 5 (mGluR5) in the pathogenesis of fragile X syndrome. J Physiol 2008;586(6):1503–8.

[39] Berry-Kravis E. Epilepsy in fragile X syndrome. Dev Med Child Neurol 2002;44(11):724–8.

[40] Musumeci SA, Hagerman RJ, Ferri R, et al. Epilepsy and EEG findings in males with fragile X syndrome. Epilepsia 1999;40(8):1092–9.

[41] Garcia-Nonell C, Ratera ER, Harris S, et al. Secondary medical diagnosis in fragile X syndrome with and without autism spectrum disorder. Am J Med Genet A 2008;146(15): 1911–6.

[42] D'Hulst C, Kooy RF. The GABAA receptor: a novel target for treatment of fragile X? Trends Neurosci 2007;30(8):425–31.

[43] Chang S, Bray SM, Li Z, et al. Identification of small molecules rescuing fragile X syndrome phenotypes in *Drosophila*. Nat Chem Biol 2008;4(4):256–63.

[44] Yan QJ, Rammal M, Tranfaglia M, et al. Suppression of two major fragile X syndrome mouse model phenotypes by the mGluR5 antagonist MPEP. Neuropharmacology 2005;49(7): 1053–66.

[45] Budimirovic DB, Bukelis I, Cox C, et al. Autism spectrum disorder in Fragile X syndrome: differential contribution of adaptive socialization and social withdrawal. Am J Med Genet A 2006;140(17):1814–26.

[46] Bailey DB Jr, Raspa M, Olmsted M, et al. Co-occurring conditions associated with FMR1 gene variations: findings from a national parent survey. Am J Med Genet A 2008;146(16):2060–9.

[47] Roberts JE, Weisenfeld LA, Hatton DD, et al. Social approach and autistic behavior in children with fragile X syndrome. J Autism Dev Disord 2007;37(9):1748–60.

[48] Hessl D, Glaser B, Dyer-Friedman J, et al. Cortisol and behavior in fragile X syndrome. Psychoneuroendocrinology 2002;27(7):855–72.

[49] Hagerman RJ, Berry-Kravis E, Kaufmann WE, et al. Advances in the treatment of fragile X syndrome. Pediatrics 2009;123(1):378–90.

[50] Roberts JE, Boccia ML, Hatton DD, et al. Temperament and vagal tone in boys with fragile X syndrome. J Dev Behav Pediatr 2006;27(3):193–201.

[51] Bailey DB Jr, Sideris J, Roberts JE, et al. Child and genetic variables associated with maternal adaptation to fragile X syndrome: a multidimensional analysis. Am J Med Genet A 2008;146(6):720–9.

[52] Berry-Kravis E, Abrams L, Coffey SM, et al. Fragile X-associated tremor/ataxia syndrome: clinical features, genetics, and testing guidelines. Mov Disord 2007;22(14):2018–30.

[53] Hagerman RJ, Hagerman PJ. Testing for fragile X gene mutations throughout the life span. JAMA 2008;300(20):2419–21.

[54] Hagerman RJ, Hall DA, Coffey S, et al. Treatment of fragile X-associated tremor ataxia syndrome (FXTAS) and related neurological problems. Clin Interv Aging 2008;3(2):251–62.

[55] Darnell JC, Mostovetsky O, Darnell RB. FMRP RNA targets: identification and validation. Genes Brain Behav 2005;4(6):341–9.

[56] Kau ASM, Tierney E, Bukelis I, et al. Social behavior profile in young males with fragile X syndrome: characteristics and specificity. Am J Med Genet 2004;126:9–17.

[57] Hatton DD, Sideris J, Skinner M, et al. Autistic behavior in children with fragile X syndrome: prevalence, stability, and the impact of FMRP. Am J Med Genet A 2006;140(17):1804–13.

[58] Loesch DZ, Bui QM, Dissanayake C, et al. Molecular and cognitive predictors of the continuum of autistic behaviours in fragile X. Neurosci Biobehav Rev 2007;31:315–26.

[59] Chiu S, Wegelin JA, Blank J, et al. Early acceleration of head circumference in children with fragile X syndrome and autism. J Dev Behav Pediatr 2007;28(1):31–5.

[60] Butler MG, Dasouki MJ, Zhou XP, et al. Subset of individuals with autism spectrum disorders and extreme macrocephaly associated with germline PTEN tumour suppressor gene mutations. J Med Genet 2005;42(4):318–21.

[61] Nowicki ST, Tassone F, Ono MY, et al. The Prader-Willi phenotype of fragile X syndrome. J Dev Behav Pediatr 2007;28(2):133–8.

[62] Buxbaum J, Dorr N, Elder G, et al. Animal models for functional evaluation of genes in autism spectrum disorders. Paper presented at: 58th Annual Meeting of the American Society of Human Genetics, November 11–15, 2008; Philadelphia.

[63] Qin M, Kang J, Burlin TV, et al. Postadolescent changes in regional cerebral protein synthesis: an in vivo study in the FMR1 null mouse. J Neurosci 2005;25(20):5087–95.

[64] Wang H, Wu LJ, Kim SS, et al. FMRP acts as a key messenger for dopamine modulation in the forebrain. Neuron 2008;59(4):634–47.

[65] Hessl D, Berry-Kravis E, Cordeiro L, et al. Prepulse inhibition in fragile X syndrome: feasibility, reliability, and implications for treatment. Am J Med Genet B Neuropsychiatr Genet 2009;150B(4):545–53.

[66] Wilson BM, Cox CL. Absence of metabotropic glutamate receptor-mediated plasticity in the neocortex of fragile X mice. Proc Natl Acad Sci U S A 2007;104(7):2454–9.

[67] Castets M, Schaeffer C, Bechara E, et al. FMRP interferes with the Rac1 pathway and controls actin cytoskeleton dynamics in murine fibroblasts. Hum Mol Genet 2005;14(6): 835–44.

[68] Nakamoto M, Nalavadi V, Epstein MP, et al. Fragile X mental retardation protein deficiency leads to excessive mGluR5-dependent internalization of AMPA receptors. Proc Natl Acad Sci U S A 2007;104(39):15537–42.

[69] McBride SM, Choi CH, Wang Y, et al. Pharmacological rescue of synaptic plasticity, courtship behavior, and mushroom body defects in a Drosophila model of fragile X syndrome. Neuron 2005;45(5):753–64.

[70] Holtmaat AJ, Trachtenberg JT, Wilbrecht L, et al. Transient and persistent dendritic spines in the neocortex in vivo. Neuron 2005;45(2):279–91.

[71] Hoeft F, Lightbody AA, Hazlett HC, et al. Morphometric spatial patterns differentiating boys with fragile X syndrome, typically developing boys, and developmentally delayed boys aged 1 to 3 years. Arch Gen Psychiatry 2008;65(9):1087–97.

[72] Gothelf D, Furfaro JA, Hoeft F, et al. Neuroanatomy of fragile X syndrome is associated with aberrant behavior and the fragile X mental retardation protein (FMRP). Ann Neurol 2008;63(1):40–51.

[73] Dalton K, Holsen L, Abbeduto L, et al. Brain function and gaze fixation during facial-emotion processing in fragile X and autism. Autism Res 2008;1(4):231–9.

[74] Hessl D, Rivera S, Koldewyn K, et al. Amygdala dysfunction in men with the fragile X premutation. Brain 2007;130(Pt 2):404–16.

[75] Rivera SM, Menon V, White CD, et al. Functional brain activation during arithmetic processing in females with fragile X syndrome is related to FMR1 protein expression. Hum Brain Mapp 2002;16:206–18.

[76] Hessl D, Rivera SM, Reiss AL. The neuroanatomy and neuroendocrinology of fragile X syndrome. Ment Retard Dev Disabil Res Rev 2004;10(1):17–24.

[77] Kabakus N, Aydin M, Akin H, et al. Fragile X syndrome and cerebral perfusion abnormalities: single-photon emission computed tomographic study. J Child Neurol 2006;21(12):1040–6.

[78] Tarkka IM. Cerebral sources of electrical potentials related to human vocalization and mouth movement. Neurosci Lett 2001;298(3):203–6.

[79] Castren M, Paakkonen A, Tarkka IM, et al. Augmentation of auditory N1 in children with fragile X syndrome. Brain Topogr 2003;15(3):165–71.

[80] St Clair DM, Blackwood DH, Oliver CJ, et al. P3 abnormality in fragile X syndrome. Biol Psychiatry 1987;22(3):303–12.

[81] Rojas DC, Benkers TL, Rogers SJ, et al. Auditory evoked magnetic fields in adults with fragile X syndrome. Neuroreport 2001;12:2573–6.

[82] Greenough WT, Klintsova AY, Irwin SA, et al. Synaptic regulation of protein synthesis and the fragile X protein. Proc Natl Acad Sci U S A 2001;98:7101–6.

[83] Braff DL, Geyer MA, Swerdlow NR. Human studies of prepulse inhibition of startle: normal subjects, patient groups, and pharmacological studies. Psychopharmacology (Berl) 2001;156(2–3):234–58.

[84] Miller LJ, McIntosh DN, McGrath J, et al. Electrodermal responses to sensory stimuli in individuals with fragile X syndrome: a preliminary report. Am J Med Genet 1999;83(4): 268–79.

[85] Hagerman PJ, Hagerman RJ. The fragile-X premutation: a maturing perspective. Am J Hum Genet 2004;74(5):805–16.

[86] Iwahashi CK, Yasui DH, An HJ, et al. Protein composition of the intranuclear inclusions of FXTAS. Brain 2006;129(Pt 1):256–71.

[87] Jacquemont S, Hagerman RJ, Leehey M, et al. Fragile X premutation tremor/ataxia syndrome: molecular, clinical, and neuroimaging correlates. Am J Hum Genet 2003;72(4):869–78.

[88] Leehey MA, Berry-Kravis E, Min SJ, et al. Progression of tremor and ataxia in male carriers of the FMR1 premutation. Mov Disord 2007;22(2):203–6.

[89] Greco CM, Tassone F, Garcia-Arocena D, et al. Clinical and neuropathologic findings in a woman with the FMR1 premutation and multiple sclerosis. Arch Neurol 2008;65(8):1114–6.

[90] Mothersead PK, Conrad K, Hagerman RJ, et al. An atypical progressive dementia in a male carrier of the fragile X premutation: an example of fragile X-associated tremor/ataxia syndrome. Appl Neuropsychol 2005;12(3):169–79.

[91] Greco CM, Berman RF, Martin RM, et al. Neuropathology of fragile X-associated tremor/ataxia syndrome (FXTAS). Brain 2006;129(Pt 1):243–55.

[92] Greco CM, Soontarapornchai K, Wirojanan J, et al. Testicular and pituitary inclusion formation in fragile X associated tremor/ataxia syndrome. J Urol 2007;177(4):1434–7.

[93] Gokden M, Al-Hinti JT, Harik SI. Peripheral nervous system pathology in fragile X tremor/ataxia syndrome (FXTAS). Neuropathology 2009;29(3):280–4.

[94] Hagerman RJ, Coffey SM, Maselli R, et al. Neuropathy as a presenting feature in fragile X-associated tremor/ataxia syndrome. Am J Med Genet A 2007;143(19):2256–60.

[95] Tassone F, Pan R, Amiri K, et al. A rapid polymerase chain reaction-based screening method for identification of all expanded alleles of the fragile X (FMR1) gene in newborn and high-risk populations. J Mol Diagn 2008;10(1):43–9.

[96] Berry-Kravis E, Potanos K. Psychopharmacology in fragile X syndrome – present and future. Ment Retard Dev Disabil Res Rev 2004;10(1):42–8.

[97] Torrioli MG, Vernacotola S, Peruzzi L, et al. A double-blind, parallel, multicenter comparison of L-acetylcarnitine with placebo on the attention deficit hyperactivity disorder in fragile X syndrome boys. Am J Med Genet A 2008;146(7):803–12.

[98] Berry-Kravis E, Hessl D, Coffey S, et al. Single dose fenobam in fragile X syndrome: safety and effects on prepulse inhibition and continuous performance measures. J Med Genet 2009;46(4):266–71.

[99] Bilousova T, Dansie L, Ngo M, et al. Minocycline promotes dendritic spine maturation and improves behavioral performance in the fragile X mouse model. J Med Genet 2009;46(2):94–102.

Advances in Pediatrics 56 (2009) 187–201

ADVANCES IN PEDIATRICS

Autism: An Update

Edward Goldson, MD

The Children's Hospital, 13123 E. 16th Avenue, Aurora, CO 80045, USA

During the last few years autism has been on the public radar. The questions frequently raised are: has there been an increase in autism? Is there an epidemic? Why are we seeing more of these children then ever before, with a prevalence now of 12.6 to 40 per 10,000 [1] or 1:150 [2] births with boys being affected four times more frequently than girls [3]? What are the causes of this disorder and can we identify children early with the disorder? The purpose of this article is to discuss the screening for and early identification of children who might fall on the autism spectrum and to address the controversy concerning the role of immunizations in autism.

SCREENING

Autism is a neurodevelopmental spectrum disorder that is characterized by three core deficits: deficits in communication, social interaction, and the presence of stereotyped patterns of behavior, restricted interests and activities [4]. Phrased another way by Aicardi, "... autism is a behavioral symptom constellation signaling underlying nervous system dysfunction [5]." The etiology of this disorder is unknown although the commonly accepted hypothesis is that there is a strong genetic basis in association with environmental factors or perturbations experienced by vulnerable children [6]. In addition, it is believed that the identification of children before 3 years of age is very important because the sooner children are identified as falling on the autism spectrum, the sooner interventions can be initiated and aimed at ameliorating the effects of this disorder. This early intervention can lead to more optimal outcomes for the child and the family. This assertion has been clearly documented by the National Research Council, which has noted that any child with an autism spectrum disorder (ASD) would benefit from appropriate early intervention [7]. Harris and Handelman [8] have noted that children starting intervention before 3 years of age make the greatest gains in their development. The American Academy of Pediatrics (AAP) recommends that all children receive autism specific screening at 18, [9], 24, and 30 months of age [10]. In a 2006 US Centers for Disease Control study [3] the average age of an ASD diagnosis was 61 months (17–205 months). In addition, there was an average delay of 13 months between the first evaluation by a professional and the diagnosis of ASD.

E-mail address: goldson.edward@tchden.org

0065-3101/09/$ – see front matter
doi:10.1016/j.yapd.2009.08.005

If we accept the proposition that early identification is essential for intervention, which would lead to a more positive outcome, we would than have to ask how we go about identifying children who might fall on the autism spectrum. One approach to identifying children in a large population is to engage in screening. Screening is a common medical practice highlighted by the mandate for newborn screening for a variety of metabolic diseases throughout the United States. There is also the federal mandate through Child Find to screen children for developmental disorders. In 2006, a provocative survey study reported on screening practices for general developmental problems and ASD in a random sample of general pediatricians in Maryland and Delaware that generated 255 responses. Most of these physicians (82%) screened for general developmental problems using a screening tool, but only 8% screened for ASD with very few using any ASD-specific tools [11]. This paucity of activity in the identification of autism on the part of pediatricians has lead the AAP to issue a strong statement encouraging pediatricians to rigorously screen for this disorder as early as 18 months [12].

There are a variety of ways that one can pursue the diagnosis of autism. The first is the use of surveillance, which is a procedure for recognizing children at risk for a disorder, be it a medical or specifically developmental problem. Surveillance involves asking parents and other caretakers if they have any concerns about the child's developmental or medical state. The physician will respond depending on the parents' answer. A formal tool to accomplish this task is the Parents' Evaluation of Developmental Status (PEDS) [13]. The PEDS consists of 10 open-ended questions designed to elicit concerns about development in children from birth to 8 years of age. The results of a recent study looking at screening strategies for children at risk for ASD [14] revealed that when using the PEDS a significant number of children with ASD were missed who had been identified by the Modified Checklist for Autism in Toddlers (M-CHAT) [15]. The M-CHAT is a modification of the Checklist for Autism in Toddlers (CHAT [discussed later in this article]) [16]. These results suggest that a surveillance tool designed to identify general developmental delays was not adequate to identify children with more specific problems, such as ASD, and that an autism-specific screen should be employed. However, the physician independent of a surveillance tool can suspect that something is not correct by refined questioning of the parent, being responsive to the parents' concern, and observation of the child. Children 9 to 12 months of age, who later met criteria for an ASD, have marked changes in their temperament ranging from marked irritability to passivity, independent of a medical illness. These children have poor eye contact, poor responses to human voices, especially to being called by one's name, poor interactive play, and more interest in objects than people. There is limited babbling and poor social reciprocity, such as a failure to orient when one's name is called or not engaging in the back-and-forth bids for attention and social interaction [17]. In this group of behaviors, not responding to one's name and poor social relatedness are of considerable concern. The Child Neurology Society practice parameter on screening for autism noted four behaviors that are of major concern and do overlap with what is noted above: no babbling or pointing or other gesture by 12 months, no single words by 16 months, no two-word spontaneous (not echolalic) phrases by 24 months, and loss of language or social skills at any age [18,19]. One of course needs to be sure that the child is not hearing impaired. The primary care provider, while using a screening algorithm [12] without any formal testing can be, and is, essential to recognizing that a child is not developing normally and might fall on the autism spectrum [20].

Surveillance is an important activity in pediatrics but one probably needs, within the context of a medical home, more formal approaches that Level I screening provides [17]. Level I screening measures can be administered to all children and are designed to differentiate children at risk for ASD, or any other disorder, from the general population. Such structured tools are designed to provide clinicians with a list of behaviors to make judgments about the risk for autism. This is an important step beyond surveillance. Essential to any screening tool is its sensitivity and specificity. The sensitivity is the proportion of children with a problem who are positively identified by the test, with a specific cut-off score. Those who have the disorder but are not identified with the test are considered to be false negatives. The specificity of a test is the proportion of children who are developing typically and are correctly identified as being typical by the test as determined by a specific cut-off score. Those who are typical but identified as being abnormal are considered to be false positives. These constructs are used as indicators of how effective the tool is at identifying the risk for the problem or if the problem exists, (eg, autism) [21].

Included in this Level I category of measures is the CHAT, an interactive interview in which there is a parent questionnaire and observation by the clinician. There is also the M-CHAT, which is a parent questionnaire that has good psychometric properties and is a reliable screen [14]. The Social Communication Questionnaire (SCQ) [22,23] is a parent questionnaire also used as a screening tool, but is frequently used in more specialized settings and is often considered a Level II screening tool.

Level II screening tools are those used in more specialized settings, such as early intervention programs or clinics. These screening tools serve to differentiate children with ASD from those with other developmental challenges, such as language delays or intellectual impairment who do not fall on the autism spectrum [17]. These tools require more specialized training and more time to administer, score, and interpret, than do Level I measures. Measures that fall into this category include the Childhood Autism Rating Scale (CARS) [24], which is a behavior checklist completed by an examiner and the Gilliam Autism Rating Scale (GARS) [25], which is also completed by an examiner.

The M-CHAT is a modified version of the CHAT that includes 23 questions including 9 parent-response questions from the CHAT and 14 additional parent-response questions relating to symptoms associated with autism in very young children. It can be used to screen children 16 to 30 months old. The authors suggest that this tool be used to screen children at 24 months of age to identify children on the autism spectrum, and those who may have re-gressed between 18 and 24 months. This is a time when parents may be noting changes in their child and when pediatricians may be more focused on devel-opmental screening. In addition, it requires only yes and no answers and does not involve a physician or other child-health worker observation [14]. Thus, it is not very time consuming for the physician and does have a reliable chance of identifying a child with an ASD.

The Level II screen, SCQ, is a parent-report screening measure for ASD based on the Autism Diagnostic Interview-Revised [26], which is an involved interview and is frequently used to make the diagnosis of an ASD. It draws on the criteria used to make the diagnosis of an ASD from the *Diagnostic and Statistical Manual* of the American Psychiatric Association [4]. It consists of 40 yes/no items that can be completed by the primary caregiver in approximately 10 minutes and scored in less than 5 minutes [27]. It is usually used to screen children above 4 years of age, but specifically to look at behaviors exhibited between 4 and 5 years of age. However, Eaves and colleagues found that this tool can be used to screen younger children for ASD. Use with children who have significant intellectual impairments is more complex as the cut-off scores for risk for autism is not applicable in this population and the some of the features associated with an ASD may be confounded by the intellectual impairment [27]. Nevertheless, Eaves and colleagues found that it was a useful tool for identifying young children in need of further evaluation by a develop-mental professional. However, they make a very important point in noting that screening tools are not diagnostic tools and no screening tool is perfect. No tool should be used alone and observation of the child and clinical judgment play critical roles in determining whether or not to pursue more extensive evalua-tions, even if the child does not meet the criteria for ASD.

Frequently there is discussion as to which screening tool is the best. In a recent paper Snow and Lecavalier [28] sought to assess the sensitivity and specificity of the M-CHAT and the SCQ. They had a sample of children with possible pervasive developmental disorders (PDD) and a group with non-PDD. The M-CHAT was used to assess children aged 18 to 48 months and the SCQ was used for children aged 30 to 70 months. There was clear diagnostic agreement between the two measures in their age ranges. The diag-nostic agreement of the two measures in the population of children that over-lapped in age was good. The conclusion however, was that the M-CHAT and the SCQ appear to more accurately identify children with PDD who have lower intellectual and adaptive functioning.

The CARS and GARS are Level II screens, which have been used exten-sively in the past but their psychometric properties have raised significant concerns [17]. Thus, there utility may be falling under question. There are a number of other Level I and Level II measures available, but their reliability and usefulness as screens remains to be further elucidated [17].

There are several tools that can be used to screen for autism early in life and more in-depth tools for measurement and evaluation. The point to be made is that whatever tool is used in the physician's office should be reliable and easy to use, within the context of the health-care setting, ideally a medical home. What is most important is that physicians put developmental screening, more specifically screening for ASD, on their well-child agenda and that it be included, early in life, as part of the well-child visit.

Finally, one can go beyond screening and pursue autism-specific diagnostic testing. The gold standard for the evaluation of children suspected of having an ASD is the Autism Diagnostic Schedule [29] and the Autism Diagnostic Interview [26], which are more complicated tools requiring training and reliability testing. These last two measures are not discussed in this article because they are in-depth evaluation tools and do not pertain specifically to screening.

IMMUNIZATIONS

Ever since the recognition and description of children with autism by Kanner in 1943 scientists and clinicians alike, have been searching for the cause of this disorder or group of disorders [30]. Initially, although Kanner in his original paper hypothesized that autism was an inborn biologic condition, misconceptions based on psychoanalytic theory led workers to view autism as a psychiatric disorder. The major proponent of the purely psychiatric approach was Bruno Bettelheim who attributed the disorder to an unnurturing mother, called the "refrigerator theory [31]." The idea of autism as a psychiatric disorder persisted until the 1960s when Rimland [32] hypothesized a neurologic basis for the disorder. Clinicians and researchers then came to recognize, as does Aicardi, that autism is a neurologic disorder expressed by a constellation of behavioral symptoms, and not infrequently, by overt neurologic symptoms, such as seizures and intellectual impairment. Several etiologies have been postulated: genetic, immunologic, infectious, toxic, environmental. There is strong evidence for a genetic influence [33,34] and more recently there has been some association of autism with low birth weight infants and with older parents [35,36].

However, the two proposed etiologies that have been the most controversial, and have had the most significant effect on the health of children, concern the possible association of toxins and vaccines with autism. The controversy is usually discussed in vaccines or immunizations, but in reality there are really three questions. First, does the measles-mumps-rubella (MMR) vaccine cause autism? Second, because we give so many vaccines, many of which are combined vaccines, does the combination cause autism? These two questions are corollaries and speak to an immunologic cause for autism, or problems associated with the administration of vaccines, such as the MMR. The third question is whether thimerosal, an ethylmercury derivative containing preservative in vaccinations, causes autism? That is to say, does mercury, a toxin, cause autism?

In 2001, Bernard and coworkers put forth the hypothesis that thimerosal in vaccines caused autism [37,38]. Thimerosal, in very low doses, was used in multidose vials of vaccines as a preservative to protect the ampules from bacterial and fungal contamination. This proposition has lead to the unyielding belief, among some, that mercury is the cause of autism. This lead to the demand that mercury be removed from vaccines, which took place several years ago. However, what is more disturbing is that parents are refusing to immunize their children even with the thimerosal removed, which speaks to the question of whether immunizations cause autism, particularly the MMR.

The issue that is clearly at stake is whether mercury, in the form of thimerosal causes autism? Nelson and Bauman conducted an extensive review of the evidence implicating thimerosal in the emergence of autism [39]. First, they compared the clinical manifestations of autism and mercury toxicity. Mercury poisoning was associated with ataxia, dysarthria, constricted visual fields, peripheral neuropathy, toxic psychosis and small head size, depression, and anxiety. Among children with autism one sees stereotypies, delayed speech and echolalia, hyper-responsiveness, social aloofness, a need for sameness, and large heads. The clinical pictures of the two disorders are entirely different. In addition, the mercury levels of children with autism, even those receiving vaccines with thimerosal, are not elevated as noted by Pichichiero [40]. Second, they evaluated the neuropathology of both disorders for which the majority of data are found in those exposed to methylmercury (MeHg), which is not used in any of the vaccines. On the contrary, ethyl mercury is the agent used in thimerosal. There is very limited information on the neuropathology associated with ethyl mercury which is metabolized differently and when there has been a rare poisoning, has a somewhat different pathologic picture. What is known about methylmercury exposure is that there is neuronal cell loss and increased gliosis in the cerebral cortex, atrophy of the calcarine cortex exposed in adults, and atrophy of the cerebellum with consistent loss of granule cells with relative sparing of the Purkinje cells. In ethyl mercury toxicity they found proliferation of glia, demyelination of the ninth and tenth cranial nerves roots, loss of nerve cells particularly in the calcarine cortex, and atrophy of the cerebellum. This is a different picture from the few studies in individuals with autism where the brains are usually large, with no cerebral loss. What has been found in the forebrain have been small, closely packed neurons and increased cell packing density in portions of the limbic system. There is loss of Purkinje cells in the posterior inferior hemispheres of the cerebellum. Thus, the neuropathologic pictures are very different in the two disorders. Finally, they did a review of the literature describing human populations exposed to mercury. Although they did identify some developmental abnormalities there were no behaviors consistent with autism. They also examined whether there had been an increase in the prevalence of autism with the introduction of thimerosal-containing vaccines. There was none. The authors concluded that there was no clear association between thimerosal in vaccines and autism.

Pichichero and colleagues [40] conducted a study in which they examined mercury concentrations and metabolism in infants less than 6 months of age receiving vaccines containing thimerosal. The vaccines administered included diphtheria-tetanus-acellular pertussis vaccine, hepatitis B vaccine and

Haemophilus influenzae type b vaccine. They administered mercury-free vaccines to a control group of infants. The authors obtained blood, urine, and stool samples 3 to 28 days after vaccination. Total mercury concentration in the samples was then measured. Overall, mercury concentrations in the mercury-exposed and nonexposed infants were below the range of quantitation in 12 out of 33 children exposed and 14 of 15 nonexposed infants. Although mercury concentrations were uniformly low, the highest levels were recorded shortly after vaccine administration, all of which were below the levels believed to be potentially toxic. Mothers' hair was measured for mercury concentration. Several of these mothers nursed, which may account for some of the mercury measured in the control group. The results of this study showed that the amounts of mercury in the blood of infants receiving mercury-containing vaccines are well below concentrations associated with potentially toxic effects. The authors concluded that thimerosal-containing vaccines posed very little risk to full-term infants.

There was also a report from the Institute of Medicine maintaining that the thimerosal in the concentrations administered in the vaccines is safe [41]. In another review it was pointed out that toxic levels of inorganic mercury and MeHg have significant neurotoxicity. Exposure to mercury vapor in adults may result in acrodynia and the classic triad of erethism (bizarre behavior, such as excessive shyness or aggression), tremor, and gingivitis. Exposure to MeHg can be fatal and involves sensory disturbances, ataxia, visual field constriction, cognitive decline, and potentially death. Neuropathology indicates that the occipital cortex and the cerebellum are affected. Prenatal exposure to MeHg resulted in diffuse central nervous system damage and disruption of cell migration. This is not the case with ethylmercury, which is found in thimerosal and has a different metabolism. The authors concluded that there is no evidence for an association between thimerosal and autism [42]. Finally, thimerosal has been removed from vaccines so the question of immunizing children, because of the presence of thimerosal, should no longer be an issue [43,44].

Despite these studies there continues to be ongoing controversy about the effect of mercury and whether it is associated with autism. Numerous parent groups advocate and demonstrate against thimerosal although it is no longer used. Many want compensation from the government and pharmaceutical companies for their children's autism, which they believe is associated with the thimerosal-containing immunizations [45]. The question emerges then as to how one can demonstrate that thimerosal is not associated with autism. One of the most logical ways is to rigorously monitor what happens once thimerosal is no longer used. Studies such as this have been performed in the United States, United Kingdom, Denmark, and Canada. Parker and colleagues [46] did an analysis of the existing literature in 2004. They looked at cohort studies and at ecologic studies, assessing the study designs and analyses and the strengths and weaknesses of the two methods. Their conclusion was that there was no link between thimerosal-containing vaccines and neurodevelopmental disorders, including autism [45]. Having stated this, and the author recommends this article to the reader, let us review several of the studies assessed.

One article reported the results of an epidemiologic study on the occurrence of autism from Danish population-based data [47]. The authors analyzed the data from the Danish Psychiatric Central Research Register which recorded all psychiatric admissions since 1971 and all psychiatric outpatient contacts in Denmark since 1995. The study population included all children aged 2 to 10 years diagnosed with autism from 1971 to 2000. The diagnosis of autism was based on criteria in the International Classification of Diseases revisions 8 and 10. A total of 956 children with a male-to-female ratio of 3.5:1 were diagnosed with autism from 1971 to 2000. The incidence rates were stable from 1971 to 1990. In the period before 1990, when thimerosal was used, there was no increase in autism. There was a mild increase in the prevalence of autism from 1990 to 1992 and a continued rise even after the discontinuation of thimerosal in 1992. The conclusion was that thimerosal use was not associated with autism.

A more recent study by Fombonne and colleagues [48] was published in 2006. The authors were interested in the relationship of trends in PDD (eg, ASD) to (1) the cumulative changes in thimerosal levels through changes in the immunization schedule, and (2) trends in MMR vaccination-use rates and the introduction of a 2 MMR dosing schedule during the study period. They evaluated a cohort of 27, 749 children born in Montreal from 1987 to 1998. With the removal of thimerosal during this time period they of course found a marked drop in the thimerosal levels from 1992 to 1995. In the cohort they identified 180 children who had a PDD; either autistic disorder, Asperger syndrome, or pervasive developmental disorder not otherwise specified (PDD-NOS). During the period of the study, they found that the prevalence of PDD had a significant linear increase. This increase continued even when the thimerosal was removed from the vaccine. In addition, when there was a decrease in the MMR-uptake rates, PDD continued to increase. After using logistic regression models of the prevalence data, the authors' found no association between the rise in PDD and thimerosal or with changes in the MMR schedule.

The prevalence of pervasive developmental disorder in Montreal was high, increasing in recent birth cohorts as found in most countries. Factors accounting for the increase include a broadening of diagnostic concepts and criteria, increased awareness, and therefore, better identification of children with PDD in communities and epidemiologic surveys, and improved access to services. The findings ruled out an association between PDD and either high levels of ethyl mercury exposure comparable with those experienced in the United States in the 1990s or 1-to 2-dose measles-mumps-rubella vaccinations [48].

In addition, the implications they drew from this study are that parents of children with PDD should be informed that there is no relationship between thimerosal and MMR and PDD and that their children and their unaffected siblings should be vaccinated. Children not vaccinated run a high risk of contracting measles with sometimes very severe sequelae. They assert that there is no relationship between thimerosal and autism and no scientific basis for the use of chelation therapies, which can be very dangerous, to treat autism. This comment relates to the fact that some individuals are suggesting that chelation of mercury is a cure for autism.

One of the initial reasons for removing thimerosal from the vaccines was that it might have adverse neurologic consequences. The original concern was not about autism but it soon evolved into a debate about autism, which was spread throughout the country and the world [45]. In a 2007 publication the neuropsychological outcomes were reported 7 to 10 years after early thimerosal exposure. Autism was not evaluated in this study. Using standardized tests 1047 children between the ages of 7 and 10 years were evaluated. Measures of speech and language, verbal memory, fine motor coordination, visual-spatial ability, general intellectual functioning attention, hyperactivity, executive functioning, the presence of motor tics, phonic tics and stuttering were employed. In addition, there was a maternal interview that included questions about vaccines, pregnancy, medications, toxin exposures, socioeconomic status, pregnancy and birth history, children's experience with computers, and a brief intelligence test was administered to the mothers. The results of this involved study did not support a causal association between exposure to thimerosal and neuropsychological functioning at the age of 7 to 10 years [49]. There are several other studies from various data banks from different countries, including the United States, none of which have identified or demonstrated an association between thimerosal and ASD [45,46]. Nevertheless, there continue to be strong advocates, ignoring the existent data, with the belief that government and the drug companies manufacturing vaccines containing thimerosal are hiding information that links thimerosal to autism. It appears that no matter what scientific information is provided, these advocates do not accept, much less believe, the results of these studies and the conclusions drawn by experts in the fields of child development, infectious disease, and public health.

The association of MMR with autism has a different origin. In 1998, Wakefield and colleagues [50] reported a new variant of autism that had been induced by the administration of MMR in the second year of life and was responsible for the increasing rates (or prevalence) of autism worldwide. There was quite a response to this report with subsequent public health consequences. It was reported in the Communicable Disease Center Weekly 2000 in the United Kingdom that MMR coverage rates in 2-year-old children fell from 92% in 1995 to 88% in 2000. This data has the potential to create significant public health problems. In a communication to the New Challenges in Childhood Immunization Conference [51], Wakefield stated his position vis a vis the MMR vaccine:

1. Atypical patterns of exposure to measles virus, including a close temporal association with another infection, are a risk factor for chronic intestinal inflammation.

2. There are factors such as age, sex and the nature of concurrent exposure(s) that influence the phenotype of the intestinal pathology that develops (ie, Crohn's disease, ulcerative colitis or autistic colitis).
3. In child with autistic colitis persistent measles virus infection of the ileal lymphoid tissues causes chronic immune mediated pathology in the intestines.
4. Associated changes in intestinal permeability and altered peptidase activity will allow neurotoxic intestinal products (eg, exorphins) to reach the brain, which is particularly susceptible to permanent damage during times of rapid cerebral development such as infancy.
5. In susceptible children (possibly for reasons of age, immune status or genetic background) MMR vaccine is an atypical pattern of measles exposure that represents a significantly increased risk for intestinal infection and associated developmental regression compared with the monovalent vaccine or natural infections.

This claim was rejected by the majority of the authors [52] of that paper approximately 6 years after its publication, after which a storm was created in the United Kingdom and in other parts of the world. Despite the retraction, the debate continues and parents feel that Wakefield's study provided the answer to autism. Parents in the United Kingdom and the United States began and continue to refuse to immunize their children. As a result, there have been surges and outbreaks of measles cases in the United Kingdom and in the United States [53–57].

Several studies have been performed around the world and have not found any association between autism and the MMR. A Finnish [58] retrospective study in 2002 reviewed the records of 535,544 1- to 7-year-old children who were vaccinated between 1982 and 1986 and sought to determine whether there was a link between the MMR and encephalitis, aseptic meningitis, inflammatory bowel disease, and autism. They found no association between MMR vaccination and encephalitis, aseptic meningitis, or autism.

Another study from Denmark reported on a retrospective cohort study of children born from 1991 to 1998. In the cohort of 537, 303 children, 440, 655 had received the MMR. The authors identified 316 children who had autistic disorder and 442 children who had another ASD. They found that the risk for ASD was not increased among children who received the MMR. They found no association between MMR vaccination and ASD and felt that their data provided strong evidence against the hypothesis that MMR caused autism [59].

The result of the controversy based on the data is that Wakefield's hypothesis does not hold, it has been retracted by most of his coauthors, there is no epidemiologic evidence from at least two countries with excellent databases on immunizations and we now have a public health problem. We are now seeing many cases of measles as reported in journals and the media and we will probably see an increase in other childhood infectious diseases as parents continue to believe that autism is caused by MMR, and by extension, other immunizations.

The final issue to be raised is the administration of many immunizations in the early years of life. Parents have the belief that the multiple vaccinations compromise their children's immune systems, thus predisposing them to infection or to weakening their immune system. In addition, one wonders if they are also concerned about autism. Offit and his coworkers have an excellent discussion of this topic [60]. They demonstrate, based on the current literature, that vaccination does not compromise the immune system, that children have the capacity, even as neonates, to mount a protective immune response. Moreover, with the administration of vaccines one is able first to prevent disease, and secondly, to prevent the bacterial complications associated with or following upon viral illness, such as pneumonia following infection with influenza and necrotizing fasciitis following varicella. Offit and Hackett also addressed the question of whether vaccines cause allergic or autoimmune diseases. They reviewed the pathogenesis of allergic diseases, autoimmune diseases, multiple sclerosis, type 1 diabetes, and chronic arthritis. There is no evidence to suggest that any of these disorders are caused by the administration of any vaccines [61].

One of the challenges for clinicians is how to educate families about autism and vaccines. It seems that parents involved in this discussion fall into three categories: (1) parents who absolutely believe that vaccines cause autism; (2) parents who are unsure about what to do, but are open minded; and (3) parents who do not believe that vaccines cause ASD. The first and third groups in many ways present no major challenge for the clinician. For group three one can provide up-to-date information about autism and vaccines and reassure them that vaccines are safe. They will immunize their children knowing they are providing good and appropriate care for their children. For group number one, no amount of data as to the safety of vaccines and a rational discussion about our level of understanding will have any effect. Trying to convince these parents that it is in their children's best interest to immunize them and discussing public health implications of not immunizing seems to have no effect on their behavior. One must not forget that this group of children needs to be cared for, but battling about immunizations will do no good, will alienate the family, and possibly lead to poor and dangerous health care. Thus, one may just need to provide good care and not get into the autism/vaccine issue, unless the parents raise it. On the other hand, the third group warrants closer attention. One needs to be open and honest about what we know and why. In the author's opinion, the data supporting the continued administration of vaccines are convincing. We also need to be open about we do not know if we are to gain trust and have credence among these families. However, we must be very firm in our convictions and the reasons for holding them [62]. Providing families with reliable information and resources that they can access and being willing to discuss the information is essential to establishing trusting relationships. Disparaging their questions and concerns is unacceptable. One needs to recognize that the field of autism is shifting and that we need to be mindful that this can be anxiety provoking for parents (and for clinicians). There is much to learn and we need to keep our minds open and help our families to do the same. Above all, we must do no harm.

SUMMARY

Screening for autism and the early identification of children with ASD is an important task for well-child care providers. Autism, as it is currently behaviorally diagnosed, is a common neuro-developmental disorder with a very broad spectrum of behaviors and medical problems. The early identification of this spectrum disorder can facilitate intervention that can lead to amelioration of the behaviors, provide support for families, and enhance the outcome for these children and their families. Thus, there is little controversy about screening other than to decide on the best tools for screening. The biggest challenge, after identification, is to provide access for these families to services and care for their children.

The larger issue in this review is the discussion of vaccines and autism. From the scientific perspective (ie, evidence based), there is no evidence to suggest either thimerosal as a toxin, or MMR and other vaccinations as immunologic agents, have any association with autism. This idea is generally accepted by most physicians and other scientists working in the field, but is not universal. Politicians, lawyers, and journalists have weighed in on the discussion and have confounded the science with emotion, belief systems, and the legal system. Parents of children with autism who received MMR or thimerosal-containing vaccines are seeking indemnity for their children's care and are turning to the courts. Also, they are not immunizing their children, thus creating a public health problem the size of which we have not seen in the more industrialized countries in decades.

As a society we have not met the diagnostic and treatment needs of children with ASD as we have not met the needs of children with other developmental disabilities. How we go about meeting the needs of these children is a major challenge for professionals caring for them. However, we must be mindful that the resolution of the scientific issues should not take place in the courts or in congress. It should take place among clinicians and scientists. How we go about providing adequate support for needy children and their families should take place in the political, legal, educational, and medical arenas. A major question confronting us now, is can these arenas work collaboratively to provide clear information scientifically to inform public policy?

References

[1] Yeargin-Allsopp M, Rice C, Krapurkar T, et al. Prevalence of autism in a US metropolitan area. JAMA 2003;289:49–55.
[2] Centers for Disease Control and Prevention. Prevalence of autism spectrum disorders - autism and developmental disabilities monitoring network, 14 Sites, United States, 2002. MMWR Surveill Summ 2007;56:12–28.
[3] Wiggins LD, Baio J, Rice C. Examination of the time between the first evaluation and first autism spectrum diagnosis in a population-based sample. J Dev Behav Pediatr 2006;27: S79–87.

[4] American Psychiatric Association. Diagnostic and statistical manual of mental disorders (DSM-IV-TR). 4th edition. Washington, DC: APA; 2000.

[5] Aicardi J. Autism and autistic-like conditions. In: Aicardi J, editor. Diseases of the nervous system in children. 2nd edition. Cambridge: University Press; 1998. p. 827.

[6] Rutter M. Autism: its recognition, early diagnosis, and service implications. J Dev Behav Pediatr 2006;27:S54–8.

[7] National Research Council. Committee on educational interventions for children with autism, Division of Behavioral and Social Sciences and Education. In: Lord C, McGee JP, editors. Educating children with autism. Washington DC: National Academy Press; 2001. p. 1–10.

[8] Harris SL, Handleman JS. J Autism Dev Disord 2000;30:137–42.

[9] American Academy of Pediatrics. Identifying infants and young children with developmental disorders in the medical home: an algorithm for developmental surveillance and screening. Pediatrics 2006;118:405–20.

[10] Gupta VB, Hyman SL, Johnson CP. Identifying children autism early? Pediatrics 2007;119: 152–3.

[11] Dosreis S, Weiner CL, Johnson L, et al. Autism spectrum disorder screening and management practices among general pediatric providers. J Dev Behav Pediatr 2006;27:S88–94.

[12] Johnson CP, Myers SM. American Academy of Pediatrics Council on children with disabilities. Identification and evaluation of children with autism spectrum disorders. Pediatrics 2007;120(5):118–215.

[13] Glascoe FP. Parents' evaluation of developmental status: how well do parents' concerns identify children with behavioral and emotional problems. Clin Pediatr (Phila) 2003;42: 133–8.

[14] Pinto-Martin JA, Young LM, Mandell DS, et al. Screening strategies for autism spectrum disorders in pediatric primary care. J Dev Behav Pediatr 2008;29:345–50.

[15] Robins DL, Fein D, Barton ML, et al. The modified checklist for autism in toddlers: an initial study investigating the early detection of autism and pervasive developmental disorders. J Autism Dev Disord 2001;31:131–44.

[16] Baron-Cohen S, Allen J, Gillberg C. Can autism be detected at 18 months? The needle, the haystack and the CHAT. Br J Psychiatry 1992;161:839–43.

[17] Johnson CP, Myers SM. Autism spectrum disorders. In: Wolraich ML, Drotar D, Dworkin P, et al, editors. Developmental and behavioral pediatrics: evidence and practice. 2nd edition. Philadelphia: Mosby Elsevier; 2008. p. 519–77.

[18] Filipek PA, Accardo PJ, Ashwal S, et al. The screening and diagnosis of autistic spectrum disorders. J Autism Dev Disord 1999;29:439–84.

[19] Filipek PA, Accardo PJ, Ashwal S, et al. Practice parameter: screening and diagnosis of autism - report of the Quality Subcommittee of the American Academy of Neurology and the Child Neurology Society. Neurology 2000;55:468–79.

[20] American Academy Pediatrics. The pediatrician's role in the diagnosis and management of autistic spectrum disorder in children. Pediatrics 2001;107:1221–6.

[21] Aylward GP, Stancin T. Measurement and psychometric considerations. In: Wolraich ML, Drotar D, et al, editors. Developmental and behavioral pediatrics: evidence and practice. 2nd edition. Philadelphia: Mosby Elsevier; 2008. p. 123–30.

[22] Berument SK, Rutter M, Lord C, et al. Autism screening questionnaire: diagnostic validity. Br J Psychiatry 1999;175:444–51.

[23] Rutter M, Bailey A, Lord C, et al. Social communication questionnaire. Los Angeles (CA): Western Psychological Services; 2003.

[24] Schopler E, Reichler R, Rochen-Renner B. The Childhood Autism Rating Scale (CARS). Los Angeles (CA): Western Psychological Services; 1988.

[25] Gillam JE. Gillam Autism Rating Scale (GARS). Austin (TX): Tex: Pro-Ed; 1995.

[26] Le Couteur A, Lord C, Rutter M. Autism diagnostic interview-revised. Los Angeles (CA): Western Psychological Services; 2003.

[27] Eaves LC, Wingert HD, Ho HH, et al. Screening for autism spectrum disorders with the social communication questionnaire. J Dev Behav Pediatr 2006;27:95–103.

[28] Snow AV, Lecavalier L. Sensitivity and specificity of the modified checklist for autism in toddlers and the social communication questionnaire in preschoolers suspected of having pervasive developmental disorders. Autism 2008;12:627–44.

[29] Lord C, Risi S, Lambrecht L, et al. The autism diagnostic schedule – generic: a standard measure of social and communication deficits associated with the spectrum of autism. J Autism Dev Disord 2000;30:205–23.

[30] Kanner L. Autistic disturbances of affective contact. Nerv Child 1943;2:217–50.

[31] Bettelheim B. The empty fortress: infantile autism and the birth of self. New York: Free Press; 1967.

[32] Rimland B. Infantile autism: the syndrome and its implications for a neural theory of behavior. New York: Appleton-Century-Crofts; 1964.

[33] Spence MA. The genetics of autism. Curr Opin Pediatr 2001;13:561–5.

[34] Rutter M. Genetic influences and autism. In: Volkmar FR, Paul R, Klim A, et al, editors. Handbook of autism and pervasive developmental disorders. 3rd edition. Hoboken (NJ): John Wiley and Sons, Inc; 2005. p. 425–52.

[35] Croen LA, Najjar DV, Fireman B, et al. Maternal and paternal age and risk of autism spectrum disorders. Arch Pediatr Adolesc Med 2007;161:334–40.

[36] Reichenberg A, Gross R, Weiser M, et al. Advancing paternal age and autism. Arch Gen Psychiatry 2006;63:1026–32.

[37] Bernard S, Enayati A, Redwood L, et al. Autism: a novel form of mercury poisoning. Med Hypotheses 2001;56:462–71.

[38] Bernard S, Enayati A, Roger H, et al. The role of mercury in the pathogenesis of autism. Mol Phys 2001;7:S42–3.

[39] Nelson KB, Bauman ML. Thimerosol and autism? Pediatrics 2003;111:674–9.

[40] Pichichero ME, Cernichiari E, Lopreiato J, et al. Mercury concentrations and metabolism in infants receiving vaccines containing thimerosal: a descriptive study. Lancet 2002;360: 1737–41.

[41] Ball LK, Ball R, Pratt RD. An assessment of thimerosol use in childhood vaccines. Pediatrics 2001;107:1147–54.

[42] Davidson PW, Myers GJ, Weiss B. Mercury exposure and child development outcomes. Pediatrics 2004;113(Suppl 4):1023–9.

[43] Freed GL, Andrea MC, Cowan AE, et al. The process of public policy formulation: the case of thimerosol vaccine. Pediatrics 2002;109:1153–9.

[44] Clarkson TW, Magos L, Myers GJ. The toxicology of mercury – Current exposures and clinical manifestations. N Engl J Med 2003;349:1731–7.

[45] Offit PA. Autism's false prophets: bad science, risky medicine, and the search for a cure. New York: Columbia University Press; 2008.

[46] Parker SK, Schwartz B, Todd J, et al. Thimerasol-containing vaccines and autistic spectrum disorder: a critical review of published original data. Pediatrics 2004;114:793–804.

[47] Madsen KM, Lauritsen MB, Pedersen CB, et al. Thimerosal and the occurrence of autism: negative ecological evidence from Danish population-based data. Pediatrics 2003;112: 604–6.

[48] Fombonne E, Zakarian R, Bennett A, et al. Pervasive developmental disorders in Montreal, Quebec, Canada: prevalence and links with immunization. Pediatrics 2006;118: e139–50.

[49] Thompson WW, Price C, Goodson B, et al. Early thimerasol exposure and neuropsychological outcomes at 7 to 10 years. N Engl J Med 2007;357:1281–92.

[50] Wakefield AJ, Murch SH, Anthony A, et al. Ileal-lymphoid-nodular hyperplasia, non-specific colitis and pervasive-developmental disorder in children. Lancet 1998;351:637–41.

[51] Halsey NA, Hyman SL, Conference Writing Panel. Measles-mumps-rubella vaccine and autistic spectrum disorder: report from the New Challenges in Childhood Immunization

Conference convened in Oak Brook, Illinois, June 12–13, 2000. Pediatrics 2001;107: e84.

[52] Murch SH, Anthony A, Casson DH, et al. Retraction of an interpretation. Lancet 2004;363: 750.

[53] McBrien J, Murphy J, Gill D, et al. Measles outbreak in Dublin. Pediatr Infect Dis J 2003;22: 580–4.

[54] Carvel J. Warning of measles epidemic as risk as cases rise. Available at: http://www.guardian.co.uk/society/2008/nov/29/health-measels-epidemic/print.

[55] Harris G. Measles cases grow in number, and officials blame parents' fear of autism. Available at: http://www.nytimes.com/2008/08/22/health/research/22measles.htm?ref=us.

[56] Rose D. Epidemic fears as MMR jab rates stall. Available at: http://www.timesonline.co.uk/tol/news/health/article4818440.ece.

[57] Walsh F. Measles cases surge to new high. Available at: http://newsvote.bbc.co.uk/2/hi/health/7753210.stm.

[58] Mäkelä A, Nuorti JP, Peltola H. Neurologic disorders after measles-mumps-rubella vaccination. Pediatrics 2002;110:957–63.

[59] Madsen KM, Hviid A, Vestergaard M, et al. A population based study of measles, mumps, and rubella vaccination and autism. N Engl J Med 2002;347:1477–82.

[60] Offit PA, Quarles J, Gerber MA, et al. Addressing parents' concerns: do multiple vaccines overwhelm or weaken the infant's immune system? Pediatrics 2002;109:124–9.

[61] Offit PA, Hackett CJ. Addressing parents concerns: do vaccines cause allergic or autoimmune diseases? Pediatrics 2003;111:653–9.

[62] Parikh RK. Fighting for the reputation of vaccines: lessons from American politics. Pediatrics 2008;121:621–2.

Advances in Pediatrics 56 (2009) 203–218

ADVANCES IN PEDIATRICS

Child Pornography: Legal and Medical Considerations

Carol D. Berkowitz, MD

Department of Pediatrics, Harbor-UCLA Medical Center, David Geffen School of Medicine at UCLA, 1000 West Carson Street Box 437, Torrance, CA 90509, USA

The spectrum of child pornography attracts public notice through newspaper headlines, drawing attention to the sensational and pervasive nature of the problem [1,2]. Child pornography has become a multimillion-dollar business, and the National Center for Missing and Exploited Children (NCMEC) reports that 20% of Internet pornography involves children and that 1 in 5 girls and 1 in 10 boys will be victimized before reaching the age of 18 years [3]. While parents attempt to address the risks to their children and to their neighborhood, the legal and medical communities are also involved in combating the problem. Of note, the issue of child pornography has assumed new dimensions in the age of the Internet [4]. Not only are children at risk for being exploited and photographed, they are also at risk for sexual victimization by predators who, using the Internet, seek them out for their personal sexual gratification.

Child pornography generally refers to images of completely or partially undressed children erotically posed or engaged in overt sexual acts. The legal community deals with issues related to a more precise definition of pornography. In addition, the legal community creates legislation to control pornography, and defines the means to enforce that legislation not only within the United States but also internationally, especially now in an age of "sexual tourism," the travel abroad for purposes of sexual escapades, often involving children [5,6]. The medical community is involved with the assessment and treatment of individuals who have been victimized by their inclusion in the production of pornography, and with assisting investigative agencies in their evaluation, particularly regarding age and sexual maturity of subjects of pornography [7].

THE ROLE OF THE LEGAL COMMUNITY
Definition of pornography
The elusiveness of defining pornography is captured in the oft-quoted 1964 comment by Justice Potter Stewart who stated, when talking about

E-mail address: carolb@pol.net

0065-3101/09/$ – see front matter
doi:10.1016/j.yapd.2009.08.002

obscenity, which is felt to be legally synonymous with hard-core pornography:

> I shall not today attempt to further define the kinds of material I understand to be embraced . . .[b]ut I know it when I see it.

Other terms linked to pornography, each have a slightly different emphasis. Obscenity relates to material that is overtly offensive to the average observer using the usual standards of modesty or decency. The *Miller test* is the United States Supreme Court's test for determining whether speech or other expression can be considered obscene. Obscene material is not covered by the First Amendment to the United States Constitution, which guarantees Freedom of Speech. The Miller test was developed following the 1973 case of *Miller v California*. The Miller test has 3 parts: [8]

> Would the average person, applying contemporary community standards, find the work, taken as a whole, appealing to prurient interest?
> Does the work depict/describe, in a patently offensive way, sexual conduct or excretory functions, specifically defined by applicable state law?
> Does the work, taken as a whole, lack serious literary, artistic, political, or scientific value? (*SLAPS* test).

To be considered obscene, the work must satisfy all 3 conditions. The Miller test allows a community to determine its own standards, rather than imposing any specific national standards, although the relevant community is not defined. Despite what may seem to be a clear legal definition, the Miller test still allows for subjectivity, and therefore may sometimes seem to be applied in a paradoxic and arbitrary manner. The community standard notion is seriously challenged by the Internet because material published on a Web server can be read by a person residing elsewhere. Which standards should apply? This matter is currently under consideration in the pending case *United States v Extreme Associates*; the District Court hearing this complex case ruled that federal antiobscenity laws were unconstitutional and that individuals had the right to view pornographic materials under the right to privacy. The case was rejected by the Supreme Court and referred back to the District Court where it was initially heard [9].

Indecent is another term that is used, and is even less precisely defined as something that is morally offensive, immodest, or lewd. Erotica is material that serves a sexual purpose when viewed within a particular context for a given individual. Nudity and erotica may represent one end of the spectrum of sexually explicit material, and illustrate how difficult a precise definition is.

Legislative approach to child pornography

International, as well as federal and state laws attempt to operationally define and regulate the distribution of pornographic material, specifically material involving children. Although the term child pornography has sometimes been restricted to prepubescent children, the expanded legal definition of "child pornography" currently extends to postpubescent adolescents up to the age of 18 years. Laws similar to United States federal laws exist in most countries in the world. Table 1 summarizes the evolution of child pornography laws in the United States. In brief, the 1970s witnessed a plethora of monthly magazines (estimated at 260 different magazines each month) containing child pornography [10]. In 1978, the Protection of Children against Sexual Exploitation Act was passed. In 1984, the act was amended to increase the age of protection of victims from 16 years to 18 years, increase penalties, and penalize the distribution of such material regardless of whether the material reached the legal definition of obscene. In 1986, the Child Sexual Abuse and Pornography Act was broadened to include transporting minors interstate or intercountry for purposes of pornography, advertising child pornography, and securing participation of a child for purposes of child pornography. In the same year, the Child Abuse Victim's Rights Act was passed, which defined civil liability for personal injuries incurred as a result of the violation of child pornography laws (within 6 years or by age 21 years). The Child Protection and Obscenity Enforcement Act, passed in 1988, prohibited the sale or receipt of child pornography on a computer, mandated that photographers maintain records of their subjects, and prohibited the sale and purchase of children for the purpose of child pornography.

Over the years, there have been challenges to the constitutionality of these laws, citing protection by the First Amendment. In *Roth v United States* in 1957 [11] and, as noted earlier, in *Miller v California* in 1973, the Supreme Court ruled that obscenity was not protected by the First Amendment. Although cases still challenge this decision, the Supreme Court in *New York v Ferber* [12] in 1982 ruled that child pornography, even if not obscene, was never protected by the First Amendment, and that states had the right to define what

Table 1
Legislative approach to child pornography

1978: Protection of Children against Sexual Exploitation Act: up to age 16 years
1984: Amended 1978 Act. Increased age of protection to 18 years; increased the penalties; didn't need to meet the legal definition of obscene
1986: Child Sexual Abuse and Pornography Act: dealt with transporting minors for the purpose of pornography
1986: Child Abuse Victim's Rights Act: Established civil liability so child could sue (within 6 years of the event or up to age 21 years)
1988: Child Protection and Obscenity Enforcement Act: Prohibited sale and receipt of child pornography on a computer; mandated that photographers maintain records of their subjects; prohibited the sale and buying of children for the purpose of child pornography
1996: Telecommunications Act: Allowed federal prosecution of obscenity on the Internet; overturned in 1997
1996: Child Pornography Act: Doesn't have to be an actual child, if the image was that of a child
2003: PROTECT Act: Multipurpose law that addresses prior legal concerns

constituted child pornography (eg, age of individuals, activity depicted), and to penalize individuals for possession of child pornography.

As a result of this ruling giving states the authority to oversee the investigation and prosecution of child pornography, penalties may vary from state to state, depending on the age of the individual portrayed within the photographs. For instance, the potential sentence for an individual convicted of possession or distribution of pornographic material varies depending on whether the portrayed individual is younger than 12 years, younger than 16 years, or younger than 18 years, and depending on the state. The age considered representative of child pornography similarly has varied among different countries.

Legal consideration regarding the Internet and child pornography

The Internet has opened up an entirely new area for the pornography industry. Pornography sites have the highest number of hits and generate the greatest amount of revenue. The amount of on-line materials is enormous. In 1995, Georgetown Law Review reported that over 450,620 pornographic images or animations were downloaded by consumers 6.4 million times, and that 83.5% of Usenet digitalized images were pornographic [13]. It is estimated that the number of child pornography images on the Internet has increased 1500% since 1997. The US Department of Justice estimates that there are more than 1 million pornographic images of children on the Internet and that 200 new images are posted every day. Much of the increase has been attributed to the ease of digital photography. Internet images have replaced the printed materials that were previously so ubiquitous. The NCMEC estimates that 58% of children used in child pornography are prepubescent and 6% are infants [3].

Attempts to regulate the distribution of material over the Internet have been fraught with claims of First Amendment infringement. The Telecommunications Act of 1996, which allowed federal prosecution of obscenity, was eventually overturned by a Supreme Court ruling in 1997. This reversal followed the determination in 1996 by US District Judge Stewart Dalzell: "The Internet may fairly be regarded as a never-ending worldwide conversation. The government may not, through the CDA (Communications Decency Act), interrupt that conversation. As the most participatory form of mass speech yet developed, the Internet deserves the highest protection from government intrusion [14]."

The PROTECT (Prosecutorial Remedies and Other Tools to end the Exploitation of Children Today) Act of 2003 again addressed some of these concerns. This law is multipurpose, not just addressing the issue of child pornography, and mandates the following: [5]

> Provides for mandatory life imprisonment of sex offenders against a minor if the offender has had a prior conviction of abuse against a minor, with some exceptions
>
> Establishes a program to obtain criminal history background checks for volunteer organizations

Authorizes wiretapping and monitoring of other communications in all cases related to child abuse or kidnapping

Eliminates statutes of limitations for child abduction or child abuse

Bars pretrial release of persons charged with specified offenses against or involving children

Assigns a national AMBER alert coordinator

Implements Suzanne's Law, named for a missing college student from the University of New York at Albany, by eliminating waiting periods before law enforcement agencies will investigate reports of missing persons aged 18 to 21 years. The reports are also filed with National Crime Information Center (NCIC)

Prohibits computer-generated child pornography when (B) such visual depiction is a computer image or computer-generated image that is, or appears virtually indistinguishable from that of a minor engaging in sexually explicit conduct; (as amended by 1466A for Section 2256(8) (B) of title 18, United States Code); (virtual child pornography)

Prohibits drawings, sculptures, and pictures of such drawing and sculptures depicting minors in actions or situations that meet the Miller test of being obscene, or are engaged in sex acts that are deemed to meet the same obscene condition

Maximum sentence of 5 years for possession, 10 years for distribution

Authorizes fines and/or imprisonment for up to 30 years for United States citizens or residents who engage in illicit sexual conduct abroad. Illicit sexual conduct as defined by the PROTECT Act refers to commercial sex with anyone under 18 years of age, and any sex with persons under 16 years of age. The law, as regards US citizens or residents, supersedes the laws of the foreign country, so that the US citizen or resident could be tried for a crime even if it occurred in a country that did not prohibit noncommercial sex with individuals under the age of 16 years.

The PROTECT Act specifically prohibits illustrations depicting child pornography even if those illustrations are computer-generated images also referred to as virtual child pornography. Thus the PROTECT Act reverses the ruling of the Supreme Court, noted above, which declared the provisions against virtual child pornography noted in the Child Pornography Prevention Act of 1996 as unconstitutional. The PROTECT Act includes the requirement of showing obscenity as defined by the Miller Test, an element not included in the Child Pornography Prevention Act of 1996.

THE ROLE OF THE MEDICAL COMMUNITY IN CHILD PORNOGRAPHY

Determining the age of individuals portrayed in child pornography

As a pediatric health care provider, one may be asked to assess the age of individuals in confiscated pornographic images and materials. Multiple agencies including the US Postal Service, US Customs, the Federal Bureau of Investigation, and local law enforcement departments may be involved in the investigation of child pornography cases, and thus may ask for assistance in the assessment of such materials. Since 2003, ICE (US Immigration and Customs Enforcement), under the Department of Homeland Security, has been delegated to investigate cases involving child pornography, particularly when cases involve sexual tourism or child exploitation overseas.

In some cases, the assessment is straightforward because the individuals are obviously prepubescent children. In one case with which the author was involved, the judge excused the author from testifying, stating: "I don't need a pediatrician to tell me these are children." Even before puberty when changes in secondary sexual characteristics evolve, there are several other recognizable characteristics that vary with age in prepubertal children. Body proportions change as a child develops. An infant's head makes up about one-third of the body (infant body equivalent to 3.5 heads). By age 3 years, the head is slightly less than 25% of the body (child's body made up of 4.5 heads). By age 6 years it is slightly less than 20% of the total body (6-year-old body made up of 5.33 heads). By age 9 years the head is about one-sixth of the body (9-year-old body made up of 6 heads), and by adulthood, age 12 years, the head is only 16% of the body (6.33 heads make up the body) [15]. The upper to lower body ratio similarly changes over time: the upper to lower segment ratio is 1.7:1 in infancy; 1.3:1 in children 3 to 4 years old, and 1:1 in older children and adults. If teeth are apparent in the images, their presence may also help with age assignment. Secondary dentition, teeth that are larger than primary dentition and scalloped, begin erupting about age 7 years. Hip broadening in females may be another clue to the entrance into puberty. Height may also be a clue if the photographs include common objects against which the stature can be gauged or the victim is standing next to the alleged perpetrator whose height can be determined [7].

Assessing the age of peri- or pubertal individuals is more challenging. Some of the photographs are apparently from an earlier time period and from different cultures. Some of these photographs are in black and white, and individuals are dressed in styles commonly seen in the 1970s. It may be difficult to pinpoint the precise time period involved (1960s or 1970s) and hence to address the mean age of puberty at the time the photographs were taken. Such older images were more commonly printed in magazines, and often appeared repeatedly from month to month, but are seen less frequently on computer-posted sites.

The basis for making the determination of the age and maturation of peri- and pubertal individuals relates to the classic work reported by Marshall and Tanner who, based on cross-sectional studies using photographs, chronicled the progression of physical growth and sexual development from childhood to adulthood [16–19]. Tanner described his data as well as that of others and noted that puberty progressed in a predicable manner, although the age at a given level of sexual maturation varied between individuals. The focus of the study was to help in the assessment of the pubertal development of an individual and to determine if such development was advanced, delayed, or age-appropriate. The highlights of pubertal development for girls involved the development of the breast and the acquisition of pubic hair. The prepubertal girl (Tanner 1) was characterized by the absence of breast tissue and pubic hair. Tanner 1 boys lacked pubic hair, and had small (1–1.5 cm) testes and a small phallus. Tanner and Marshall never commented on the appearance of the hymen or labia minora in females.

In 1969, Huffman [20] reported on the effects of estrogen on female genitalia and divided these effects into 4 stages: stage 1, postnatal regression (0–2 months); stage 2, early childhood (2 months to 7 years); stage 3, late childhood (7–11 years); stage 4, premenarche (11–12 years). The effect of estrogen on the hymen and external genitalia has been further appreciated with additional publications related to the assessment of girls for physical evidence of child sexual abuse [21–23]. When available, close-up images clearly delineating the genitalia (including the hymen) are most helpful when determining the age of girls in some pornographic images.

In 1995, Herman-Giddens and Bourdony refined and further characterized pubertal development in girls in their monograph on Sexual Maturity Rating in Girls based on an American Academy of Pediatrics PROS (Pediatric Research in Office Settings) study [24,25]. The key features regarding breast development as noted in the PROS studies are as follows: change in contour of the areola, separation of the contour of the areola and nipple, and movement of the breasts from lateral to a more medial position. Pubic hair progression was similarly categorized. The study did not define the age or average age of individuals at various stages of breast development. The monograph is a mini-atlas, and the photos that are included are useful for purposes of comparison with the images being assessed.

The PROS study on the pubertal development of boys is not yet complete, but will assess development across ethnic and racial lines for individuals between the ages of 6 and 16 years residing in the United States. Male pubertal development is characterized by enlargement of the testes, enlargement of the penis, and progressive development of pubic hair [19]. There are additional changes, such as linear growth, muscular development, facial and axillary hair, and voice deepening, but these changes are not always apparent in images nor are they usually considered when assessing the age of an individual in a photograph.

Stages of pubertal development are variously referred to as Tanner stages, sexual maturity rating (SMR), and sexual maturity index (SMI). More specifically, breast development may be designated as B1 to B5 (for the sexual maturity of the breast); pubic hair as PH 1 to 5, and genital stage as G 1 to 5.

Ethnic considerations in pubertal development

In looking at a photograph, the assessor will comment on the degree of sexual maturity, and then attempt to assign an age based on secondary sexual characteristics if present, while taking into account other morphologic findings. Assigning an age to an individual is therefore contingent on information regarding the age of pubertal development in that individual's population or racial or ethnic group. There have been numerous studies over the past 40 years examining the age of puberty in different parts of the world [26–70].

Stathopulu and colleagues [7], using a review of the literature, examined the average age of menarche in girls from Southeast Asia. Variation in the age of menarche was associated with factors such as socioeconomic status, maternal nutrition during pregnancy, and nutrition during childhood. Age of onset of pubertal development was more difficult to assess, and variability was noted. It appeared that at least 10% of Chinese girls had achieved an SMR of 2 for breast development (B2) before the age of 8 years. The investigators also noted that the secular trend for earlier onset of menarche had slowed down. The median age of menarche in London, England in 1969 was 13.0 years; by 1999, the age was 12.9 years, younger, though significantly not different when determining the age of girls in pornographic photographs. Overall, the investigators concluded that 97.5% of Southeast Asian girls achieve B2 breast development by age 13.7, and if breast development was below B2, one could conclude with 97.5% certainty that the individual was under that age (ie, younger than 13.7 years).

There is now a plethora of studies addressing the age of menarche throughout the world, and though there are some differences, the mean age of menarche seems to be about 12.2 ± 1.2 years [66]. The impact of other health considerations has been noted in some studies. Abolfotouh [71] reported a delay in pubertal maturation in blind and deaf male students in Saudi Arabia. He specifically noted that only 79% of blind students and 70% of deaf students had achieved a sexual maturity rating of 4 or 5 by age 16 years. There were no comparison groups of normally sighted or hearing students to observe how divergent this was from the ethnic population with which he was working. Abolfotouh concludes, however, that blind and deaf children attain sexual maturity at an older age than the reference population.

Although there are some data suggesting a further decrease in the age of puberty in the United States in recent years, the trend seems to be toward earlier breast development but not menarche, and this trend may be related to the increasing incidence of child hood obesity [72]. From a forensic perspective, a trend toward earlier puberty would lead to an overestimation of the age of children in the images, rather than an underestimation (eg, estimating a 9-year-old girl with B4 to be 16 years old).

In 1998, Rosenbloom and Tanner [73], in a letter published in *Pediatrics*, criticized the practice of assigning age-based sexual maturity rating as an "illegitimate use" of the data. Detective James F. McLaughlin [74], in a letter to Dr Rosenbloom, noted that experts did not use the Tanner Scale in isolation but rather in the context of rendering an expert opinion based on "knowledge, skill, experience, training, or education." Rosenbloom responded to Detective McLaughlin that indeed such assessments were not simply related to Tanner rating [75]. The California Court of Appeals, in *People v Thomas Joseph Kurey*, determined that testimony regarding age using the Tanner scale was admissible

[76]. Defense attorneys, however, continue to use the 1998 letter of Tanner and Rosenbloom to question the validity of the age assignment, and expert consultants should therefore be familiar with both the medical literature and the legal opinions related to these discussions. The numerous studies defining the age range of pubertal development around much of the world have to some extent addressed the criticism of Rosenbloom and Tanner, and have led to a purposeful avoidance of using the term "Tanner staging" and use of the replacement terms SMR or SMI, or the designation with the specific ratings B, PH, G for breast, public hair, and genitals.

Validity and reliability of age assessments

In 1997, Berkowitz and colleagues [77] reported on the ability of 3 pediatricians who served as consultants on aging children to each examine confiscated pornographic photos, and assign an SMI and age to the image. The 3 pediatricians (2 with expertise in adolescent medicine) reviewed 33 confiscated photographs involving 44 nude children and adolescents, and assigned an age and sexual maturity rating to each individual. The photographs, some in color and others in black and white, included males and females. Results showed a high degree of agreement among the evaluators, with a greater degree of agreement on male subjects. In 5 of 25 (20%), all 3 evaluators agreed on the exact same age; in 19 of 25 (76%), evaluators agreed on the age within 2 years. Evaluator 3 generally judged girls to be 2 years younger than either of the other 2 evaluators, who agreed on the age of female subjects within 1 year in 13 of 18 (72%). There was also a high degree of agreement on the SMI within 1 stage, as follows: males, pubic hair 19 of 22 (86%); genitalia 14 of 22 (64%); females, breast 9 of 18 (50%); pubic hair 12 of 16 (75%). Different evaluators often assigned the same age despite disparate SMI, because features other than SMI were used to determine age. The study concluded that there was a high degree of agreement in assigning age and SMI to both male and female subjects in sexually explicit photographs.

Example of the application of the assessment process

When photographs are assessed, each image should be specifically identified. Usually computer files are stored under unique titles and images are specifically labeled. These labels can serve to identify the image being evaluated. If printed copies are presented, they can be labeled directly on the photograph or on the back of the photograph, initialed, and dated, to maintain a chain of evidence showing that the specific image was reviewed. Such photographs are often presented to the expert in court with a query: "Have you seen this photograph before? Are these your initials?"

It is helpful to keep personal notes from the review because photographs are kept by the agency seeking the consultation, and are generally not available at the time a letter or report is generated. It is equally helpful to note any unique features of the individual that might serve to verify who was in the photograph and to also trigger a recollection for the examiner. For instance, the presence of tattoos, unique body piercing, or physical features can be recorded (eg, an individual with prominent thoracic tattoos in a weblike pattern). The number of photographs or videos reviewed in a single session may range from several to several hundred, though the same individual is frequently present in multiple images. It is therefore often difficult to independently remember the details of the photographs without one's notes.

It is also important to carefully describe the physical features, particularly relating to the pubertal development, and to not simply note the SMI (eg, scrotum not thin or pendulous; sparse pubic hair 1–2). Separate data are recorded on each victim, noting if the same victim appears in multiple photographs as would be evidenced by the same appearance and distinctive features of the individual. Usually the final assessment is determined by multiple different images. It is also appropriate to comment on whether the absence of pubic hair relates to the hair having been shaved, often done to make the individual appear younger. Sometimes there are images in which individuals have pubic hair in some but not all of the images.

The age is then estimated based on the SMI published for individuals from that ethnic background [67,68]. For instance, in a case involving 7 males from Southeast Asia, some victims were felt to have adult (SMI 5) appearance based on their genitalia and pubic hair. Their age was judged to be adult (older than 18 years) although one of the victims had been located and was actually only 14 years old. Published data note the mean age for a Southeast Asian male with PH 4 ranges from 13.6 to 15 years depending on the study. In most studies the standard deviation is approximately 1.5 years. Using the upper mean age noted, 15 years, 84% (1 standard deviation above the mean) of individuals would have achieved PH 4 by 16.5 years and 97.7% by age 18 years. One could conclude with reasonable medical certainty that Southeast Asian males with PH 3 are younger than 18 years. This type of analysis has proved helpful in the evaluation of cases, particularly those involving children from other countries, and has been accepted in both federal and state courts.

PROTECTING CHILDREN FROM SEXUAL EXPLOITATION
International efforts to combat child pornography

International efforts exist to help identify the victims of child pornography and child prostitution. The National Child Victims Identification Program preserves the world's largest database of child pornography. This database is maintained in the United States Department of Justice. When cases involve sexual tourism—that is, child prostitution—in addition to having images, the victims may be located and their age established. Correlating the professed age of the victim and the estimated age based on the photographs helps improve the diagnostic skills of the consultant and also helps corroborate the statements of the child as to their age. In general, when victims of sexual tourism are transported to the United States to testify, they are not subjected to a separate physical examination. Often, not all victims seen in confiscated photographs can be located [6]. Victims can usually self-identify their own images.

There is a unified international effort to prevent child pornography. The effort initiated in 2002 and referred to as The Dublin Plan is funded in part through a $1 million donation from Microsoft [78]. The Dublin Plan is a global campaign against child pornography, which has created an international monitoring and oversight system. A significant focus of the plan is to develop and promote systems for identifying victims of child pornography. The plan attempts to enhance the capacity of law enforcement to investigate and prosecute child pornography cases. The plan includes international efforts to craft model legislation and foster consistency of laws between different countries. Lastly, the plan strives to increase public awareness of the problem.

Despite the cooperative efforts of Interpol, the US Department of Justice, and other governments, it is estimated that less than 1% of children in pornographic images can be located.

Impact of child pornography on children

Children suffer on multiple levels as a result of child pornography, even if they are not involved in the production of the images. First, there is a significant link between the possession of child pornography and child molestation [79]. One report noted that 85% of individuals prosecuted for child pornography were also child molesters. For many pedophiles, collecting child pornography becomes an obsession, and serves to link individuals together through sharing materials and experiences. Child pornography serves to sexually stimulate individuals with a propensity to engage in sex with children, and to normalize the activity in their minds [10].

Children may be exposed to child pornography in an effort to engage them in subsequent sexual abuse. The images serve to both arouse the child and to normalize sex between children and adults. This process is referred to as "child grooming."

Children who are photographed are almost always sexually abused also, and are at risk for both the medical and psychological consequences of the abuse [80]. These children also experience humiliation when their images continue to be circulated worldwide. The personal devastation of the experience has been described by victims of child pornography during the Congressional hearing on the subject [81].

Caring for victims of sexual exploitation

When children or adolescents who have been sexually exploited are identified, they should undergo a comprehensive medical as well as psychological assessment. The medical assessment must include a detailed history related to preexisting medical conditions as well as any symptoms that may be related to sexual abuse. A menstrual history is appropriate, as is a careful history related to genitourinary symptoms or surgeries. The presence of a vaginal or urethral discharge suggests the possibility of a sexually transmitted infection (STI). Stool patterns as well as episodes of hematochezia should be noted. Fecal incontinence may result from injury to the rectum during a sexual assault, or to the emotional trauma following the event. Information about ano-genitourinary symptoms is not only relevant to the medical care of the individual but also has implications from a forensic perspective, validating the history or delineating sequelae from any sexual assault. Human immunodeficiency virus (HIV) should always be considered, especially in an individual diagnosed with another STI or with any symptom suggestive of HIV/AIDS.

A complete physical examination should be included in the assessment. The examination must include an evaluation of the anogenital area. The anogenital examination may reveal evidence of antecedent trauma, or of an STI including human papilloma virus or syphilis. The presence of scars or disruptions should be noted, mainly for forensic considerations. However, the anogenital examination is often normal in sexually abused children, and the absence of abnormal findings does not preclude prior abuse [82].

Most children who have been exploited benefit from psychological counseling, even if they seem well-adjusted and functioning. Group counseling often offers the benefit of interacting with other youngsters who have had similar experiences. Such interactions help address the concern of the child or adolescent that they are alone or unique in their traumatic event.

It is equally important to be vigilant concerning the long-term sequelae of sexual exploitation. The primary physician is in a unique position to monitor the health of the patient over time. In a series of now classic articles, Felitti [83,84], in association with the Centers for Disease Control and Prevention, clearly delineated the long-term consequences of such experiences. The work, performed as part of the Adverse Childhood Experiences (ACE) study, has involved over 50,000 adult subjects. Individuals who had experienced neglect, household dysfunction, and abuse, including sexual abuse, are at increased risk for depression, suicide attempts, somatization, smoking, alcoholism, illicit drug use, obesity, and high-level promiscuity. There was also evidence that organic diseases such as coronary heart disease and chronic obstructive lung disease are associated with ACEs. It is hoped that early detection, intervention, and counseling may reduce the heightened medical and psychological risks from even the most adverse childhood experience.

Counseling families about the risk of the Internet

In addition to serving as a valuable resource for information and access to a host of resources, the Internet has served as a "superhighway" for the dissemination of pornographic materials. Throughout the world, Internet cafés serve as a site for viewing pornographic materials by youth, particularly in countries such as India, Pakistan, and Senegal. Again, viewing such material desensitizes youth to sexual matters and facilitates the engagement in adult activities; it also increases the risk of child exploitation, especially in developing countries.

Even in industrialized nations, the Internet has served as a mechanism by which children may be enticed into sexual encounters, both real and virtual. Pediatricians should counsel parents about the potential for exposure of their youngsters to pornography and to predators on the Internet. There are numerous strategies that parents can access to reduce the risk of such exposure

[85,86]. Parents can use filters that may be purchased through the server or by the client. Parents may also install software to allow them to track Internet use. There are multiple web-based resources for parents related to Internet safety. The Federal Bureau of Investigation site is replete with general information and specifics on what to do if one's child is being engaged in inappropriate sexual advances through the Internet, telephone, or mail [87]. The American Academy of Pediatrics also has numerous free resources that parents can access to assist in making the Internet a safe and educational place for their children [88].

SUMMARY

The pediatric health care provider has an important role in the investigation of cases of child pornography and child exploitation. Familiarity with normal child physical development, particularly during puberty, allows the clinician to render an opinion about the degree of sexual maturation and offer an approximation of the child's age. Recent collaboration between nations has facilitated the apprehension and prosecution of suspected offenders. The clinician can also advocate for legislation aimed at protecting children, and assist families about the safe use of the Internet.

Acknowledgments

The author thanks Dr. Carole Jenny for sharing information as well as her extensive bibliography related to pubertal development of children around the world.

References

[1] Clair Stacy St. 'Worst imaginable' child porn. Daily Herald Thursday, March 16, 2006;c7.

[2] Wendy Koch. Child porn suspects include a teacher. USA Today March 17, 2006;3A.

[3] Available at: www.missingkids.com.

[4] Kurt Eichenwald. From their own online world, pedophiles extend their reach. NY Times (Print) August 26, 2006;A1:A14.

[5] PROTECT Act of 2003. Available at: www.usdoj.gov/opa/pr/2003/April/03_ag_266. Accessed August 31, 2009.

[6] United States v Michael Joseph Pepe. Available at: http://www.usdoj.gov/usao/cac/pressroom/pr2008/074.html. Accessed August 31, 2009.

[7] Stathopulu E, Hulse JA, Canning D. Difficulties with age estimation of Internet images of south-east Asian girls. Child Abuse Rev 2003;12:46–57.

[8] Miller v California 413 U.S. 15. Available at: http://caselaw.lp.findlaw.com/scripts. 1973. Accessed August 31, 2009.

[9] United States v Extreme Associates. Available at: http://www.ca3.uscourts.gov/opinarch/051555p.pdf. Accessed August 31, 2009.

[10] Watson DE. Child pornography flourishes on the internet. NCIS Bulletin 1998;II:16–26.

[11] Roth v United States. Available at: http://laws.findlaw.com/us/354/476.html.

[12] New York v Ferber. Available at: http://laws.findlaw.com/us/458/747.html.

[13] Rimm M. Marketing pornography on the information superhighway: a survey of 917,410 images, descriptions, short stories, and animations downloaded 8.5 million times by consumers in over 2000 cities in forty countries, provinces and territories. Georgetown Law Review 1995;83(5):1849–73.

[14] Available at: http://news.cnet.com/2009-1023-21448.html. Accessed August 31, 2009.

[15] Raynes J. A Step-by-step guide to drawing the figure. Cincinnati (OH): F & W Media, Inc; 1997. p. 58.

[16] Marshall WA, Tanner JM. Variations in pattern of pubertal changes in girls. Arch Dis Child 1969;44:291–303.

[17] Marshall WA, Tanner JM. Variations in the pattern of pubertal changes in boys. Arch Dis Child 1970;45:13–23.

[18] Tanner JM, Whitehouse RH, Marubini E, et al. The adolescent growth spurt of boys and girls of the Harpenden growth study. Ann Hum Biol 1976;3:109–26.

[19] Tanner JM. Growth at adolescence. 2nd edition. Blackwell Science, Ltd; 1978. p. 28–54.

[20] Huffman JW. Principles of pediatric gynecology. Obstet Gynecol Annu 1979;3: 407–24.

[21] Berenson A, Heger A, Andrews S. Appearance of the hymen in newborns. Pediatrics 1991;87:458–65.

[22] Berenson AB, Heger AH, Hayes JM, et al. Appearance of the hymen in prepubertal girls. Pediatrics 1992;89:387–94.

[23] Chadwick DL, Berkowitz CD, Kerns D, et al. Color atlas of child sexual abuse. Chicago: Year Book Medical Publisher, Inc; 1989.

[24] Herman-Giddens ME, Bourdony CJ. Assessment of sexual maturity stages in girls. Pediatric Research in Office Settings. Elk Grove Village (IL): American Academy of Pediatrics; 1995.

[25] Herman-Giddens ME, Slora EJ, Wasserman RC, et al. Secondary sexual characteristics in young girls seen in office practice: a study from the Pediatric Research in Office Settings Network. Pediatrics 1997;99:505–12.

[26] Agarwal DK, Agarwal KN, Upadhyay SK, et al. Physical and sexual growth pattern of affluent Indian children from 5 to 18 years of age. Indian Pediatr 1992;29:1203–82.

[27] Antony TP, Sarasa G, Cherian G, et al. Sexual and physical growth in Kerala boys. J Assoc Physicians India 1992;40:669–70.

[28] Ayatollahi SM, Dowlatabadi E, Ayatollahi SA. Age at menarche in Iran. Ann Hum Biol 2002;29:355–62.

[29] Bai KI, Vijayalakshmi B. Sexual maturation of Indian girls in Andhra Pradesh (South India). Hum Biol 1973;45:695–707.

[30] Belmaker E. Sexual maturation of Jerusalem schoolgirls and its association with socioeconomic factors and ethnic group. Ann Hum Biol 1982;9:321–8.

[31] Bhargava SK, Duggal S, Ramanujacharyula TK, et al. Pattern of pubertal changes and their interrelationship in boys. Indian Pediatr 1979;16(10):849–53.

[32] Bhargava SK, Duggal S, Ramanujacharyulu TK, et al. Pubertal changes and their interrelationship in Indian girls. Indian Pediatr 1980;17:657–65.

[33] Bielicki T, Koniarek J, Malina RM. Interrelationships among certain measures of growth and maturation rate in boys during adolescence. Ann Hum Biol 1984;11:201–10.

[34] Buckler JM, Wild J. Longitudinal study of height and weight at adolescence. Arch Dis Child 1987;62:1224–32.

[35] Chumlea WE, Schubert CM, Roche AF, et al. Age at menarche and racial comparisons in US girls. Pediatrics 2003;111:110–3.

[36] Engelhardt L, Willers B, Pelz L. Sexual maturation in East German girls. Acta Paediatr 1995;84:1362–5.

[37] Flugg D, Largo RH, Prader A. Menstrual patterns in adolescent Swiss girls: a longitudinal study. Ann Hum Biol 1984;11(6):495–508.

[38] Hafez AS, Salem SI, Cole TJ, et al. Sexual maturation and growth pattern in Egyptian boys. Ann Hum Biol 1981;8:461–7.

[39] Hagg U, Karlberg J, Taranger J. The timing of secondary sex characters and their relationship to the pubertal maximum of linear growth in girls. Swed Dent J 1991;15(6):271–8.

[40] Hesketh T, Ding QJ, Tomkins A. Growth status and menarche in urban and rural China. Ann Hum Biol 2002;29:348–52.

[41] Huen KF, Leung SS, Lau JT, et al. Secular trend in the sexual maturation of southern Chinese girls. Acta Paediatr 1997;86(10):1121–4.

[42] Jauratanasirikul S, Lebel L. Ages at thelarche and menarche: study in southern Thai school-girls. J Med Assoc Thai 1995;78:517–20.

[43] Katiyar GP, Sehgal D, Khare BB, et al. Physical growth characteristics of upper socio-economic adolescent boys of Varanasi. Indian Pediatr 1985;22:915–22.

[44] Kaul KK, Sundaram KR, Rajput VJ, et al. Influence of socio-economic deprivation on physical and sexual growth during adolescence in school and college boys. Indian J Med Res 1982;75:624–31.

[45] Largo RH, Prader A. Pubertal development in Swiss boys. Helv Paediatr Acta 1983;38: 211–28.

[46] Largo RH, Prader A. Pubertal development in Swiss girls. Helv Paediatr Acta 1983;38: 229–43.

[47] Lee MM, Chang KS, Chan MM. Sexual maturation of Chinese girls in Hong Kong. Pediatrics 1963;32:389–98.

[48] Lee PA. Normal ages of pubertal events among American males and females. J Adolesc Health Care 1980;1:26–9.

[49] Low WD, Kung LS, Leong JC. Secular trend in the sexual maturation of Chinese girls. Hum Biol 1982;54:539–51.

[50] Mahachoklertwattana P, Suthutvoravut U, Charoenkiatkul S, et al. Earlier onset of pubertal maturation in Thai girls. J Med Assoc Thai 2002;85(suppl 4):S1127–34.

[51] Neyzi O, Alp H, Orhon A. Sexual maturation in Turkish girls. Ann Hum Biol 1975;2(1):49–60.

[52] Papadimitriou A, Stephanou N, Papantzimas K, et al. Sexual maturation of Greek boys. Ann Hum Biol 2002;29:105–8.

[53] Prabhakar AK, Sundaram KR, Ramanujacharyulu TK, et al. Influence of socio-economic factors on the age at the appearance of different puberty signs. Indian J Med Res 1972;60:789–92.

[54] Prader A, Largo RH, Wolf C. Timing of pubertal growth and maturation in the first Zurich longitudinal growth study. Acta Paediatr Hung 1984;25:155–9.

[55] Qamra SR, Mehta S, Deodhar SD. A study of relation between physical growth and sexual maturity in girls—V. Indian Pediatr 1991;28:265–72.

[56] Roede MJ, Van Wieringen JC. Growth diagrams, 1980. Tijdschr Soc Gezondheidsz 1985;63:1–34.

[57] Singhi S, Lall KB, Gurnani M, et al. Age of appearance of secondary sex characters in Ajmer school children. Indian J Pediatr 1982;49(399):547–52.

[58] Spurr GB, Reina JC, Barac-Nieto M. Marginal malnutrition in school aged Colombian boys: anthropometry and maturation. Am J Clin Nutr 1983;37:119–32.

[59] Taranger J, Engstrom I, Lichtenstein H, et al. VI. Somotac pubertal development. Acta Paediatr Scand Suppl 1976;258:121–35.

[60] Thomas F, Renaud F, Guegan J, et al. International variability of ages at menarche and meno-pause: patterns and main determinants. Hum Biol 2001;73:271–90.

[61] Tripathi AM, Perierra P, Khare BB, et al. Development of sexual characteristics in upper so-cio-economic girls. Indian Pediatr 1985;22:883–9.

[62] Villarreal SF, Martorell R, Mendoza P. Sexual maturation of Mexican-American adolescents. Am J Hum Biol 1989;1:87–95.

[63] Waaler PE, Thorsen T, Stoa KF, et al. Studies in normal male puberty. Acta Paediatr Scand Suppl 1974;249:1–36.

[64] Wheeler MD. Physical changes of puberty. Endocrinol Metab Clin North Am 1991;20: 1–14.

[65] Willers B, Engelhardt L, Pelz L. Sexual maturation in East German boys. Acta Paediatr 1996;84:785–8.

[66] Whincup PH, Gilg JA, Cook DG, et al. Age of menarche in contemporary British teenagers: survey of girls born between 1982 and 1986. BMJ 2001;322:1095–6.

[67] Wong GW, Leung SS, Law WY, et al. Secular trend in the sexual maturation of southern Chinese boys. Acta Paediatr 1996;85:620–1.

[68] Boon WH, Woon F. Anthropometric studies on Singapore children: III: pubertal studies on Singapore children. J Singapore Paediatr Soc 1977;19:217–32.

[69] World Health Organization Task Force on Adolescent Reproductive Health. World Health Organization multicenter study on menstrual and ovulatory patterns in adolescent girls. II. Longitudinal study of menstrual patterns in the early postmenarcheal period, duration of bleeding episodes and menstrual cycles. J Adolesc Health 1986;7:236–44.

[70] Wyshak G, Frisch RE. Evidence for a secular trend in age of menarche. N Engl J Med 1982;306:1033–5.

[71] Abolfotouh MA. Growth and sexual maturation of blind and deaf male students in Abha City, Saudi Arabia. Ann Saudi Med 2000;20:447–9.

[72] Slyper AH. The pubertal timing controversy in the USA, and a review of possible advance in timing of puberty. Clin Endocrinol 2006;65:1–8.

[73] Rosenbloom AL, Tanner JM. Misuse of tanner puberty stages to estimate chronologic age. Pediatrics 1998;102:1494.

[74] McLaughlin JF. City of Keene New Hampshire Police Department. Letter to Dr. Arlan Rosenbloom, December 16, 1998.

[75] Rosenbloom AL. Letter to Detective McLaughlin, January 21, 1999.

[76] People v Thomas Joseph Kurey (2001) DJDAR 4173. Available at: www.courtinfo.ca.gov/opinions/archive/B141119.pdf. Accessed August 31, 2009.

[77] Berkowitz CD, Johnson RL, Rimsza ME. Child pornography: an assessment of subject sexual maturity index and age. Ambul Child Health 1997;3:220.

[78] Available at: www.microsoft.com/presspass/press/2004/apr04/04–22ICMECGlobal) PR.asp. Accessed August 31, 2009.

[79] Nutter DE, Kearns ME. Patterns of exposure to sexually explicit material among sex offenders, child molesters, and controls. J Sex Marital Ther 1993;19:77–85.

[80] Rubin D, Feinstein JA, Berkowitz CD. Medical and psychological sequelae of child abuse and neglect. In: Reece RM, Christian C, editors. Child abuse: medical diagnosis and management. 3rd edition. Elk Grove Village (IL): American Academy of Pediatrics; 2008. p. 853–75.

[81] Brochman J. Child sex as internet fare, through the eyes of a victim. NY Times (Print), April 5, 2006, Available at: http://www.nytimes.com/2006/04/05/washington/05porn.html. Accessed August 31, 2009.

[82] Adams JA, Harper K, Knudson S, et al. Examination findings in legally confirmed child sexual abuse: it's normal to be normal. Pediatrics 1994;94:310–7.

[83] A parent's guide to internet safety. US Department of Justice, Available at: www.fbi.gov/publications/pguide/pguidee.htm. Accessed August 31, 2009.

[84] Felitti VJ, Anda RF, Nordenberg D, et al. The relationship of adult health status to childhood abuse and household dysfunction. Am J Prev Med 1998;14:245–58.

[85] Dube SR, Anda RF, Felitti VJ, et al. Childhood abuse, neglect, and household dysfunction and the risk of illicit drug use: the Adverse Childhood Experiences Study. Pediatrics 2003;111:564–72.

[86] Available at: http://onecare.live.com/familysafety. Accessed August 31, 2009.

[87] Interactive Internet Safety Presentations. CD-ROM. Available through the National Center for Missing and Exploited Children. 2004.

[88] Available at: http://aap.org/parents.html. Accessed August 31, 2009.

Advances in Pediatrics 56 (2009) 219–248

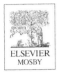

ADVANCES IN PEDIATRICS

ELSEVIER
MOSBY

Advances in the Care of Children with Burns

Renata Fabia, MD, PhD, Jonathan I. Groner, MD*

Department of Pediatric Surgery, The Ohio State University College of Medicine, Nationwide Children's Hospital, 700 Children's Drive, Columbus, OH 43205, USA

B urns remain a significant cause of death and disability in the pediatric population. According to the Centers for Disease Control and Prevention (CDC), there were 1168 burn-related deaths among 77,546,344 children ages newborn to 18 years in the United States in 2005, for a crude rate of 1.5 per 100,000. A review of 5 years of data from the authors' burn center, which serves a total population of approximately 1.5 million people, reveals that there are on average 135 admissions to the pediatric burn unit and 2 pediatric burn deaths per year. The mean age for burn admissions is 5 years old, and the mean length of stay is 2.5 days. Approximately 44% of the patients admitted to the burn unit are transferred from other hospitals in the region.

BURN EPIDEMIOLOGY AND ETIOLOGY

Seventy-nine patients age birth to 4 years are admitted to the burn unit each year, and the leading injury mechanisms in this age group are hot liquids (scalds), followed by hot objects and outdoor fires (bonfires, camp fires, trash fires). Nineteen admissions per year occur in the 5- to 9-year age group, and the mechanisms for this age are (in order) hot liquids, house fires, and ignition of flammable materials. There were 22 admissions per year among the 10- to 14-year age group, and hot liquids also leads the mechanisms in this group, followed by ignition of flammable materials and outdoor fires. These statistics indicate that injury prevention programs directed toward scald injuries and reducing outdoor fires could reduce thermal injuries in children.

There are also significant ethnic disparities in the rate of burn injury. Data collected from Ohio's 6 pediatric trauma centers in 2005 indicated that African American children had a burn admission rate that was 7.70 times greater than the admission rate for white children. The admission rate for all minorities was 6.64 times greater than the white admission rate. Furthermore, data from this study demonstrates that thermal injury is a disease of poverty. A zip code analysis of the rate of burn injuries in the minority population found that the rate of burn hospitalizations correlates with the number of vacant housing units, the

*Corresponding author. E-mail address: gronerj@chi.osu.edu (J.I. Groner).

0065-3101/09/$ – see front matter
doi:10.1016/j.yapd.2009.08.020

percentage of people with education below the ninth grade, the rate of unemployment, and the population density; however, burn admissions had an inverse correlation with median income [1].

Treadmill injuries are also included in the burn data, and between 2 and 4 cases are seen per year. These injuries sometimes require skin grafting. Intravenous (IV) infiltration, particularly in infants and small children, can cause deep (but usually small) burns, but these are not included in burn registry data. Skin-destructive diseases, such as toxic epidermal necrolysis (TEN) and epidermolysis bullosa, can also result in extensive partial and deep partial skin loss in children and, although not counted in the burn registry, are treated by the multidisciplinary burn team in conjunction with pediatric colleagues.

ADVANCES IN TREATMENT OF MAJOR BURNS
Transfer to a burn center and unique challenges
Burn centers are specialized treatment facilities designed to manage challenging patients with burn injury. Pediatric patients represent a special management challenge for various reasons. Children have a larger body surface area (BSA) to weight ratio, hence are more susceptible to water loss and hypothermia. Their renal immaturity causes problems with handling of fluid overload, and an immature immune system places them at increased risk for infection. Furthermore, pediatric patients are also prone to multisystem injuries. Children are also at increased risk of inhalational injury and carbon monoxide exposure, as they are often not able to escape flames and have increased minute ventilation [2]. In addition; there are specific psychological challenges with children.

Criteria to transfer to specialized burn centers have been established by the American Burn Association and the American College of Surgeons. The transfer criteria for the pediatric population are similar to those of adults and include the following: patients with 10% and more of total body surface area (TBSA) second-degree burns, third-degree burns greater than 1%, smoke inhalation, chemical and electrical burns, burns involving critical, esthetic, or functional areas (face, hands, genitalia, major joints), coexisting trauma, very young age (younger than 2 years), significant medical condition, and children of special needs. Also, children with burn injuries in hospitals without qualified personnel or equipment for the care of children and cases of suspected abuse should be transferred to specialized burn centers [2,3].

Burn assessment
After assuring adequate airway, breathing, and circulation, burn wounds are carefully inspected and their severity assessed, based on depth and TBSA. Depth of injury is characterized as superficial (first degree, not included in calculation of TBSA), partial thickness (second degree), or full thickness (third degree). Superficial wounds involve the most superficial aspect of the skin—the epithelium. The classic superficial burn is sunburn. Partial-thickness burns involve the dermis and the epidermis. Superficial and intermediate-depth

partial-thickness burns are characterized by painful, moist, red, and often blistered surfaces. Deeper partial-thickness burns are paler in color and usually drier [2]. Full-thickness burn is identified by a dry and leathery appearance, sometimes with hemorrhagic or purpuric pattern.

The degree of tissue damage after a thermal injury depends primarily on the temperature of the heat source and the duration of the exposure. The younger the patient, the more sensitive is his or her skin to burn injury. For example, immersion time needed to induce burn if exposed to water heated to 130°F (54.4°C), is 30 seconds for an adult, 10 seconds for a child, and less than 5 seconds for an infant. It takes only 1 second for an infant's skin to burn when exposed to water at 140°F (60°C). In addition to thermal exposure, burn injuries can also result from chemical and electrical contact.

An accurate quantification of the extent of surface area involved is an essential part of assessment, treatment, and care for the patient with thermal injury. There are several methods available to calculate TBSA. Among these, the most common are "pediatric rule of nines," which modifies the adult method described by Wallace and colleagues according to patient age, and the Lund and Browder Normogram [4]. In the pediatric population, the values assigned to the certain body regions change with age, to represent the disproportionate growth of the head and extremities, assuming their adult values usually at age 15 years. A useful tool for estimating smaller and scattered surfaces of burn is to assign a value of 1% TBSA to the area represented by the patient's hand and fingers.

The full breath of the patient's burn injuries may not be revealed until after the initial debridement [2]. The magnitude and severity of a thermal injury often can be deceiving, being addressed as a local insult, while the 3-dimensional pattern of injury and the systemic consequences of deeper and more extensive injuries are not fully appreciated.

Local response to a burn can be characterized into 3 zones of injury: central zone of coagulation and, extending peripherally, zones of stasis and hyperemia. The intermediate zone of stasis has particular clinical relevance because it represents a potentially salvageable area. Without proper initial management, this zone may progress from superficial partial-thickness to deep partial or full-thickness injury. Therefore, most modern burn care efforts focus on this zone, as it has the potential to epithelialize if optimized [3]. Cells in this zone require fluid administration in the first 24 to 48 hours to increase their chance of survival.

Evaluation of the dermal injury depth and estimation as to whether it will heal within the 3 weeks is difficult, particularly on presentation, as wound appearance changes over the first days, and depends on patient age, mechanism of injury, and quality of care. Several old and newly emerging technologies are being tested for accuracy and effectiveness of burn assessment. These techniques include burn wound biopsy, ultrasound, vital dyes, fluorescein fluorometry, laser Doppler fluorometry, thermography, light reflectance, and magnetic resonance imaging [3,5–10]. To date there is no optimal technology that has been proved to be reproducible, accurate, cost-effective, and clinically practical [3,5].

Advances and current expectation

Morbidity and mortality of pediatric burn victims have improved with advances in emergent and multidisciplinary care [3]. The concept of a multidisciplinary approach has been proved to provide good-quality care for these difficult patients with complex needs. Management of the burned child requires a coordinated response of emergency department burn services and pediatric intensive care unit as well as complex interaction among medical, surgical, critical care, and rehabilitation approaches.

Size of burn, age, and worst base deficit in first 24 hours remain the predictors of mortality [11]. The data comparing pediatric death during 7-year intervals separated by 10 years documented significant improvement of survival for children, including young children and large burns [12]. Factors that contributed to increased survival include improved fluid resuscitation and nutrition, advances in wound coverage and antimicrobial therapy, earlier wound excision, and improved critical care management of inhalation injury [2]. Better understanding of shock and metabolic response along with emerging technologies has made burn care more precise. Use of modern occupational and physical medicine techniques have reduced long-term complications.

Psychosocial support and new pain control strategies have dramatically improved the quality of life for patients during and after the acute course of care [3].

Initial treatment of injury

Airway management

Most severely burned patients require intubation for airway management and respiratory support. The major predictor of morbidity and mortality after burn injury is the presence of inhalational injury. The pathogenesis can be differentiated into direct pulmonary and upper airway inhalation injury, and secondary (indirect) pulmonary injury due to activation of the systemic inflammatory response [13]. In addition, secondary delayed pulmonary injury can be caused by sepsis and pneumonia. Ventilator-associated lung injury may be an important contributing iatrogenic factor.

Deposition of mucus and fibrin in the airways has been identified as a major component of lung dysfunction [14]. Early administration of aerosolized heparin and acetylcysteine has been shown to reduce pulmonary dysfunction. However, heparin is unable to dissolve already formed thrombus, and many patients do not arrive at burn centers for several hours [10] Experimental studies have demonstrated high efficacy of aerosolized tissue plasminogen activator in improvement of gas exchange and pulmonary compliance, without major bleeding complications [15]. The clinical study, however, is still unaccomplished. Other adjunct therapies such as nitric oxide have proved useful in treating hypoxic vasoconstriction in burn patients [16].

The reduced pulmonary compliance and chest wall rigidity of burn patients often require aggressive ventilatory management with high airway pressures that by itself exacerbates acute lung injury. Techniques of low tidal ventilation and permissive hypercapnia have been used with success in such cases [17]. Despite optimal early care, many patients progress to develop acute respiratory distress syndrome, with associated high morbidity and mortality. The optimal strategy for mechanical ventilation in these patients remains unknown. Use of high-frequency oscillatory ventilation and high-frequency percussive ventilation has been shown to be beneficial, especially in the young pediatric population but also in selected adult patients [10,13]. The major drawback is the need for deep sedation and chemical paralysis. Extracorporeal membrane oxygenation has also been used with success as an ultimate salvage option in pediatric patients [18].

Fiberoptic bronchoscopy traditionally was the gold standard for the diagnosis of inhalation injury, but it requires the availability of a skilled endoscopist, is invasive, and may worsen hypoxia or cause progression of airway obstruction [10].With the availability of high-resolution computed tomography (CT) scanners, a virtual bronchoscopy technique has been developed to diagnose suspected inhalational injury [19]. Due to a potential risk associated with transportation, this technique may be useful to rule out occult trauma in selected patients already going for CT scan.

Controversy still exists regarding tracheotomy need, optimal timing, and technique [13]. Recent studies demonstrated that translaryngeal intubation is a safe and effective method of providing long-term ventilatory support in severely burned children [20]. There is, however, no obvious proof of superiority of either technique [21]. For many years in children younger than 8 years, a standard technique of intubation was the use of an uncuffed tube, to avoid potential risk of tracheal injury. It has been shown recently that in critically burned children expected to require prolonged mechanical ventilatory support, low-pressure cuffed endotracheal tubes should be placed, regardless of the child's age [22].

Resuscitation fluids: anything new?
Advancements in fluid resuscitation of critically burned patients have made a major impact on patient survival and decreased complication rate, as it helps to minimize the occurrence of burn shock. Burn injury leads to a combination of hypovolemic and distributive shock by means of generalized microvascular injury and interstitial third spacing due to collagen and matrix degeneration [13]. Various available fluid resuscitation formulas are based on percentage of TBSA burn and weight, as they are targeted to address dynamic and ongoing fluid shifts occurring during such an insult. Perhaps the most widely used formulas include evolutions of the Parkland formula, which estimates 2 to 4 mL/kg per % TBSA burn with half of the calculated crystalloid fluid administered in the first 8 hours and the second half in the next 16 hours. Different physiologic demands in children of various ages as well as the size

of burn required even more modification of this guideline formula. For burn wounds of less than 10% TBSA, oral fluids or maintenance IV fluid is usually sufficient. Children with burns between 10% and 15% TBSA generally respond appropriately to 1.5 maintenance fluid. For burns larger than 15% TBSA in children weighing more than 20 kg, a modified Parkland (or other) formula is necessary. For children with more than 15% TBSA burn and weight less than 20 kg, an additional maintenance fluid containing glucose should be administered [2,23]. Infants younger than 2 years may easily become hypoglycemic due to limited glycogen stores. These children also tend to lose more fluid after thermal insult, as they have greater evaporative water loss due to large BSA/weight ratio and thinner skin.

Even with these mathematical formulas for guidance, burn resuscitation remains inconsistent and unpredictable. According to a multicenter meta-analysis, actual volumes of administered resuscitation fluid appear generally higher than predicted by the calculated formulas [11,24–26]. Of note, there was no close correlation between fluid requirement and TBSA burned, but an impact was more affected by patient weight, depth of burn, and need for mechanical ventilation. Inhalation injury increases fluid demand by an extra 1.1 mL/kg/% TBSA [24]. In addition, the increased use of sedative and analgesic medication may contribute to increased fluid volumes given to burned patients [10].

Large volume resuscitation has been shown to correlate with higher morbidity and even increased mortality [25,27,28]. In addition to the well-known extremity compartment syndrome, overresuscitation may lead to development of abdominal compartment syndrome and orbital compartment syndrome [28,29], as well as pulmonary edema.

Crystalloid solutions, such as lactated Ringer solution and normal saline, are still first-line fluid replacements in burn resuscitation, and an appropriate urine output remains the main goal of resuscitation. Recent studies have focused on hypertonic saline (HTS) resuscitation, because the theoretically beneficial use of colloids as an alternative has not demonstrated expected improvement in patient outcomes [30–32]. With an ability of rapid restoration of blood pressure and cardiac output, improved cerebral perfusion, and even modulation of systemic inflammatory response, HTS resuscitation has been shown in burn animal models to improve organ perfusion and outcomes [30,33,34]. The effectiveness of HTS resuscitation in the clinical setting, however, has been inconsistent in preventing organ damage [35], therefore it is not routinely used in burn patients and requires further investigation.

Shifting the focus of resuscitation from fluids to adequate end-point monitoring, more precise factors than just urine output have been postulated in recent years. With the availability of more advanced invasive cardiovascular monitoring, the goals of a cardiac index of more or equal to 3.5 $L/min/m^2$ and an intrathoracic blood volume index greater than 800 mL/m^2 have been used as a guide for fluid resuscitation [36]. Unfortunately, in addition to receiving more fluid, the hemodynamically guided patients did not show any change in morbidity and mortality compared with those receiving Parkland formula [36].

Other end-point goals like tissue pH and CO_2 and gastric CO_2, as well as serum lactate levels, seem to be related to changes in actual burn perfusion in a more timely fashion [37]. When encountered, new strategies of conservative treatment of intra-abdominal hypertension can be applied, avoiding abdominal decompression by laparotomy. Medical therapies include narcotic pain medication and benzodiazepines, paralytics, and diuretics. High doses of ascorbic acid (66 mg/kg/h) during the first 24 hours after thermal injury may significantly reduce resuscitation volumes [38]. In some cases, large amounts of intraperitoneal fluid are the cause of abdominal compartment syndrome, and simply tapping this or percutaneously draining it through a large-bore hemodialysis catheter placed into the intra-abdominal space can improve the situation enough to avoid laparotomy.

Recent analyses found an increased mortality in burn patients associated with blood transfusion [39]. Furthermore, a restrictive strategy of red cell transfusion (hemoglobin concentration maintained at 7.0–9.0 g/dL) has been shown to be superior to a liberal transfusion strategy (hemoglobin at 10.0–12.0 g/dL) in critically ill patients (with the possible exception of patients with compromised coronary artery flow), including the pediatric population [13,40].

Nutrition

A modern concept of nutritional support is thought to be one of the most significant advances in burn care in the last 20 years [3]. Burn injury significantly increases energy expenditure by induction of an exaggerated catabolic state. Concomitant sepsis further exaggerates the catabolic process. Significant hypermetabolism observed in response to burn injury is associated with protein catabolism and decreased hepatic protein synthesis [41,42]. For pediatric patients with TBSA burn grater than 40%, the resting metabolic rate increases to 160% to 200%.

The use of high-calorie nutritional support may attenuate the catabolic response after thermal injury [13]. Enteral nutrition is a preferred route for burn victims, with parenteral nutrition reserved for those unable to tolerate the former. Inadequate feeding leads to delayed wound healing and increased morbidity such as immunodeficiency, sepsis, loss of lean body mass, and cardiac ischemia [41,43]. On the other hand, overfeeding is associated with complications such as fatty liver, hyperglycemia, and ventilator dependence due to increased carbon dioxide production [43,44]

High carbohydrate diet may improve the net balance of skeletal muscle protein [45]. The glucose level, however, needs to be well controlled, as hyperglycemia may be detrimental in critically ill patients [46]. Adequate protein intake is essential, as the protein requirement is increased to 1.5 to 2.0 g/kg/d for severely burned patients due to increased oxidation of amino acids [42]. Hypoalbuminemia complicates most major burn injuries, causing visceral edema when levels decrease to less than 2.6 g/dL. The use of peptide-containing formulas may result in greater absorption than achieved by free amino acids. Excessive protein intake has a calciuretic effect, which may predispose to renal stones and nephrotoxicity. Protein intake therefore should not exceed 4 g/kg preinjury weight in the child.

Patients with burns metabolize fat at normal or increased rates. Careful balance of ω-6 and ω-3 fatty acids is recommended to achieve the highest benefit. Formulas using ω-6/ω-3 fatty acid in a ratio of less than 3:1, accounting for 10% to 15% of the patient calories, has been recently proposed [3].

Vitamins A and C as well as zinc should be supplemented in patients suffering from burns [47]. To ensure the intake of other nutrients involved in wound healing, one multivitamin with minerals should be supplemented daily [48]. Similarly to fluid resuscitation, there are numerous formulas available to calculate caloric needs in pediatric burn patients. After reviewing the predictive value of resting energy expenditure, it has been concluded that indirect calorimetry remains the standard of care.

A calorie count, serum prealbumin, transferrin, and C-reactive protein levels, as well as nitrogen balance (obtained by 24-hour urinary urea nitrogen) can be beneficial. However, in the context of clinical progress these trends, rather than actual values, and wound healing must be monitored [2].Weight monitoring is important, as the ultimate goal is to assure that patients do not lose more than 10% of their preinjury weight [3].

Discontinuation of enteral tube feeding is not recommended until patients can reliably and comfortably consume orally 70% of nutritional requirements. If this goal cannot be met, nocturnal feeding with approximately 50% of patient's need is warranted [3].

Hormonal and metabolic manipulation to improve healing

Burn injury is associated with increased levels of catecholamines and catabolic hormones. Modulation of catecholamines is therefore under intensive investigation in an attempt to attenuate the catabolic response after burn injury [13].

β-Adrenergic receptor blockade can attenuate hypermetabolism, decrease oxygen demand and resting energy expenditure, heart rate, and cardiac oxygen demand [42]. In addition, it may decrease catecholamine-induced muscle metabolism and lipolysis, and even improve the immune response [49,50]. Some studies in children with severe burns showed that treatment with propranolol (a nonselective β-antagonist) attenuates hypermetabolism and reverses muscle protein catabolism, as well as reducing release of free fatty acids from adipose tissue [51,52]. There are no large randomized studies evaluating the use of β-blockers in modulating morbidity and mortality. Furthermore, some studies in adults suggest that benefit can be achieved only in patients who have already been treated with β-blockers prior to a burn [53]. Nevertheless, many burn centers use β-blockers as the most effective catabolic treatment in burn patients [13].

Insulin, in addition to preventing hyperglycemia, has been found to decrease the level of proinflammatory cytokines, increase levels of anti-inflammatory cytokines, and decrease acute phase proteins [54]. In addition, children receiving insulin required less albumin administration to maintain appropriate levels [55]. Treatment of burn victims with insulin and metformin were shown to improve muscle kinetics [56]. Therefore, insulin may act directly to achieve anti-inflammatory and anticatabolic effects, not simply through the lowering of the serum glucose [57]. However, there are no studies on the correlation between these physiologic effects and incidence of infection, or on other morbidity and mortality.

The anabolic steroid oxandrolone has been shown to have similar effects to those of insulin on acute-phase protein and albumin synthesis, as well as improving muscle protein metabolism when used in severely burned children [58,59]. Several studies have shown that oxandrolone significantly decreases weight loss, restores lean body mass, and increases donor site wound healing [60,61]. Adequate protein intake is required during treatment with oxandrolone; dosing adjustment is necessary for patients with renal insufficiency, and diabetes and liver function must be monitored [3,13].

Growth hormone, in the form of recombinant human growth hormone (rhGH), used in severely burned children has been shown to be effective in enhancing wound healing and decreasing protein loss [62]. Demonstration of its accelerating effects on donor-site healing times allow reharvesting of skin from the same site, further supporting its usefulness in children with extensive burns in need of large surface autografts [63,64]. Administration of the hormone, however, may be associated with deleterious side effects such as hyperglycemia and increased triglycerides, which may contribute to mortality in critically ill patients. It has been demonstrated recently that rhGH in combination with the β-blocker propranolol attenuates hypermetabolism and inflammation without the adverse side effects found with rhGH alone [65].

Erythropoietin, which despite expectations did not prevent the development of postburn anemia or decrease transfusion requirement, has been shown in experimental studies to improve healing of burn wounds [66,67]. This repair is obtained through increased epithelial proliferation, maturation of the extracellular matrix, and angiogenesis [67]. Future clinical studies are warranted before routine clinical use is possible.

Increased risk of infection in a portion of burn victims can be genetically predetermined. There are at least 2 subgroups of patients that are recognized as those with increased risk: patients with specific polymorphism in the tumor necrosis factor and in the bacterial recognition genes [68]. Although this defect cannot be corrected, early recognition of it may allow more aggressive treatment [10].

Immunotherapy for the treatment of burned patients has gained considerable attention in the era of its substantial research. Immune-enhancing diets and agents including arginine, glutamine, ω-3 fatty acids, and antioxidants have been studied extensively [13]. Clinical studies, however, have not to date confirmed the beneficial findings of experimental studies [69,70].

Use of high doses of ascorbic acid and α-tocopherol may reduce the rate of organ failure in critically ill patients [71]; however, further clinical trials are needed for assessment of its effectiveness in the burn patient. Similarly, recombinant human activated protein C (activated drotrecogin-α), approved for the treatment of sepsis, may be potentially useful in burn patients with severe sepsis [13,72].

Topical immunotherapy, including activated kinase inhibitor p38 mitogen, have been demonstrated experimentally to decrease dermal inflammation, systemic inflammatory response, and secondary pulmonary complications [73]. At present, however, these agents are not clinically approved.

Anesthesia and pain management

Following the initial resuscitation of burn patients, the pain experienced may be divided into a "background" pain and a "breakthrough" pain associated with painful procedures. Whereas background pain may be treated with intravenous opioids via continuous infusion or patient-controlled analgesia (PCA), or less potent oral opioids, breakthrough pain may be treated with a variety of interventions. Current techniques of sedation and analgesia include different approaches, from a slight increase in background pain therapy (eg, morphine PCA) to PCA with rapid-onset opioids, to multimodal drug combinations, nitrous oxide, regional blocks, or nonpharmacologic approaches such as hypnosis and virtual reality. The most reliable way to administer drugs is intravenously. Fast-acting opioids can be combined with ketamine, propofol, or benzodiazepines. Adjuvant drugs such as clonidine, or nonsteroidal anti-inflammatory drugs and paracetamol (acetaminophen) have also been used [74].

Ketamine is particularly suited for the sedation of pediatric patients undergoing procedures away from the operating room. Pediatric patients have fewer adverse emergent reactions than adults [75]. In general, a subanesthetic dose ($\leq$1.0 mg/kg IV) is used for dressing changes; this dose gives adequate operating conditions but a rapid return to normal function, including the resumption of eating, which is important in maintaining proper nutrition in burn patients.

Resistance to the effects of nondepolarizing neuromuscular blocking drugs is usually seen in patients with greater than 25% TBSA burns [76,77]. Recovery of neuromuscular function to preburn levels may take several months or even years after the burn injury [78,79]. The increase in serum potassium that normally follows succinylcholine administration is markedly exaggerated in burned victims [80,81]. Potassium concentrations as high as 13 mEq/L resulting in ventricular tachycardia, fibrillation, and cardiac arrest have been reported [81,82]. The magnitude of the hyperkalemic response does not seem to closely correlate with the magnitude of the burn injury. Potentially lethal hyperkalemia was seen in a patient with only an 8% TBSA burn [83]. Succinylcholine has been safely administered within 24 hours of a burn injury. After this initial 24 hours, however, sufficient alteration in muscle response may have occurred, and the use of succinylcholine is best avoided.

Pain management is of crucial importance in pediatric burn patients who are exposed to multiple dressing changes, surgical manipulation of the wound, and diagnostic examination. Accurate prediction of medication concentration in plasma of the severely burned patient is impossible due to altered pharmacokinetics secondary to fluid fluxes, changes in cardiac output, decreased organ perfusion, loss of renal function, and loss of protein [84]. Furthermore, the regeneration of nerve fibers in healing burn wounds cause paresthesias resistant to opiates [84]. An additional challenge is caused by the difficult interpretation of pain in small children unable to verbalize. Therefore, sedation and pain management must be approached on an individual basis chosen from a broad spectrum of available analgesics and sedatives, carrying different risks and benefits [2].

Methadone is often used in the recovery phase to allow for gradual weaning from narcotic therapy while ensuring adequate pain management. The specialized Pain Team is invaluable in assisting with pain therapy in the severely (>15% TBSA) burned patient.

Fear and anxiety in burned children, also more pronounced than in the adult, may be addressed with benzodiazepines. Child Life assistance is an important additive as a distractive therapy, proven to be effective in children. Multiple new techniques are arising, including Virtual reality that uses 3-dimensional interactive tools [85].

Psychological and social support
A burn injury represents one of the most stressful events for a patient and family. Excessive pain, frightening wounds, potential deformities, disfiguring scars, and limited motion have an enormous impact on a patient's emotions, including self-image. The severely burned patient may experience depression and social withdrawal following hospital discharge [3].

Judicious use of psychopharmacologic agents in pediatric critical care, using the limited but growing evidence base and a clinical best practices approach, can reduce anxiety, sadness, disorientation, and agitation, improve analgesia, and save lives of children who are suicidal or delirious. In addition to pain, other disorders or indications for psychopharmacologic treatment are affective disorders: posttraumatic stress disorder (PTSD); post suicide attempt patients; disruptive behavior disorders (especially attention deficit hyperactivity disorder [ADHD]); and adjustment, developmental, and substance use disorders. Treating children who are critically ill with psychotropic drugs is an integral component of comprehensive pediatric critical care in relieving pain and delirium, reducing inattention, agitation, or aggressive behavior, relieving acute stress, anxiety, or depression, and improving sleep and nutrition [86].

Clinically significant distress experienced in the hospital predicts severe distress up to 2 years later. Early assessment and intervention for acute stress disorder during the burn recovery may be an important first step in the prevention of PTSD. Clinicians should be aware and vigilant of symptoms of PTSD, such as hyperalertness, nightmares, and chronic fearfulness [87]. Psychological support, patient and family education, social networking, counseling, comprehensive support, and involvement in a burn survivor program can be helpful and rewarding [3].

Surgical techniques
Debridement techniques
Debridement of the burn wound initially is performed by cleaning and removing debris to allow assessment of the depth and extent of the injury. Care is conducted in a warm environment to protect patients from temperature loss and improve their comfort. Wounds are cleaned with mild dilute detergents, and loose debris is removed gently. Large blisters are removed carefully, minimizing exposure of the underlying wound to vasoconstrictor-rich blister fluid [3].

Planning of the excision of extensive surface burns is the one of most challenging aspects of burn care, to the point that it has been called "the art and philosophy unto itself" [3]. When, how, and in how many stages excision has to be performed all have to be determined. The decision depends on several factors, including patient hemodynamic stability, existence of concomitant injuries, pulmonary considerations, and availability of resources [3]. Although early excision of large burns is beneficial and is advocated to be performed as soon as the patient is deemed stable, the treating team is exposed to particular confrontations in claiming whether the patient is safe for operation during the first or second week after a serious burn. Massive fluid shifts, critical airways, and concomitant traumatic or inhalational injury causing systemic effects on the patient have to be carefully reflected in the decision. Mixed distributions of burn depth as well as indeterminate-depth burn injuries add to the challenge. Burn wound sites should be excised and covered if they have not or are not estimated to heal within 14 days of injury, to prevent the risk of scarring or infection. On the other hand, premature or aggressive excision poses a risk of permanent loss of functional and esthetic tissue for which no perfect replacement is possible [3].

The common practice of the experienced burn center is to excise and provisionally cover the largest area of burn injury as soon as possible, usually from the trunk and areas critical for vascular and pulmonary access. Critical esthetic and functional areas that require a longer, meticulous approach can be addressed in the second surgical intervention [3,88].

Tangential excision, which involves the sequential and layered excision of devitalized tissue to a vital bed that is recognized by punctuate bleeding, remains a standard technique that has replaced full excision of the skin. Full (down to the fascia) excision, although avoiding massive blood loss that could be critical in hemodynamically unstable patients, results in major deformities. Tangential excision, more cosmetically appropriate, carries the risk of significant bleeding and inadequate excision, leading to infection. Several methods have been applied to minimize blood loss, including maintaining the patient's core temperature (warm environment, warm intravenous fluids, warm humidified air circuits for anesthesia), the use of electrocautery, the application of topical hemostatic agents (epinephrine or thrombin solution), injecting dilute epinephrine solution at the donor sites and below the eschar, the use of topical fibrin sealant, and the use of a tourniquet for extremity excision [3,88].

A recently developed water-jet debridement device, VersaJet (Smith & Nephew, Largo, FL) has demonstrated several benefits, including improved precision and control of debridement as well as decreased blood loss [89]. This device uses the technique of a controlled tight beam of sterile saline that travels parallel to the wound, and can be used in the operating room as well as at bedside. Figs. 1 and 2 depict a debridement of a full-thickness burn injury with hydrosurgery.

New techniques of graft stabilization, such as a fibrin sealant, showed satisfactory efficacy, safety, decreased incidence of hematoma/seroma, and decreased pain by the elimination of staples or stitches [90].

Coverage technique
Approaches for topical coverage of the burn wound have recently undergone significant changes. Many burn centers have replaced topical antimicrobials, historically providing the first line of therapy, by the early application of biosynthetic dressings or cytoprotective factors for intermediate-depth burn injuries. Enzymatic debriding agents (collagenase and urea derivatives), oat-derived agents, hydrogels, biochemical skin substitutes, and various moisturizers are used with increasing enthusiasm for noninfected wounds.

Even more evolution has taken place over the last half-century regarding the treatment of deep or extensive thermal injuries. Until the 1970s deep burn wounds were treated with topical antimicrobials that allowed for autolytic debridement of devitalized eschar and granulation over a period of weeks. A concept of early excision has had a significant impact on patient survival and decreased morbidity [3].

A deep partial or full-thickness burn will heal with application of a skin graft, but functional and cosmetic results are variable. Autografts may be limited by

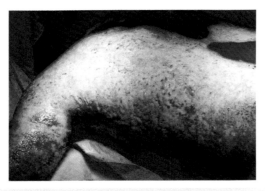

Fig. 1. Full-thickness scald injury of back and arm (toddler).

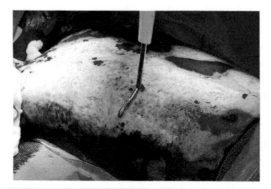

Fig. 2. Debridement of full-thickness burn injury with hydrosurgery.

available donor site in patients with a large burn. Requiring harvesting, split-thickness skin grafts create new wound sites, bleeding, and potential for scar formation. Figs. 3 and 4 depict coverage of a full-thickness burn with a split-thickness skin graft.

Tissue engineering and advancements in biotechnology have provided several novel modalities to address such issues. A variety of products are available, including skin, dermal, and epithelial substitutes. Temporary skin substitutes include biologic dressings (allograft and xenograft) and the biosynthetic products Apligraf, Biobrane, and TransCyte.

Allograft, which is harvested from human donors, can be used temporarily in patients with limited donor sites for autografting. An allograft provides excellent coverage, but is rejected in 1 to several weeks [3,91]. Xenograft, skin received from adult pigs, is a true biologic dressing, rich in growth factors, which similarly undergoes a rejection process. Both types of graft allow prompt coverage and result in a good wound bed, suitable for skin autografting or even epithelial autografting. The drawbacks include the fact that their quality varies

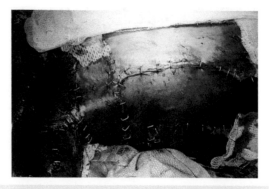

Fig. 3. Coverage of full-thickness burn with split-thickness skin graft.

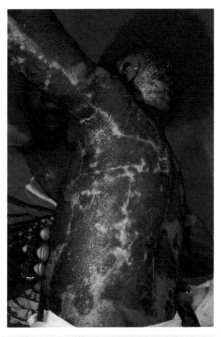

Fig. 4. Three weeks following split-thickness skin graft to back and arm.

depending on donor age and harvesting technique, both have to be removed, and both carry the potential risk for viral infection transmission [92,93].

Apligraf (Novartis International AG, Switzerland) is an allogeneic bilayered skin equivalent, which consists of human keratinocytes and human fibroblasts in a lattice of bovine type I collagen (Ho). Apligraf helps to restore a healing environment by providing a covering barrier and multiple growth factors, cytokines, and angiogenic factors [94].

Biobrane (Bertek Pharmaceuticals, Sugarland, TX) consists of a nylon mesh coated with porcine collagen type I peptides, bonded to silicone rubber membrane [95]. Biobrane is easy to use as it comes in various shapes, including that of a glove. This dressing requires meticulous preparation of the wound bed, and although used with excellent results for partial-thickness burns, it has not been accepted universally as a skin substitute for excised or full-thickness wounds [3]. TransCyte (Smith & Nephew) represents human neonatal fibroblasts seeded on coated nylon of Biobrane, which allows a proliferating form of dense cellular tissue [96,97]. This tissue substitute contains multiple growth factors and secreted matrix molecules. TransCyte has been shown to be very effective in the treatment of partial-thickness wounds and as a temporary closure of excised wounds [98,99]. TransCyte is easy to handle and to remove, with reduced bleeding compared with an allograft [99]; its drawback is its significant cost of production.

Dermal substitutes include Integra, AlloDerm, and Matriderm. Integra (Integra LifeScience Corp., Plainsboro, NJ) is a bilaminate membrane that consists of bovine collagen-based dermal analogue covered with silastic sheeting. The collagen matrix placed on an excised wound bed serves as a template for fibrovascular ingrowth. After several weeks, when the material is vascularized, the silastic membrane is peeled away and replaced with a thin split-thickness autograft. Integra is used as a biologic skin replacement system when autograft is unavailable or cannot be used due to the patient's condition, and it is indicated for treatment of life-threatening full-thickness or deep partial-thickness burns [91]. Despite prolonged times for biointegration, the use of Integra has been shown to be associated with reduced length of stay in severely burned patients, with 2 or more mortality risk factors [100]. The product has a favorable outcome in scarring formation [3]. Integra has, however, poor resistance to infection, requiring meticulous dressing change and local antimicrobial control. Long-acting silver coating dressings or negative-pressure wound therapy is frequently used [3]. Integra can be used in wounds consisting of exposed bone and tendon, and cavitary defects can be treated with multiple layers of the product placed sequentially [3,101]. New formulations and combinations of products with Integra are under evaluation.

AlloDerm (LifeCell Corp., Branchburg, NJ) is an acellular dermal substitute processed from cryopreserved human cadaver skin that is deprived of cells of the epidermis and dermis, leaving dermal matrix and basement membrane [3]. AlloDerm is used simultaneously with thin split-thickness autograft (making the donor site less deep) or cultured keratinocytes, with good results in full-thickness burns [102,103]. Although scar results are not superior, the skin texture appears to be superior when treated with AlloDerm [103]. The product is easy to store and apply, but meticulous attention to dressing is critical. Matriderm (Dr. Suwelack Skin and Health Care, Billerbeck, Germany) is a bovine noncross-linked collagen/elastin matrix. Matriderm can be applied simultaneously with a split-thickness autograft, yielding good dermal regeneration and a reduction in wound contraction [104].

Cultured epithelial and composite (epidermal-dermal) substitutes are available in different forms; as keratinocyte sheet grafts, keratinocytes in suspension, and keratinocytes inoculated on a dermal substrate. Cultured epithelial sheets (Epicel, Genzyme Tissue Repair, Cambridge, MA) are single-cell suspensions of keratinocytes on an irradiated mouse fibroblast line coupled with mitogens [3]. Epicel is used in the treatment of extensive skin loss and the absence of sufficient autologous donor skin. In addition, it is used in the treatment of partial-thickness wounds of the face, where it accelerates healing with subsequent reduction of the scar. There are several drawbacks in using the technique: it needs significant biopsy, requires prolonged time (average 3 weeks) to produce a stable sheet graft, it is expensive and difficult to handle, and the graft take rate varies considerably [105]. New advances in the sheet-handling technique could enhance the use of the product.

The attempt to overcome technical difficulties with enzymatic separation of cell sheets from culture vessels as well as shortening the period of culture has led to the development of new lines of products: keratinocyte suspension in fibrin glue (Bioseed) and in a liquid medium (CellSpray, C3, Coral Springs, FL). Both products have been reported to be successful in reepithelialization of deep partial and full-thickness wounds [106,107]. Of note is the success of restoration of melanocytes into the culture, suggesting a potential for the restoration of skin color after burn wound treatment [108]. The composite grafts combining keratinocyte cultures on dermal substitute have demonstrated good results in experimental studies; however, they are not yet commercially available [109].

Dressings

Dressing of the burn wound constitutes a mainstay of daily burn care, whose goals include optimizing of healing and prevention of wound progression, preparation of the area for closure, and control of microorganisms to reduce the potential for invasive wound infection [91,110]. Synthetic dressings, classically used for burn care, have undergone modifications paralleling advances in other technologies. New dressings are designed to preserve wound moisture, for example, Adaptic (Johnson & Johnson, Arlington, TX; cellulose acetate impregnated with a petrolatum) and Aquaphor (Smith & Nephew Healthcare Ltd, UK; gauze coated with Aquaphor ointment), or they are designed to absorb excessive exudates such as foam dressings (Lyofoam, Seton Healthcare Group, Oldham, UK). Polyurethane dressings, which are permeable to water vapor and oxygen while being impermeable to microorganisms, may be useful for superficial wounds and donor sites [91].

Xeroform (Kendall Co., Mansfield, Massachusetts), in addition to containing petrolatum that helps to keep moisture, also has antimicrobial properties due to bismuth tribromophenate. Acticoat (Smith & Nephew) is a dressing that uses the technology of slow release of broadly antimicrobial silver ion from synthetic material composed of polyethylene mesh and rayon/polyester core, which can be changed every 3 to 7 days [111]. New techniques include the Silon-TSR temporary skin replacement (BioMed Sciences, Allentown, PA), made from a complex weave of polymers. As a dual dressing (additional absorbing foam), it may be used directly on burn wounds, autografted sites, donor sites, or laser resurfacing areas.

Biosynthetic dressings are composed of both synthetic and biologic elements. Biobrane, mentioned earlier, is one of the examples. Calcium alginate (mixed calcium/sodium salts of alginic acid from seaweed) can be used in heavily exudative wounds, as it creates a hydrophilic gel on contact with wound exudate [91,112]. Glucan II (Brennen Medical, St. Paul, MN), a biosynthetic dressing, contains a gas-permeable layer and β-glucan, a healing-stimulating carbohydrate derived from oats [113]. Glucan II is useful in donor site covering. Glucan II Matrix consists of silver-impregnated material, which in addition is mixed with β-glucan. A variety of other commercially available dressings exist that are proven to be beneficial in the treatment of burn wounds; however, a description of all products exceeds the capacity of this article.

In addition to advancements in topical dressings, a technology of hypobaric treatment has been adopted to aid in burn wound care. Wound VAC (Vacuum Application Closure) is a negative (subatmospheric) pressure dressing consisting of a close-cell polyurethane or polyvinyl alcohol foam sponge cut to the shape of the wound, sealed with adhesive tape, and connected to a pump. The adhesive drape is gas-permeable to avoid anaerobic conditions. Negative pressure induces movement of blood, lymph, and interstitial fluid, reducing peripheral edema and bacterial load. These movements in turn lead to an increase in formation of granulation tissue and facilitate epidermal migration. Wound VAC can be used in the direct treatment of burn wounds or as a dressing for a skin graft [114,115]. In addition, it has been shown that by decreasing edema and preserving better blood flow to the injured area, early VAC application may prevent the progression of a partial-thickness burn to a full-thickness injury [116].

Rehabilitation

Progressive rehabilitation of the patient with a severe burn begins early after admission and may continue for years after hospital discharge. The goal is to preserve a maximum range of motion, prevent disabling contractures, and facilitate return to normal daily activity with reintegration to home and society.

Inpatient care consists of range-of-motion (ROM) exercises, splinting, and assisting with ambulation and activity, as well as scar care if wounds are already healing. In general, most of the scar treatment is performed in an outpatient setting.

ADVANCES IN THE TREATMENT OF MINOR AND OUTPATIENT BURNS

Criteria for outpatient burn management

Burns can be managed in the outpatient setting when they are not meeting previously discussed criteria for admission, hence of lesser surface affected (<10% TBSA), more superficial, uncomplicated, not crossing major joints, not circumferential, and not on special areas like the face, hands, and genitalia. However, the rule does not apply rigidly and therefore exceptions need further elaboration.

The treatment of minor facial, feet, or hand burns can be well performed in an outpatient setting as long as it is done under direction of a specialized team that includes occupational therapy and physical therapy. Similar rules apply to very small (<0.25%) full-thickness burns, chemical burns, and minor burns over joints.

Patients with special needs, such as ADHD or developmental delay, with minor burns can be treated in an outpatient setting as long as there is a reliable support system arranged. However, patients with a suspected child abuse etiology of their burn injury should be admitted to the hospital until child safety is assured.

Minor trauma that does not require hospitalization, in addition to trauma that is minor, superficial, and remote from the burn site, may also be appropriate for outpatient care. Nevertheless, all inhalational injuries and the majority of electrical burns should be treated as inpatients. The criteria for outpatient management vary based on the center's experience and resources [117].

Outpatient dressings

New advances in burn care are possible thanks to the availability of a variety of burn wound care products and dressings. The most desirable burn dressing used in the outpatient setting should, in addition to all properties needed to assure safe and prompt healing, be relatively easily applicable and manageable in the home environment [3,91,118]. Detailed instructions should be available to caregivers regarding the technique of cleaning the wound and dressing changes. Helping-hand written and illustrated instructions provided by specialized care centers are useful.

Advances in understanding and educating the principles of burn care among community medical care centers and parents allow for eliminating a significant misconception regarding burn care, precluding burn wounds from being inappropriately washed and dressed. The burned area should be washed with water and preferably unscented soap once or twice a day before application of burn ointment. The washing can be accomplished along with bathing of the entire body, provided there is no other open, infected wound. Inadequate washing and failure to remove old ointment before applying the new are the major reasons for wound infection in an outpatient setting.

Dressings should be applied in a way that prevents slipping and exposure of the wound, However, care should be taken to not compromise ROM. In the case of a hand burn, the dressing should be wrapped around each finger separately to allow for their independent motion. These simple measures have a significant impact on burn healing and scar prevention [119].

Advances in topical antimicrobial agents

Topical antimicrobial agents traditionally have been applied to a burn wound debrided of devitalized skin in a form of ointment, cream, or solution. These agents include neosporin, bacitracin, silver sulfadiazine, and mafenide acetate [3,91,120]. Although very effective as antimicrobial agents against surface infection, these agents usually require wound washing and reapplication twice daily. Secondary dressings should be applied to a burn wound over antimicrobial agents. Those include gauze, Xeroform (3% bismuth tribromophenate in a petrolatum-blend on fine gauze), Aquaphor gauze, foam dressings, and polyurethane dressings.

These types of dressings are painful and, particularly in children, associated with a significant anxiety. In addition, the willingness and ability of caretakers to effectively participate in wound care requiring frequent dressing changes is highly variable [120,121]. This variation often leads to prolonged hospitalization of children with minor burns that otherwise could be treated on an outpatient basis.

Recent developments of new silver-based antimicrobial delivery systems have eliminated the disadvantages of daily dressing change. Examples of available products include (among many) Acticoat, Aquacel Ag (ConvaTec, Princeton, NJ) Mepilex Ag (Mölnlycke Health Care, PA), and Glucan Silver Matrix (Brennen Medical) [111,120,122].

These products consist of silver-containing pads or hydrocolloid fiber sheets that provide a sustained delivery mechanism for silver and, in addition, function to absorb excessive exudate from a wound [122]. Applied to the debrided wound surface, these products can be left in place for several days. Elimination of the need for daily dressing changes decreases pain and anxiety in patients, and reduces the responsibility of caretakers. In addition, it reduces cost as well as length of hospital stay of burned patients [123,124].

Although topical antimicrobial agents do not contain growth factors, they provide an environment conducive to healing by helping prevent infection. These agents have wide activity against pathogenic organisms, delay colonization of organisms, and keep wound flora to a minimum, while not interfering with wound healing, and having minimal systemic absorption and toxicity [91,125].

Other techniques use substances that stimulate wound healing, such as oat β-glucan (Glucan-Pro, Brennen Medical), which is manufactured in several forms including a cream, gel, or carbohydrate dressing. β-Glucan is a cell-wall carbohydrate derived from oats that has the ability to activate and stimulate macrophages. β-Glucan can be used in a pure form or as a mixture with antimicrobial silver, such as Glucan-Silver Matrix.

Another concept helpful in outpatient burn care is biosynthetic dressings which, despite lack of antimicrobial properties, provide temporary wound closure, mechanical protection, a moist environment, and promotion of epithelial regeneration [3,91,125,126]. EZ-derm (Brennen Medical) is an example of such a product. EZ-derm is a porcine-derived xenograft in which the collagen is chemically cross-linked with aldehyde to provide strength and durability. This dressing is nonantigenic, conforms to irregular skin surfaces, and is easy to apply, care for, and remove as underlying skin is healing.

These products allow easier, less stressful, and less painful dressing changes, making it more appropriate for the outpatient setting. Figs. 5–8 depict the use of a porcine xenograft to deep partial-thickness burns in a 4-year-old.

USE OF BURN TREATMENT TECHNIQUES FOR NONTHERMAL INJURIES

The experience and techniques learned and resources gathered during the care of burn injuries can be used in the treatment of soft tissue wounds, IV infiltrations, and open skin lesions typically seen in immunosuppressed patients (eg, patients after bone marrow transplant), epidermolysis bullosa,

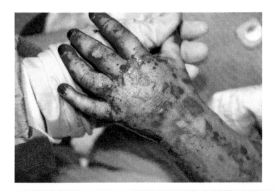

Fig. 5. Deep partial-thickness grease burn to fingers, hand, and arm in a 4-year-old.

Stevens-Johnson syndrome, and TEN. Patients affected by these conditions, in addition to disease-specific intervention (eg, immunoglobulin and steroid treatment of Steven-Johnson syndrome), require meticulous skin care and coverage to prevent infection and accelerate healing.

ADVANCEMENTS IN SCAR MANAGEMENT

Comprehensive scar care constitutes an integral part of burn care. Development of abnormal scarring is one of the most devastating sequels of a deep burn, as its progression may lead to disfiguration, pain, and functional restriction. Scars tend to be mostly located on the chin, neck, chest, and upper thighs, but can develop anywhere in the body. Early evidence of scar formation can be observed as early as 2 weeks post burn [127]. The process may continue for 1 to 2 years. Over time scars may subside, an outcome that is more likely if there is a reduction in burn wound tension.

Early scar modification therapies include massage aimed to desensitize and help collagen alignment, ultrasound and sclerotherapy for ablation of

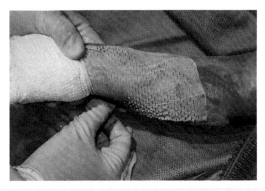

Fig. 6. Application of porcine xenograft to deep partial-thickness burn in a 4-year-old.

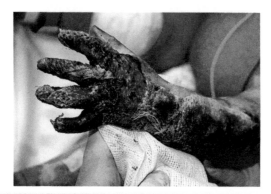

Fig. 7. Five days after application of porcine xenograft.

hypervascularity, pressure garment therapy, and the topical application of silicone. Compression therapy, which is believed to devascularize scar by applying pressure equal to wound capillary pressure, therefore flattening and softening the scar, has become a common adjunctive therapy for burn scar deformities [128,129]. A new generation of see-through facial masks, created by 3-dimensional scanning devices, may result in improved compliance and efficacy.

A variety of pharmacologic agents, including chemotherapeutic agents, calcium channel blockers, collagenolytics, and anti-inflammatory drugs injected intralesionally have been used with various, wide-ranging results [3,130].

Surgical interventions, proven to be beneficial in decreasing scar tension, are generally performed when inflammatory and hypervascular patterns diminish or tissue integrity improves; but nonsurgical methods fail in improving scar hypertrophy. Various surgical techniques are used, including interlesional geometric rearrangements of tissue (Z, W, and Y-V-plasty) and the release of

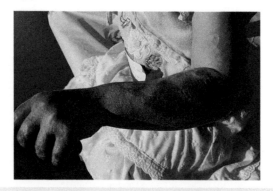

Fig. 8. Three months following treatment with porcine xenograft.

augmenting areas of tension (scar excision with full-thickness skin graft, or biosynthetic, skin flap, free flap, and tissue expanders) [3,131,132]. Other surgical techniques include dermal abrasion (optional adjunct to scar excision that removes epidermis and partial-thickness dermis, smoothing surface irregularities); scalpel sculpturing (uses a scalpel blade to micro-shave and feather the skin edges); cryosurgery (applies nitrous oxide once a month for over 3 months); and laser (removes injury precisely). These methods are reported to have modest to good success [133–135]. Increased efficacy of surgery may be achieved when it is combined with radiation or intralesional therapy [3,136].

Heterotropic ossification, a late complication, can occur in children with burns located close to joints by the development of new bone growth in nonosseous tissue [137]. Most commonly affected joints are the elbows, but shoulders, hips, knees, and forearms can be affected as well. Heterotropic ossification can cause severe impairment in activity, and can be treated by surgical excision. However, intensive physical therapy and passive motion devices should be used postoperatively, as recurrences have been observed.

Hypopigmentation (leukoderma) is one of the most common abnormalities occurring after partial-thickness burns. The etiology of leukoderma likely lies in the fact that the scar tissue prevents migration of melanocytes and melanin transfer. Several reported methods have been used, with similar success, for treatment of leukoderma. Such methods include superficial dermabrasion with melanocyte transplantation, CO_2 laser-assisted dermabrasion, use of micropigmentation, and dermatome deepithelialization with thin skin grafting [138].

THE FUTURE IN BURN CARE

Progressive improvement in the understanding of the pathophysiology of burn injury, advancements in critical care, and rapid development of biotechnology assure high expectations regarding future advancements in burn care. New effective methods of assessment of burn wound and extent of tissue injury may contribute to burn care planning and increased efficacy of treatment. The development of adequate and easily applicable end-point monitoring of burn fluid resuscitation with more precise parameters than just urine output may prevent progression of tissue damage and organ failure, while at the same time preventing the morbidity of overresuscitation. A better understanding of nutritional needs and metabolic and immune disarrangements after burn injury may lead to the development of more ideal nutritional and pharmacologic interventions. The early recognition of genetically predetermined risk factors for infection (eg, polymorphism of tumor necrosis factor) may allow more aggressive treatment with antibiotics or immunomodulators [139]. The traditional means of caring for large partial-thickness burns may no longer be optimal, because skin substitutes have been proven to shorten the time of healing and require fewer autografting processes [140].

An ideal skin substitute would closely mimic the natural functions of the skin and possess the following qualities: nonantigenic, durable, flexible, inexpensive, easy to prepare and apply, conforms to irregular wound surfaces, requires one operation, does not become hypertrophic, and grows with children [141]. Current research is focused on creating skin equivalents that could be used for temporary and permanent wound coverage. Understanding keratinocyte-matrix interaction may lead to additional matrix molecule treatment that enhances keratinocyte or epithelial take [142]. New modalities to protect cells after thermal injury may reduce the need to graft wounds [3]. With the development of stem cell research, it may be possible to generate a complete skinlike substitute from bone marrow derived cells [143]. Finally, pediatric burn and plastic reconstructive surgeons will continue to improve both the functional and esthetic outcome for patients with this devastating injury.

References

[1] Hayes JR, Groner JI. Minority status and the risk of serious childhood injury and death. J Natl Med Assoc 2005;97(3):362–9.

[2] Pizano LR, Davies J, Corallo JP, et al. Critical care and monitoring of the pediatric burn patient. J Craniofac Surg 2008;19(4):929–32 [review].

[3] Tenenhaus M, Rennekampff HO. Burn surgery. Clin Plast Surg 2007;34(4):697–715.

[4] Demling RH. Fluid resuscitation. In: Boswick JA Jr, editor. The art and science of burn care. Rockville (IN): Aspen; 1987. p. 189–202.

[5] Bishop JF. Burn wound and surgical management. Crit Care Nurs Clin North Am 2004;16: 145–77.

[6] Wachtell TL, Leopold GR, Frank HA, et al. Mode ultrasonic echo-determination of depth of thermal injury. Burns Incl Therm Inj 1986;12:432–7.

[7] O'Reilly TJ, Spence RJ, Taylor RM, et al. Laser Doppler flowmetry evaluation of burn wound depth. J Burn Care Rehabil 1989;10(1):1–6.

[8] Liddington MI, Shakespeare PG. Timing of the thermographic assessment of burns. Burns 1996;22(1):26–8.

[9] Svaasand LO, Spott T, Fishkin JB, et al. Reflectance measurements of layered media with diffuse photon-density waves: a potential tool for evaluating deep burns and subcutaneous lesions. Phys Med Biol 1999;44(3):801–13.

[10] Cone JB. What's new in general surgery: burns and metabolism. J Am Coll Surg 2005;200(4):607–15 [review].

[11] Cancio LC, Chavez S, Alvrado-Ortega M, et al. Predicting increased fluid requirements during the resuscitation of thermally injured patients. J Trauma 2004;56:404–14.

[12] Sheridan RL, Remensnyder JP, Schnitzer JJ, et al. Current expectations for survival in pediatric burns. Arch Pediatr Adolesc Med 2000;154(3):245–9.

[13] Ipaktchi K, Arbabi S. Advances in burn critical care. Crit Care Med 2006;34(9 Suppl): S239–44 [review].

[14] Suter PM. Nebulised heparin: a new approach to the treatment of acute lung injury? Crit Care 2008;12(4):170 [Epub 2008 Jul 25].

[15] Enkhbaatar P, Murakami K, Cox R, et al. Aerosolized tissue plasminogen inhibitor improves pulmonary function in sheep with burn and smoke inhalation. Shock 2004;22(1):70–5.

[16] Westphal M, Cox RA, Traber LD, et al. Combined burn and smoke inhalation injury impairs ovine hypoxic pulmonary vasoconstriction. Crit Care Med 2006;34(5):1428–36.

[17] Hanson JH, Flori H. Application of the acute respiratory distress syndrome network low-tidal volume strategy to pediatric acute lung injury. Respir Care Clin N Am 2006;12(3): 349–57.

[18] Kane TD, Greenhalgh DG, Warden GD, et al. Pediatric burn patients with respiratory failure: predictors of outcome with the use of extracorporeal life support. J Burn Care Rehabil 1999;20(2):145–50.

[19] Gore MA, Joshi AR, Nagarajan G, et al. Virtual bronchoscopy for diagnosis of inhalation injury in burnt patients. Burns 2004;30(2):165–8.

[20] Kadilak PR, Vanasse S, Sheridan RL. Favorable short- and long-term outcomes of prolonged translaryngeal intubation in critically ill children. J Burn Care Rehabil 2004;25(3):262–5.

[21] Pelosi P, Severgnini P. Tracheostomy must be individualized! Crit Care 2004;8(5):322–4 [Epub 2004 Sep 8].

[22] Sheridan RL. Uncuffed endotracheal tubes should not be used in seriously burned children. Pediatr Crit Care Med 2006;7(3):258–9.

[23] Schulman CI, King DR. Pediatric fluid resuscitation after thermal injury. J Craniofac Surg 2008;19(4):910–2.

[24] Kramer G, Hoskins S, Copper N, et al. Emerging advances in burn resuscitation. J Trauma 2007;62(6 Suppl):S71–2 [Review].

[25] Klein MB, Hayden D, Elson C, et al. The association between fluid administration and outcome following major burn: a multicenter study. Ann Surg 2007;245(4):622–8.

[26] Engrav LH, Colescott PL, Kemalyan N, et al. A biopsy of the use of the Baxter formula to resuscitate burns or do we do it like Charlie did it? J Burn Care Rehabil 2000;21(2):91–5.

[27] Baxter CR, Shires T. Physiological response to crystalloid resuscitation of severe burns. Ann N Y Acad Sci 1968;150(3):874–94.

[28] O'Mara MS, Slater H, Goldfarb IW, et al. A prospective, randomized evaluation of intraabdominal pressures with crystalloid and colloid resuscitation in burn patients. J Trauma 2005;58(5):1011–8.

[29] Sullivan SR, Ahmadi AJ, Singh CN, et al. Elevated orbital pressure: another untoward effect of massive resuscitation after burn injury. J Trauma 2006;60(1):72–6.

[30] Arbabi S. Hypovolemic shock. In: Mulholland MW, Doherty GM, editors. Complications in surgery. Philadelphia: Lippincott Williams and Wilkins; 2005. p. 136–43.

[31] Oda J, Ueyama M, Yamashita K, et al. Hypertonic lactated saline resuscitation reduces the risk of abdominal compartment syndrome in severely burned patients. J Trauma 2006;60(1):64–71.

[32] Cooper AB, Cohn SM, Zhang HS, et al. ALBUR Investigators. Five percent albumin for adult burn shock resuscitation: lack of effect on daily multiple organ dysfunction score. Transfusion 2006;46(1):80–9.

[33] Bulger EM, Cuschieri J, Warner K, et al. Hypertonic resuscitation modulates the inflammatory response in patients with traumatic hemorrhagic shock. Ann Surg 2007;245(4): 635–41.

[34] Murao Y, Loomis W, Wolf P, et al. Effect of dose of hypertonic saline on its potential to prevent lung tissue damage in a mouse model of hemorrhagic shock. Shock 2003;20(1):29–34.

[35] Murao Y, Hoyt DB, Loomis W, et al. Does the timing of hypertonic saline resuscitation affect its potential to prevent lung damage? Shock 2000;14(1):18–23.

[36] Holm C, Mayr M, Tegeler J, et al. A clinical randomized study on the effects of invasive monitoring on burn shock resuscitation. Burns 2004;30(8):798–807.

[37] Jeng JC, Jaskille AD, Lunsford PM, et al. Improved markers for burn wound perfusion in the severely burned patient: the role for tissue and gastric Pco2. J Burn Care Res 2008;29(1): 49–55.

[38] Tanaka H, Lund T, Wiig H, et al. High dose vitamin C counteracts the negative interstitial fluid hydrostatic pressure and early edema generation in thermally injured rats. Burns 1999;25(7):569–74.

[39] Palmieri TL, Caruso DM, Foster KN, et al. Effect of blood transfusion on outcome after major burn injury: a multicenter study. Crit Care Med 2006;34(6):1602–7.

[40] Lacroix J, Hébert PC, Hutchison JS, et al. Transfusion strategies for patients in pediatric intensive care units. N Engl J Med 2007;356(16):1609–19.

[41] Hart DW, Wolf SE, Herndon DN, et al. Energy expenditure and caloric balance after burn: increased feeding leads to fat rather than lean mass accretion. Ann Surg 2002;235(1): 152–61.

[42] Herndon DN, Tompkins RG. Support of the metabolic response to burn injury. Lancet 2004;363(9424):1895–902 [review].

[43] Suman OE, Mlcak RP, Chinkes DL, et al. Resting energy expenditure in severely burned children: analysis of agreement between indirect calorimetry and prediction equations using the Bland-Altman method. Burns 2006;32(3):335–42 [Epub 2006 Mar 10].

[44] Wolf SE, Debroy M, Herndon DN. The cornerstones and directions of pediatric burn care. Pediatr Surg Int 1997;12(5–6):312–20 [review].

[45] Hart DW, Wolf SE, Zhang XJ, et al. Efficacy of a high-carbohydrate diet in catabolic illness. Crit Care Med 2001;29(7):1318–24.

[46] Gore DC, Chinkes D, Heggers J, et al. Association of hyperglycemia with increased mortality after severe burn injury. J Trauma 2001;51(3):540–4.

[47] ASPEN. The science and practice of nutrition support. Dubuque (IA): Kendall/Hunt; 2001 271–4.

[48] Rodriguez D. Nutrition in major burn patients. Support Line 1995;17(4):1–8.

[49] Herndon DN, Nguyen TT, Wolfe RR, et al. Lipolysis in burned patients is stimulated by the beta 2-receptor for catecholamines. Arch Surg 1994;129(12):1301–4 [discussion: 1304–5].

[50] Louis SN, Jackman GP, Nero TL, et al. Role of beta-adrenergic receptor subtypes in lipolysis. Cardiovasc Drugs Ther 2000;14(6):565–77.

[51] Herndon DN, Hart DW, Wolf SE, et al. Reversal of catabolism by beta-blockade after severe burns. N Engl J Med 2001;345(17):1223–9.

[52] Morio B, Irtun O, Herndon DN, et al. Propranolol decreases splanchnic triacylglycerol storage in burn patients receiving a high-carbohydrate diet. Ann Surg 2002;236(2): 218–25.

[53] Arbabi S, Ahrns KS, Wahl WL, et al. Beta-blocker use is associated with improved outcomes in adult burn patients. J Trauma 2004;56(2):265–9 [discussion: 269–71].

[54] Jeschke MG, Klein D, Herndon DN. Insulin treatment improves the systemic inflammatory reaction to severe trauma. Ann Surg 2004;239(4):553–60.

[55] Klein D, Schubert T, Horch RE, et al. Insulin treatment improves hepatic morphology and function through modulation of hepatic signals after severe trauma. Ann Surg 2004;240(2):340–9.

[56] Gore DC, Herndon DN, Wolfe RR. Comparison of peripheral metabolic effects of insulin and metformin following severe burn injury. J Trauma 2005;59(2):316–22 [discussion: 322–3].

[57] Jeschke MG, Klein D, Thasler WE, et al. Insulin decreases inflammatory signal transcription factor expression in primary human liver cells after LPS challenge. Mol Med 2008;14 (1–2):11–9.

[58] Miller JT, Btaiche IF. Oxandrolone in pediatric patients with severe thermal burn injury. Ann Pharmacother 2008;42(9):1310–5 [Epub 2008 Aug 5] [review].

[59] Pham TN, Klein MB, Gibran NS, et al. Impact of oxandrolone treatment on acute outcomes after severe burn injury. J Burn Care Res 2008;29(6):902–6.

[60] Demling RH, DeSanti L. Oxandrolone induced lean mass gain during recovery from severe burns is maintained after discontinuation of the anabolic steroid. Burns 2003;29(8): 793–7.

[61] Demling RH, DeSanti L. Oxandrolone, an anabolic steroid, significantly increases the rate of weight gain in the recovery phase after major burns. J Trauma 1997;43(1):47–51.

[62] Ramirez RJ, Wolf SE, Barrow RE, et al. Growth hormone treatment in pediatric burns: a safe therapeutic approach. Ann Surg 1998;228(4):439–48.

[63] Losada F, García-Luna PP, Gómez-Cía T, et al. Effects of human recombinant growth hormone on donor-site healing in burned adults. World J Surg 2002;26(1):2–8 [Epub 2001 Oct 25].

[64] Herndon DN, Barrow RE, Kunkel KR, et al. Effects of recombinant human growth hormone on donor-site healing in severely burned children. Ann Surg 1990 Oct;212(4):424–9 [discussion: 430–1].

[65] Jeschke MG, Finnerty CC, Kulp GA, et al. Combination of recombinant human growth hormone and propranolol decreases hypermetabolism and inflammation in severely burned children. Pediatr Crit Care Med 2008;9(2):209–16.

[66] Still JM Jr, Belcher K, Law EJ, et al. A double-blinded prospective evaluation of recombinant human erythropoietin in acutely burned patients. J Trauma 1995;38(2):233–6.

[67] Galeano M, Altavilla D, Bitto A, et al. Recombinant human erythropoietin improves angiogenesis and wound healing in experimental burn wounds. Crit Care Med 2006;34(4):1139–46.

[68] Barber RC, Aragaki CC, Rivera-Chavez FA, et al. TLR4 and TNF-alpha polymorphisms are associated with an increased risk for severe sepsis following burn injury. J Med Genet 2004;41(11):808–13.

[69] Kieft H, Roos AN, van Drunen JD, et al. Clinical outcome of immunonutrition in a heterogeneous intensive care population. Intensive Care Med 2005;31(4):524–32 [Epub 2005 Feb 10].

[70] Briassoulis G, Filippou O, Kanariou M, et al. Temporal nutritional and inflammatory changes in children with severe head injury fed a regular or an immune-enhancing diet: a randomized, controlled trial. Pediatr Crit Care Med 2006;7(1):56–62.

[71] Nathens AB, Neff MJ, Jurkovich GJ, et al. Randomized, prospective trial of antioxidant supplementation in critically ill surgical patients. Ann Surg 2002;236(6):814–22.

[72] Bernard GR, Vincent JL, Laterre PF, et al. Recombinant human protein C Worldwide Evaluation in Severe Sepsis (PROWESS) study group. Efficacy and safety of recombinant human activated protein C for severe sepsis. N Engl J Med 2001;344(10):699–709.

[73] Ipaktchi K, Mattar A, Niederbichler AD, et al. Topical p38MAPK inhibition reduces dermal inflammation and epithelial apoptosis in burn wounds. Shock 2006;26(2):201–9.

[74] Gregoretti C, Decaroli D, Piacevoli Q, et al. Analgo-sedation of patients with burns outside the operating room. Drugs 2008;68(17):2427–43.

[75] Sussman DR. A comparative evaluation of ketamine anesthesia in children and adults. Anesthesiology 1974;40:459–64.

[76] Marathe PH, Dwersteg JF, Pavlin EG, et al. Effect of thermal injury on the pharmacokinetics and pharmacodynamics of atracurium in humans. Anesthesiology 1989;70:752–5.

[77] Martyn JA, Szyfelbein SK, Ali HH, et al. Increased d-tubocurarine requirement following major thermal injury. Anesthesiology 1980;52:352–5.

[78] Cronan T, Hammond J, Ward CG. The value of isokinetic exercise and testing in burn rehabilitation and determination of back-to-work status. J Burn Care Rehabil 1990;11:224–7.

[79] St-Pierre DM, Choiniere M, Forget R, et al. Muscle strength in individuals with healed burns. Arch Phys Med Rehabil 1998;79:155–61.

[80] Gronert GA, Theye RA. Pathophysiology of hyperkalemia induced by succinylcholine. Anesthesiology 1975;43:89–99.

[81] Schaner PJ, Brown RL, Kirksey TD, et al. Succinylcholine-induced hyperkalemia in burned patients. 1. Anesth Analg 1969;48:764–70.

[82] Belin RP, Karleen CI. Cardiac arrest in the burned patient following succinyldicholine administration. Anesthesiology 1966;27:516–8.

[83] Viby-Mogensen J, Hanel HK, Hansen E, et al. Serum cholinesterase activity in burned patients. II: anaesthesia, suxamethonium and hyperkalaemia. Acta Anaesthesiol Scand 1975;19:169–79.

[84] Beushausen T, Mucke K. Anesthesia and pain management in pediatric burn patients. Pediatr Surg Int 1997;12:327–33.

[85] Sharar SR, Miller W, Teeley A, et al. Applications of virtual reality for pain management in burn-injured patients. Expert Rev Neurother 2008;8(11):1667–74, 78.

[86] Stoddard FJ. Psychopharmacology in pediatric critical care. Child Adolesc Psychiatr Clin N Am 2006;15(3):611–55.

[87] Dyster-Aas J, Willebrand M, Wikehult B, et al. Major depression and posttraumatic stress disorder symptoms following severe burn injury in relation to lifetime psychiatric morbidity. J Trauma 2008;64(5):1349–56.

[88] Cartotto R, Musgrave MA, Beveridge M, et al. Minimizing blood loss in burn surgery. J Trauma 2000;49(6):1034–9.

[89] Kimble RM, Mott J, Joethy J. Versajet hydrosurgery system for the debridement of paediatric burns. Burns 2008;34(2):297–8 [author reply 299].

[90] Foster K, Greenhalgh D, Gamelli RL, et al. FS 4IU VH S/D Clinical Study Group. Efficacy and safety of a fibrin sealant for adherence of autologous skin grafts to burn wounds: results of a phase 3 clinical study. J Burn Care Res 2008;29(2):293–303.

[91] Honari S. Topical therapies and antimicrobials in the management of burn wounds. Crit Care Nurs Clin North Am 2004;16:1–11.

[92] Kealey GP. Disease transmission by means of allograft. J Burn Care Rehabil 1997;18(1 Pt 2):S10–1.

[93] Kobayashi H, Kobayashi M, McCauley RL, et al. Cadaveric skin allograft-associated cytomegalovirus transmission in a mouse model of thermal injury. Clin Immunol 1999;92(2): 181–7.

[94] Jimenez PA, Jimenez SE. Tissue and cellular approaches to wound repair. Am J Surg 2004;187(5A):56S–64S.

[95] Lang EM, Eiberg CA, Brandis M, et al. Biobrane in the treatment of burn and scald injuries in children. Ann Plast Surg 2005;55(5):485–9.

[96] Zapata-Sirvent R, Hansbrough JF, Carroll W, et al. Comparison of Biobrane and Scarlet Red dressings for treatment of donor site wounds. Arch Surg 1985;120(6):743–5.

[97] Pham C, Greenwood J, Cleland H, et al. Bioengineered skin substitutes for the management of burns: a systematic review. Burns 2007;33(8):946–57 [Epub 2007 Sep 7]. [review].

[98] Pape SA, Byrne PO. Safety and efficacy of TransCyte for the treatment of partial-thickness burns. J Burn Care Rehabil 2000;21(4):390.

[99] Purdue GF, Hunt JL, Still JM Jr, et al. A multicenter clinical trial of a biosynthetic skin replacement, Dermagraft-TC, compared with cryopreserved human cadaver skin for temporary coverage of excised burn wounds. J Burn Care Rehabil 1997;18(1 Pt 1):52–7.

[100] Ryan CM, Schoenfeld DA, Malloy M, et al. Use of Integra artificial skin is associated with decreased length of stay for severely injured adult burn survivors. J Burn Care Rehabil 2002;23(5):311–7.

[101] Bhavsar D, Tenenhaus M. The use of acellular dermal matrix for coverage of exposed joint and extensor mechanism in thermally injured patients with few options. Eplasty 2008;8: e33.

[102] Munster AM, Smith-Meek M, Shalom A. Acellular allograft dermal matrix: immediate or delayed epidermal coverage? Burns 2001;27(2):150–3.

[103] Rennekampff HO, Pfau M, Schaller HE. Acellular allograft dermal matrix: immediate or delayed epidermal coverage? Burns 2002;28(1):100–1.

[104] Van Zuijlen PP, Vloemans JF, van Trier AJ, et al. Dermal substitution in acute burns and reconstructive surgery: a subjective and objective long-term follow-up. Plast Reconstr Surg 2001;108(7):1938–46 [Links].

[105] Desai MH, Mlakar JM, McCauley RL, et al. Lack of long-term durability of cultured keratinocyte burn-wound coverage: a case report. J Burn Care Rehabil 1991;12(6):540–5.

[106] Horch RE, Bannasch H, Kopp J, et al. Single-cell suspensions of cultured human keratinocytes in fibrin-glue reconstitute the epidermis. Cell Transplant 1998;7(3):309–17.

[107] Atiyeh BS, Costagliola M. Cultured epithelial autograft (CEA) in burn treatment: three decades later. Burns 2007;33(4):405–13 [Epub 2007 Apr 2] [review].

[108] Navarro FA, Stoner ML, Lee HB, et al. Melanocyte repopulation in full-thickness wounds using a cell spray apparatus. J Burn Care Rehabil 2001;22(1):41–6.

[109] Boyce ST, Goretsky MJ, Greenhalgh DG, et al. Comparative assessment of cultured skin substitutes and native skin autograft for treatment of full-thickness burns. Ann Surg 1995;222(6):743–52.

[110] Staley M, Richard R. Management of the acute burn wound: an overview. Adv Wound Care 1997;10(2):39–44.

[111] Cuttle L, Naidu S, Mill J, et al. A retrospective cohort study of Acticoat versus Silvazine in a paediatric population. Burns 2007;33(6):701–7 [Epub 2007 Jul 17].

[112] Kneafsey B, O'Shaughnessy M, Condon KC. The use of calcium alginate dressings in deep hand burns. Burns 1996;22(1):40–3.

[113] Delatte SJ, Evans J, Hebra A, et al. Effectiveness of beta-glucan collagen for treatment of partial-thickness burns in children. J Pediatr Surg 2001;36(1):113–8.

[114] Adámková M, Tymonová J, Zámecníková I, et al. First experience with the use of vacuum assisted closure in the treatment of skin defects at the burn center. Acta Chir Plast 2005;47(1):24–7.

[115] Scherer LA, Shiver S, Chang M, et al. The vacuum assisted closure device: a method of securing skin grafts and improving graft survival. Arch Surg 2002;137(8):930–3 [discussion: 933–4].

[116] Kamolz LP, Andel H, Haslik W, et al. Use of subatmospheric pressure therapy to prevent burn wound progression in human: first experiences. Burns 2004;30(3):253–8.

[117] Kassira W, Namias N. Outpatient management of pediatric burns. J Craniofac Surg 2008;19(4):1007–9.

[118] Atiyeh BS, Gunn SW, Hayek SN. State of the art in burn treatment. World J Surg 2005;29(2):131–48.

[119] Hunter GR, Chang FC. Outpatient burns: a prospective study. J Trauma 1976;16(3): 191–5.

[120] Duffy BJ, McLaughlin PM, Eichelberger RM. Assessment, triage, and early management of burns in children. Clin Pediatr Emerg Med 2006;7(2):82–93.

[121] Klein GL, Herndon DN. Burns. Pediatr Rev 2004;25:411–7.

[122] Mishra A, Whitaker IS, Potokar TS, et al. The use of aquacel Ag in the treatment of partial thickness burns: a national study. Burns 2007;33(5):679–80 [Epub 2007 May 18].

[123] Paddock HN, Fabia R, Giles S, et al. A silver impregnated antimicrobial dressing reduces hospital length of stay for pediatric patients with burns. J Burn Care Res 2007;28(3): 409–11.

[124] Paddock HN, Fabia R, Giles S, et al. A silver-impregnated antimicrobial dressing reduces hospital costs for pediatric burn patients. J Pediatr Surg 2007;42(1):211–3.

[125] Patel PP, Vasquez SA, Granick MS, et al. Topical antimicrobials in pediatric burn wound management. J Craniofac Surg 2008 Jul;19(4):913–22 [review].

[126] Feng X, Shen R, Tan J, et al. The study of inhibiting systematic inflammatory response syndrome by applying xenogenic (porcine) acellular dermal matrix on second-degree burns. Burns 2007;33(4):477–9 [Epub 2007 Feb 28].

[127] Scott PG, Ghahary A, Tredget EE. Molecular and cellular aspects of fibrosis following thermal injury. Hand Clin 2000;16(2):271–87 [Review].

[128] Wienert V. Compression treatment after burns. Curr Probl Dermatol 2003;31:108–13 [review].

[129] Puzey G. The use of pressure garments on hypertrophic scars. J Tissue Viability 2002;12(1):11–5 [review].

[130] Grisolia GA, Danti DA, Santoro S, et al. Injection therapy with triamcinolone hexacetonide in the treatment of burn scars in infancy: results of 44 cases. Burns Incl Therm Inj 1983;10(2):131–4.

[131] Ulkur E, Acikel C, Evinc R, et al. Use of rhomboid flap and double Z-plasty technique in the treatment of chronic postburn contractures. Burns 2006;32(6):765–9 [Epub 2006 Jul 11].

[132] Lin TM, Lee SS, Lai CS, et al. Treatment of axillary burn scar contracture using opposite running Y-V-plasty. Burns 2005;31(7):894–900 [Epub 2005 Jul 11].

[133] Holmes JD, Rayner CR, Muir IF. The treatment of deep dermal burns by abrasion. Scand J Plast Reconstr Surg Hand Surg 1987;21(3):237–40.

[134] Muti E, Ponzio E. Cryotherapy in the treatment of keloids. Ann Plast Surg 1983;11(3): 227–32.

[135] Kawecki M, Bernad-Wiśniewska T, Sakiel S, et al. Laser in the treatment of hypertrophic burn scars. Int Wound J 2008;5(1):87–97, 34.

[136] Donelan MB, Parrett BM, Sheridan RL. Pulsed dye laser therapy and z-plasty for facial burn scars: the alternative to excision. Ann Plast Surg 2008;60(5):480–6.

[137] Davoodi P, Fernandez JM, O SJ. Postburn sequelae in the pediatric patient: clinical presentations and treatment options. J Craniofac Surg 2008;19(4):1047–52 [review].

[138] Onur Erol O, Atabay K. The treatment of burn scar hypopigmentation and surface irregularity by dermabrasion and thin skin grafting. Plast Reconstr Surg 1990;85(5):754–8.

[139] Shalhub S, Pham TN, Gibran NS, et al. Tumor necrosis factor gene variation and the risk of mortality after burn injury: a Cohort study. J Burn Care Res 2009;30(1):105–11.

[140] Kumar RJ, Kimble RM, Boots R, et al. Treatment of partial-thickness burns: a prospective, randomized trial using Transcyte. ANZ J Surg 2004;74(8):622–6.

[141] Sheridan RL, Tompkins RG. Skin substitutes in burns. Burns 1999;25:97–103.

[142] Takeda A, Kadoya K, Shioya N, et al. Pretreatment of human keratinocyte sheets with laminin 5 improves their grafting efficiency. J Invest Dermatol 1999;113(1):38–42.

[143] Kataoka K, Medina RJ, Kageyama T, et al. Participation of adult bone marrow cells in reconstruction of skin. Am J Pathol 2003;163:1227–31.

Advances in Pediatrics 56 (2009) 249–269

ADVANCES IN PEDIATRICS

Pediatric Brain Tumors

Ronald T. Grondin, MD, FRCSC[a],*, R. Michael Scott, MD[b], Edward R. Smith, MD[b]

[a]Department of Pediatric Neurosurgery, Nationwide Children's Hospital, The Ohio State University, 700 Children's Drive, Columbus, OH 43205, USA
[b]Department of Neurosurgery, Children's Hospital Boston/Harvard Medical School, 300 Longwood Avenue, Boston, MA 02115, USA

B rain tumors are the most common solid cancer of childhood and are currently the leading cause of death in children, excluding trauma [1–3]. The number of primary and metastatic brain tumors is steadily increasing, whereas mortality rates for many central nervous system (CNS) tumor types have remained essentially unchanged [4]. Many of these tumors remain difficult to detect before the onset of symptoms. Once identified, rapid referral to an appropriate specialist for treatment is often critical to obtaining an optimal outcome.

One major advantage in treating brain tumors in children is that significant improvements in outcome can be achieved in many cases with early diagnosis. The relationship between children and pediatricians, with the established routine of regular visits, provides an opportunity for identifying worrisome symptoms at their initial presentation. This article has 2 objectives: to outline signs and symptoms that may indicate the presence of a brain tumor in a child, and to provide primary care physicians with information about the major categories of pediatric brain tumors, including common problems, treatment options, prognoses, and recent advances.

GENERAL PRINCIPLES IN THE DIAGNOSIS AND EVALUATION OF BRAIN TUMORS IN CHILDREN

Identification and diagnosis of brain tumors in children can be difficult. Sometimes these lesions are effectively undetectable, despite excellent care, and may not be recognized until a tumor is large or disseminated. Rarely, imaging of the brain obtained for other reasons (such as trauma) may reveal a lesion incidentally, but this is the exception rather than the rule. However, there are some general screening questions and findings on clinical examination that may help to identify patients at risk for harboring intracranial masses.

*Corresponding author. E-mail address: ronald.grondin@nationwidechildrens.org (R.T. Grondin).

0065-3101/09/$ – see front matter
doi:10.1016/j.yapd.2009.08.006

Family history

Family history may be important in the process of screening patients for the presence of brain tumors. Although most tumors are believed to arise from spontaneous mutations, a small number of genetic conditions are known to have an increased risk of brain tumors (Table 1). If a family history of one of these disorders is present, screening with magnetic resonance imaging (MRI) should be considered.

Review of systems

A careful review of systems may provide clues to the presence of intracranial tumors in children. Headaches, seizures, focal neurologic deficits (weakness, numbness, visual field problems), or cognitive decline may be present. The presence of certain findings in the patient history should raise the level of concern for an intracranial process (Table 2). Evidence of syndromes known to be associated with brain tumors should be addressed in the patient interview.

Special note should be made of vomiting as a symptom of brain tumors in the pediatric population. It is one of the most common presenting symptoms in children and, unlike adults, may not always be found in association with headache [5,6]. Although other causes of vomiting may be far more common in children (gastrointestinal disorders, migraines), the possibility of a brain tumor should not be overlooked, particularly if the vomiting occurs on waking in the morning or if other interventions do not alleviate the symptoms. Careful re-evaluation of children with persistent emesis may be warranted if no proximate cause is readily identified.

Children with brain tumors may also present with endocrine deficiencies, especially if the tumors are located near the hypothalamus or involve the pituitary gland. These lesions, commonly craniopharyngiomas or pituitary adenomas, may be smaller in size than hemispheric tumors and, as such, not produce the more easily recognized symptoms of headache, vomiting, or neurologic deficit. Patients with tumors in this location may have growth disturbances, irregular menstrual cycles, precocious puberty, hypothyroidism, or diabetes insipidus. The presence of a bitemporal visual field cut in association with an endocrinopathy may assist the clinician in making a diagnosis.

Examination

Obvious neurologic deficits can serve to cue the examiner to the potential of a brain tumor; focal weakness or numbness in a cortical distribution, visual field deficits, or papilledema (see Table 2). However, beyond the common,

Table 1
Genetic conditions associated with brain tumors

Neurofibromatosis 1 (NF1) and neurofibromatosis 2 (NF2)
Turcot syndrome (APC)
Gorlin syndrome/basal cell nevus syndrome (PTCH)
Tuberous sclerosis (TSC1 and TSC2)
Li-Fraumeni syndrome (TP53)

Table 2
Findings suggestive of an intracranial lesion

Sleep-related headache
No family history of migraine
Vomiting
Absence of visual symptoms (migraine scotoma)
Headache of less than 6 months' duration
Confusion
Abnormal neurologic examination findings
A positive correlation between number of predictors and risk of surgical lesion [7]

but not universal, complaints of vomiting and headache, the typical patient with a brain tumor may not have any obvious findings on general physical examination to suggest an underlying problem. Even a detailed neurologic examination may not always reveal deficits, particularly in early stages of tumor development, making the diagnosis of brain tumor in the clinic a difficult task.

Once the tumor has progressed beyond a critical threshold, there are certain findings on physical examination that may be present and are often associated with neurologic emergencies (Table 3). If an emergency is detected, transfer to a tertiary care center with pediatric neurosurgeons should be arranged.

Radiographic evaluation

In general, the diagnosis of a brain tumor is made with an imaging study. A variety of methods are available; each with advantages and shortcomings. This article does not review the means of establishing the diagnosis of systemic disorders, such as neurofibromatosis I or tuberous sclerosis, but does describe the workup relevant to each insofar as there is a need to screen for brain tumors. This section serves as an overview of the general categories of imaging studies relevant to brain tumors, with greater detail provided in the specific sections for each individual tumor type.

Intracranial ultrasonography is easy, fast, and essentially without risk. However, it is limited to use in infants with an open fontanel, is operator-dependent, and has limited usefulness beyond revealing large tumors, hydro-cephalus, or hemorrhage. It is generally a good screening test in infants, but can miss smaller tumors or lesions in the posterior fossa. If the index of

Table 3
"Red flags" on examination

Bradycardia, hypertension, decreased respirations (Cushing response)
Dilated pupil, hemparesis (uncal herniation)
Fixed downward gaze (Parinaud syndrome)
Lethargy, tense open anterior fontanelle
Ataxia with nausea and vomiting
Sudden onset of a third nerve palsy, including involvement of the pupil (dilated)
Sudden onset of "the worst headache of my life"

suspicion is high, an alternative imaging modality (such as MRI) should be considered.

Computerized tomography (CT) is an excellent initial study for brain tumors. CT can detect large masses, hemorrhage, hydrocephalus, and can identify the presence of calcium within lesions, which is important for the diagnosis of several tumor types. CT may serve as an important complementary study to MRI. However, CT studies expose children to radiation, and the use of contrast is associated with a small but real risk of allergic reaction. The presence of braces or other metal objects such as piercings may produce artifacts (in CT and MRI) and should be removed if possible. In the setting of an emergency, an axial CT of the brain is the most common screening modality.

MRI has revolutionized the diagnosis of brain tumors in children. There is little risk other than the rare reaction to gadolinium, the need for sedation/general anesthesia to reduce motion artifact in children unable to tolerate the confines of the scanner, and, in infants, the potential for hypothermia in the cooled MRI suite. MRI can provide exquisitely detailed images of the brain, excellent reconstructions of lesions in 3 planes, and magnetic resonance (MR) spectroscopy may help ascertain the identity of a tumor. If a brain tumor is detected, spine imaging should be considered to detect disseminated disease.

Once a tumor has been identified, the next step is a referral to a tertiary care center experienced in the care of brain tumors. A brief phone consultation with a neurosurgeon, as soon as a diagnosis is made, can sometimes be helpful in determining the urgency of an appointment. Some children need an immediate transfer, whereas others may be completely elective. Every effort should be made to provide copies of any imaging studies, not just written reports, to colleagues in neurosurgery. A preliminary diagnosis can often be made from the initial images, although definitive pathology may not be available until several days after surgery. The following section reviews common brain tumor subtypes with an emphasis on information relevant to the primary care physician, including recent advances in the diagnosis and treatment of these challenging lesions [7].

SPECIFIC DISEASE ENTITIES

This section describes most of the tumors that present in childhood (Fig. 1)

Supratentorial brain tumors

Supratentorial gliomas

Introduction. Gliomas are primary brain tumors of glial origin. This is a broad category of tumors with different cell lineages. Some of the more common tumors of this class found in children include fibrillary astrocytomas, juvenile pilocytic astrocytomas, oligodendrogliomas, ependymomas, glioblastoma multiforme, and pleomorphic xanthoastrocytomas.

Gliomas represent most of the brain tumors found in the cerebral hemispheres in children. Astrocytomas (of all types) represent approximately half

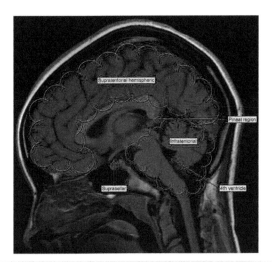

Fig. 1. Common tumor types by location. Supratentorial hemispheric: astrocytoma, ganglioglioma, DNET. Suprasellar: craniopharyngioma, optic pathway glioma, germ cell tumor, pituitary adenoma. Pineal region: germ cell tumor, pineal parenchymal tumor (pineocytoma, pineoblastoma), astrocytoma. Infratentorial: cerebellar astrocytoma, medulloblastoma, brainstem tumor, ependymoma. Fourth ventricle: medulloblastoma, ependymoma, brainstem glioma, choroid plexus tumor.

of the gliomas in this location. In contrast to adults, in whom most supratentorial gliomas are of higher grades, most of these tumors in children are low grade [8,9].

Epidemiology. Recent data suggest an overall incidence of pediatric brain tumors of about 3.5/100,000 [10] Supratentorial tumors account for 40% to 60% of this group. They are twice as common in infants as they are in older children [11]. About 20% are malignant (World Health Organization [WHO] grade III or IV). The cause is usually unclear; although some tumors arise in association with defined tumor syndromes. About one-third of optic pathway/hypothalamic gliomas are associated with neurofibromatosis type 1 (NF1) [12] and 10% to 30% of NF1 patients develop optic gliomas [13].

Presentation. Because most supratentorial gliomas in children are low grade and grow over a period of months to years, their presentation is manifested by a gradual progression of symptoms. Supporting this hypothesis, a recent study revealed that the average time from symptom onset to diagnosis of brain tumors in children was greater than 7 months [14]. The symptoms and signs of presentation are determined by tumor location and by patient age.

Tumors obstructing cerebrospinal fluid (CSF) flow may present with enlarging head circumferences in children younger than 2 years of age, whereas headaches and ataxia are more common in older children. Suprasellar lesions may present with endocrine abnormalities or visual field deficits. Tumors of the optic system may present with insidious visual loss which may go unrecognized by the parents and caregivers for months. Thalamic tumors may present with failure to thrive. Cortical tumors may also present with seizures or with the development of a focal deficit, such as weakness or sensory changes.

Diagnosis. MRI is the single most important investigation for the diagnosis and management of brain tumors. This is often the first investigation performed in a symptomatic child. However, CT is still a useful adjunct for identification of calcification in a tumor. This information can be helpful in the diagnosis of a tumor and in the surgical planning.

Treatment

Surgery. A surgical procedure is often a first step following the diagnosis of a supratentorial brain tumor. Surgery has 2 goals. The first, and most important, is to obtain a tissue diagnosis that will guide further management. The second objective is resection, if it is possible. In some cases, tumor location may prohibit a complete resection because of the risk of injuring critical neural or vascular structures. For deep lesions or lesions in eloquent cortex where an extensive resection would result in unacceptable morbidity, it is still often possible to obtain a diagnostic stereotactic needle biopsy.

For accessible, well-circumscribed lesions, surgical resection may be the only treatment necessary to achieve long-term progression-free survival. However, when the tumor is left behind, or for higher-grade lesions, patients may require adjuvant therapy with either chemotherapy, radiation therapy, or both. Due to the particular susceptibility of the brain to radiation injury in early development, the use of radiotherapy is often limited to children more than 3 years old. In some cases, the use of chemotherapy may serve as a means to control tumor growth until a child becomes old enough to become a candidate for radiotherapy.

Low-grade gliomas. Radiation therapy in the setting of an incompletely resected low-grade glioma may prolong progression-free survival, but has been shown to have little impact on overall survival [15]. Furthermore, it is associated with significant morbidity, particularly in younger children. Therefore, its use is often limited to patients with progressive or recurrent disease, or for palliation of highly symptomatic patients.

Chemotherapy can provide good disease control for many low-grade gliomas. For example, vincristine and actinomycin D have demonstrated long-term progression-free survival for nearly two-thirds of patients with optic pathway gliomas [16]. There are currently ongoing trials using a variety of chemotherapeutic regimens including lomustine, procarbazine, cisplatin, and carboplatin.

High-grade gliomas. Most high-grade gliomas are treated with surgical resection and postoperative radiation. Postoperative radiation therapy for high-grade gliomas has been shown to increase survival compared with surgery alone [17]. The effectiveness of chemotherapy for high-grade gliomas is less clear. Chemotherapy is rarely used as a stand-alone treatment, and is often used in conjunction with radiation. An example of this is temazolamide, an agent which has been shown to prolong survival in a subset of adult patients with glioblastoma multiforme, and is, therefore, increasingly used in the pediatric population with high-grade gliomas.

Outcomes. Patient age and histologic subtype are the most important predictors of patient outcome. The ability to achieve a complete resection with acceptable morbidity is also widely accepted to provide a longer progression-free survival [11]. As a general guideline, under optimal conditions, patients with low-grade gliomas have a 10-year survival rate of up to 90%, children with anaplastic gliomas have up to a 50% 5-year survival rate, and of those with glioblastoma, fewer than 20% will be alive 5 years after diagnosis [18–21].

Table 4 Supratentoral gliomas: key points
Most are low-grade astrocytomas with insidious presentation
May arise in association with tumor syndromes (eg, neurofibromatosis type 1)
Surgery usually required for resection or tissue diagnosis
Many tumors responsive to chemotherapy/radiation
Older patients and lower-grade tumors associated with more favorable outcomes

Neuronal tumors

Introduction. In contrast to gliomas, neuronal tumors have (as their name suggests) cells derived from neural lineages. These tumors are generally found supratentorially and are slow growing [22]. The most common tumor types are gangliogliomas, gangliocytomas, dysembryoplastic neuroepithelial tumors (DNET), and central neurocytomas. They are low-grade, well-circumscribed tumors whose primary clinical significance is that they may cause medically refractory seizures.

Epidemiology. Gangliogliomas and gangliocytomas account for approximately 7% of brain tumors in the pediatric population [23]. There is a slight male predominance with a male/female ratio of 1.1:1 to 1.9:1. The median age at presentation is 9 years [24]. DNETs usually present with seizure, and their incidence among patients with epilepsy is 1% to 5% [25,26]. Central neurocytomas represent about 0.25 to 0.5% of brain tumors in adolescents and young adults [27]. Their mean age at presentation is later than other neuronal tumors at 29 years, and they occur approximately equally in men and women.

Presentation. The most common presentation for gangliogliomas, gangliocytomas, and DNETs is medically refractory focal epilepsy. The semiology of the seizures depends on the tumor location. Occipital lobe tumors may present with seizures preceded by visual auras, frontal lobe tumors can present with motor seizures, and temporal lobe lesions (the most common location), often present with complex partial seizures. Central neurocytomas usually occur within the ventricles and therefore frequently present with symptoms attributable to raised intracranial pressure (headaches, nausea, and vomiting.). Duration of symptoms is typically less than 6 months, and most patients have symptoms attributable to hydrocephalus at the time of presentation [22].

Diagnosis. Gangliogliomas, gangliocytomas, and DNET are identified on MRI as well-circumscribed lesions adjacent to the cortex. Central neurocytomas are intraventricular lesions located in the lateral ventricle close to the foramen of Monro. The enhancing patterns of neuronal tumors vary. Although some lesions (such as gangliogliomas) may have nodular enhancement, others may have patchy or absent uptake of contrast. Lesions may be solid or may have cystic components. Calcification is occasionally seen on CT and is considered to indicate a slow-growing lesion that has been present for a long time, which is an especially common finding in central neurocytomas (50%–70%) [28].

Treatment. The treatment of symptomatic gangliogliomas, gangliocytomas, and DNETs is surgical resection of the lesion. They typically do not require adjuvant therapy. Consideration must also be given to treatment of their associated seizure disorder. Usually, resection of the lesion alone is sufficient to cure the seizures. However about 30% of these lesions are also associated with adjacent focal cortical dysplasia [29] which may warrant a more extensive resection if indicated by intraoperative electrocorticography.

Complete surgical resection is also the treatment of choice for central neurocytomas. This treatment also re-establishes CSF pathways in patients with hydrocephalus. Following successful surgery, most patients do not require CSF shunting. Recurrence is best treated with repeat surgery. However, stereotactic radiosurgery may be considered for small, residual, or recurrent tumors in selected patients [22].

Outcomes. The long-term outcome for neuronal tumors is favorable. These tumors rarely progress and their associated symptoms are often well controlled after complete resection of the lesions. Surgery provides for good long-term tumor control in 80% to 100% of patients [22].

Table 5
Neuronal tumors: key points

Slow-growing tumors with neuronal elements
Often present with history of medically refractory seizures for cortically located tumors
Central neurocytomas occur within lateral ventricle and may cause symptoms associated with hydrocephalus
Good outcome with complete surgical resection

Sellar and pineal brain tumors
Intracranial germ cell tumors
Introduction. Germ cell tumors are of germ cell origin, and their occurrence in the CNS is uncommon. They are more commonly found outside the CNS, with primary sites arising from the testes and ovaries. Within the CNS, they

most frequently arise near midline structures such as the pineal gland, the pituitary gland, and the third ventricle. Subtypes include germinomas and nongerminomatous germ cell tumors (NGGCT) such as teratomas (mature and immature), endodermal sinus tumor, choriocarcinoma, embryonal carcinoma, and mixed germ cell tumors [30].

Epidemiology. In North America, intracranial germ cell tumors account for 1% to 2% of all CNS tumors, and 2% to 4% of pediatric CNS tumors [28]. They are more common in Asian countries; accounting for up to 11% of brain tumors in those populations. There is a male predominance for all germ cell tumors with a male/female ratio of 2.5:1. Germinomas account for most germ cell tumors, comprising 50% to 70% of the total [30].

Presentation. Presenting symptoms depend on the size and location of the tumor. Pineal region tumors may present with hydrocephalus and extraocular muscle disorders from compression of the tectum. Patients with suprasellar tumors often present with endocrinopathies such as diabetes insipidus or precocious puberty.

Diagnosis. Diagnosis is made with MRI and laboratory investigations for the biochemical markers α-fetoprotein (AFP) and β-human chorionic gonadotropin (β-HCG). Elevations in either of these markers in either the CSF or in blood indicate an NGGCT. Human placental alkaline phosphatase (PLAP) is often elevated in germinomas. However, this test is not routinely available at most institutions.

Tissue diagnosis is often required before initiation of treatment, although some institutions treat based on imaging and biomarker profiles alone. Tissue diagnosis can often be achieved endoscopically at the time of performing a third ventriculostomy, or by stereotactic or open biopsy.

Treatment. Germ cell tumors are sensitive to chemotherapy and radiation therapy. In many cases, the role of surgery is limited to tissue diagnosis, management of hydrocephalus, and treatment of residual disease. Teratomas may be treated with surgical resection. Germinomas are remarkably sensitive to radiotherapy and are often treated by radiotherapy alone. In contrast, NGGCTs are not as radiosensitive, and therefore are also treated with chemotherapy.

Outcomes. The cure rate of germinomas is greater than 90% with radiotherapy alone. Similar outcomes for teratomas treated with surgical resection are also possible. The prognosis for other NGGCTs, however, is far worse, with 20% to 50% 5-year survival rates [30].

Table 6
Intracranial germ cell tumors: key points

Most commonly arise adjacent to midline structures: sella turcica, pineal region, and third ventricle

Role of surgery in many tumor types is primarily for tissue diagnosis and management of hydrocephalus

Germinomas are often sensitive to radiotherapy alone

NGGCTs are treated with a combination of radiation and chemotherapy

Craniopharyngiomas

Introduction. Craniopharyngiomas arise from squamous cells along the primitive craniopharyngeal duct and anterior pituitary gland. They are found in the sellar/suprasellar region, but may extend into, or reside entirely within, the third ventricle. They are histologically benign; however, their clinical course is often dictated by the associated tissue destruction that ensues. There are 2 subtypes: papillary and adamantinomatous. The adamantinomatous subtype is the type most frequently encountered in the pediatric population [31].

Epidemiology. The annual incidence is 0.13 per 100,000 population and affects males and females equally [32,33]. There is a bimodal age distribution with a peak incidence during childhood between 5 and 14 years. A second peak occurs in late adulthood. Craniopharyngiomas account for more than 50% of pediatric sellar and suprasellar tumors [32].

Presentation. Because craniopharygiomas occur in the sellar/suprasellar region, their most common presentation is as a result of compression or destruction of adjacent tissues. Patients may present with headaches, progressive visual loss, or endocrine abnormalities, such as growth delay.

Diagnosis. MRI and CT are useful for the diagnosis of craniopharyngiomas, with complementary imaging characteristics. Calcification is present in 80% of pediatric craniopharyngiomas and is best seen on CT [34]. MRI provides better detail of the relationship between the tumor and adjacent neural structures, and can also assist surgical planning.

Treatment. Complete surgical resection is the best treatment of craniopharyngiomas. However, this is sometimes not possible if the tumor is adherent to adjacent tissues such as cranial nerves and vascular structures. Radiosurgery, with either linear accelerator or γ knife, is another option for treatment, and has been reported to provide excellent long-term tumor control. Conventional radiation therapy may be used as adjuvant therapy for incomplete resections or for tumor recurrences. Intracavitary chemotherapy with bleomycin is sometimes used for recurrent tumor with a significant cystic component.

In addition to treatments for tumor control, endocrine replacement is a critical component of patient management as most patients have significant pituitary dysfunction following surgery or radiation therapy. Patients with craniopharyngiomas should be evaluated by an endocrinologist. Steroids may be necessary for patients subjected to physiologic stresses, such as surgery or systemic illness.

Outcomes. Because craniopharyngiomas are relatively benign tumors, they are associated with 10-year survival rates of better than 90%. Recurrence-free survival rates are somewhat lower and are mainly determined by the completeness of initial surgical resection [32]. Nonetheless, these tumors can follow a relentless course and long-term follow-up is warranted, as recurrence can occur years after treatment.

Pituitary tumors. In general, pituitary tumors are rare in children. Most common are adenomas, including those that secrete hormones (functional) and those that do not (nonfunctional). When symptomatic, these lesions frequently present with endocrinologic or visual symptoms. Diagnosis is made by endocrine and visual testing, coupled with dedicated imaging such as MRI. Some lesions, such as prolactinomas, can be successfully treated with medical therapy. Others require surgical intervention, often with a transsphenoidal approach. Long-term prognoses for these lesions are usually good, although the cumulative morbidity of endocrinopathies can be overlooked.

Table 7
Craniopharyngiomas: key points

Most commonly arise in sellar/suprasellar region and cause mass effect on pituitary gland and optic chiasm

Often present with visual field loss, endocrine abnormalities, or mass effect—usually hydrocephalus from third ventricle obstruction

Treated by multiple modalities including surgery, stereotactic radiosurgery, radiation therapy, and intracavitary chemotherapy

Patients may require long-term pituitary hormone replacement after treatment, including stress-dose steroids

Infratentorial brain tumors

Cerebellar astrocytomas

Introduction. Cerebellar astrocytomas are tumors of astrocytic origin that usually occur in the cerebellar hemisphere and may have extension into the brainstem and adjacent structures. They are the most common posterior fossa tumors in children, and most (>80%) of these tumors are pilocytic astrocytomas (WHO grade I) [35].

Epidemiology. Cerebellar astrocytomas are among the most common type of pediatric brain tumor. Their incidence is approximately 0.4 per 100,000 children per year [36]. The incidence peaks between 4 and 10 years of age. The male/female ratio is about 1:1 [35,37].

Presentation. The duration of symptoms before diagnosis can be lengthy: up to 5 months in one series [13]. This duration is longer than for patients with other posterior fossa tumors such as ependymomas and medulloblastomas, presumably due to the slow growth of pilocytic astrocytomas [35].

Most children present with symptoms of increased intracranial pressure, including headache, nausea and vomiting, gait disturbance, and, in infants, increasing head circumference. Signs at diagnosis often include papilledema, ataxia, and nystagmus. These signs and symptoms may be due to direct compression of neural structures, or secondary to hydrocephalus caused by tumor obstruction of the fourth ventricle.

Diagnosis. CT and MRI can be useful in detecting a cerebellar astrocytoma, although MRI is generally most helpful in making the radiographic diagnosis, and is useful for surgical planning. Classic imaging findings include a cystic lesion of the cerebellar hemisphere with an enhancing mural nodule. However, these tumors may also be solid without any cystic component. CT appearance is usually hypodense, whereas MRI typically reveals a lesion that is bright on T2, indicating the high water content of these tumors. The solid component usually enhances uniformly, whereas cystic areas may not take up contrast. Greater than 85% of patients also have evidence of hydrocephalus, usually secondary to CSF obstruction at the level of the fourth ventricle.

Treatment. Gross total resection is the single best treatment of cerebellar astrocytomas and may be achieved in up to 80% of operative cases. Postoperative MRI within 72 hours of resection is commonly obtained to evaluate the extent of surgical resection. If residual tumor remains, the surgeon may decide to attempt further resection, depending on the location of the tumor and the clinical status of the patient.

Recurrence of cerebellar astrocytomas may occur years after treatment. When identified, most can be managed with reoperation. Similar to primary surgery, a gross total resection at a second operation is associated with a good long-term prognosis.

Outcomes. Long-term survival after surgery is common and dependent on the extent of tumor resection. With gross total resection, outcomes are excellent, with 5- and 10-year progression-free survival of greater than 80% [38]. With subtotal resection, about 75% have progression during follow-up [37].

Table 8
Cerebellar astrocytomas: key points
Most common posterior fossa tumor of childhood
Present with progressive symptoms over several months
Excellent outcome with complete surgical resection

Brainstem gliomas
Introduction. Brainstem gliomas had historically been considered a homogenous group of neoplasms with a dismal prognosis. However, the understanding of these lesions has changed with the advent of MRI and improved surgical techniques. Today, it is recognized that tumors of glial origin that arise from the brainstem vary in histology, location, and prognosis [39].

Glial-based tumors of the brainstem can be broadly classified as either diffuse or focal. The diffuse intrinsic gliomas (the subtype most commonly attached to the name "brainstem glioma") have uniformly poor prognoses. Although these diffuse lesions may have variable histologic subtypes (WHO grades II, II or IV), differing grades do not correlate with clinical course or response to therapy; the outcome is poor in nearly all cases (see section on Outcome later). In contrast, focal tumors, often found in the midbrain or cervicomedullary junction as dorsally exophytic lesions, are slower growing and have a more favorable prognosis. Histologic subtypes of these lesions commonly include pilocytic astrocytoma or ganglioglioma.

Epidemiology. Brainstem gliomas represent about 25% of pediatric posterior fossa tumors and 10% to 20% of all CNS tumors in children [39]. The median age at presentation is 7 years and the male/female ratio is approximately 1:1 [39].

Presentation. Presentation of brainstem gliomas is related to the location and type of tumor. Physical findings in patients with diffuse brainstem gliomas often include cranial nerve palsies, ataxia, and long-tract signs such as weakness, hyperreflexia, and spasticity. Focal midbrain tumors may present with extraocular motor palsies and hydrocephalus secondary to obstruction of the cerebral aqueduct. Dorsal exophytic tumors with extension into the fourth ventricle may present with symptoms of raised intracranial pressure including nausea, vomiting, ataxia, headaches, and ataxia. Cervicomedullary tumors may present with torticollis, nystagmus lower cranial nerve palsies resulting in dysphagia, dysarthria, and apnea.

Diagnosis. MRI is the diagnostic modality of choice for brainstem tumors; however brainstem tumors can often be identified on CT. Diffuse pontine gliomas are characterized by an enlarged pons with minimal or patchy enhancement, whereas focal lesions are well circumscribed on imaging, often with intense uptake of contrast.

Treatment. Treatment must be tailored to the specific type of tumor. Diffuse pontine gliomas are diagnosed by MRI and there is frequently no need for tissue diagnosis. The current treatment of these is fractionated radiotherapy, but the prognosis is poor [40]. The role of systemic and intrathecal chemotherapy via a ventricular reservoir remains a topic of debate. Treatment of obstructive hydrocephalus may be achieved through endoscopic third ventriculostomy (ETV) or ventriculoperitoneal (VP) shunting.

For focal tumors, surgery may be an option. With midbrain gliomas involving the tectum, CSF diversion via ETV or VP shunting may be the only treatment necessary, as some of these tumors follow an indolent course. For other focal tumors, surgical resection of accessible tumor may be indicated to confirm diagnosis and relieve symptoms from mass effect or CSF obstruction. If possible, gross total resections may be curative, although subtotal resection is common due to the risk of injury to surrounding structures. With focal lesions, recurrences may be amenable to reoperation. Some institutions have used chemotherapy for focal lesions, either as a primary treatment or as a precursor to an attempt at an aggressive surgical resection.

Outcomes. The outcome for diffuse brainstem gliomas remains poor despite the use of radiation and chemotherapy. Most patients have some response to radiation; however, median survival is 5 to 6 months, with less than 10% survival after 2 years [41].

Outcomes for focal brainstem tumors are considerably better than for diffuse tumors. Patients with tectal gliomas usually require little more than management of hydrocephalus and periodic neuroimaging (ultimately many transition from a scan every 3–6 mo to annual studies). Patients with other focal tumors also fare well after treatment. With current treatment modalities, 5-year tumor control is seen in 90% of patients with focal brainstem tumors (Table 9–11) [42].

Table 9
Brainstem gliomas: key points

Heterogeneous group of tumors with variable prognosis
Often present with cranial nerve palsies and ataxia
Diffuse tumors have worst prognosis, with median survival of 6 months
Focal tumors are more indolent, with good long-term survival

Ependymomas
Introduction. Ependymomas are tumors arising from the ependymal lining of the ventricular system. They can be found throughout the CNS. Two-thirds of intracranial ependymomas arise within the posterior fossa and often extend out the foramina of the fourth ventricle, and only one-third of ependymomas present supratentorially [28]. Ependymoma cells have the capacity to disseminate throughout the neuraxis, and patients may already have distal seeding on presentation [43].

Epidemiology. Ependymomas represent the third most common pediatric brain tumor, behind medulloblastoma and astrocytoma, and have an annual incidence of 0.2 to 0.3 per 100,000 children. The median age at diagnosis is between 4 and 6 years. There is a second, smaller peak in the mid-30s. There is a male predominance, with a male/female ratio of 2:1 [43].

Presentation. Patients with ependymomas usually present with symptoms related to increased intracranial pressure secondary to hydrocephalus resulting from obstruction of CSF pathways. Common symptoms include headaches, nausea, vomiting, and gait disturbances. However, focal deficits may occur if a tumor compresses specific nuclei or spinal cord tracts.

Diagnosis. Ependymomas are included in the differential diagnosis of a fourth ventricle tumor on either CT or MRI. Extension of tumor through the foramina of Lushka or Magendie raises the suspicion of an ependymoma. Given the capacity of these tumors to seed the CNS, dissemination into the spinal canal may be present, and MRI of the entire neuraxis should be performed. Enhancement of these lesions is often patchy.

Treatment. The recommended treatment of ependymoma is gross total resection. Unfortunately, this is not always possible because tumor invasion into the brainstem, and infiltration around cranial nerves, prevents complete resection in many patients. Radiation therapy is a standard adjuvant to surgical resection in children older than 3 years, and has been shown to reduce the risk of recurrence [43]. In some cases, especially infants for whom radiation may not be an option, a combination of systemic and intrathecal chemotherapy may be used. Commonly, this includes cisplatin as a key agent [43].

Outcomes. With a combination of surgical resection, adjuvant radiotherapy, and chemotherapy, progression-free survival is 30% to 45%. Overall survival is slightly better at 50% to 60% [43]. Long-term outcomes are significantly influenced by the long-term effects of treatment. One major concern, especially in younger children, is long-term cognitive impairment. The degree of cognitive impairment has been shown to correlate with the dose of craniospinal radiation and the age of the child at time of treatment [44].

Table 10
Ependymomas: key points

Arise from ependymal lining of ventricular system
Third most common posterior fossa tumor of childhood
Mainstays of treatment include surgical resection and radiotherapy

Medulloblastoma and other embryonal tumors
Introduction. This group of tumors accounts for a large proportion of pediatric brain tumors, of which medulloblastoma is the most common. They are often referred to as primitive neuroectodermal tumors (PNET) and include medulloblastoma, atypical teratoid/rhabdoid tumors (ATRT), pineoblastoma, and ependymoblastoma. They are often also collectively referred to as "small blue cell tumors" along with other primitive tumors, such as Ewing sarcoma, because of their histologic appearance [45].

Epidemiology. Medulloblastomas account for about 20% of all pediatric brain tumors and are the second most common type of brain tumor after pilocytic astrocytomas. Median age at presentation is 4 years. Male/female ratio is 1.5:1 [45].

Presentation. Medulloblastomas most often occur in the midline cerebellum at the level of the fourth ventricle. Similar to ependymomas, they may present with symptoms related to CSF obstruction and hydrocephalus, such as headache, nausea, vomiting, and gait disturbance.

Diagnosis. CT demonstrates a hyperdense tumor, usually in the midline cerebellum with relatively homogenous enhancement. Hydrocephalus is present in 95% of patients. As with most brain tumors, MRI provides higher resolution imaging than CT and should generally be obtained for surgical planning. Medulloblastomas exhibit patchy contrast enhancement in more than 90% of cases. Because of the tendency of medulloblastomas to disseminate within the CNS, MRI of the spine should be performed as part of the staging evaluation.

Treatment. Surgical resection is the primary treatment of medulloblastomas. The goals of treatment are tissue diagnosis, re-establishment of CSF flow, and cytoreduction. After resection, patients are stratified according to standard risk or increased risk. This risk stratification is based on the presence of distant metastases and the amount of residual tumor. The stratification is then used to determine the type of adjuvant radiation and chemotherapy that patients receive, with higher risk patients receiving more intensive therapy [46]. Nearly all patients need adjuvant therapy postoperatively.

Some patients may need VP shunting even after restoration of normal CSF pathways. This need for shunting may be due to elevated protein in the CSF, but regardless of the cause, it is important for the clinician to be cognizant of the possibility of delayed hydrocephalus. Diagnosis can usually be made clinically, with the findings of headache or vomiting, and radiographically, with CT or MRI, looking for ventricular enlargement. Placement of a shunt entails the risk of introducing tumor cells outside of the CNS, although this is a largely theoretical risk.

Outcomes. Overall survival for patients with medulloblastoma is now greater than 60% at 5 years, and up to 50% at 10 years [45]. As with ependymomas, the need for cranial radiation may be associated with cognitive decline in long-term survivors. Younger patients may also have growth retardation secondary to the effects of irradiation to the pituitary gland and spine.

Table 11
Medulloblastoma and other embryonal tumors: key points

Second most common posterior fossa tumor of childhood
Belong to larger category of aggressive "small blue cell tumors"
Require aggressive surgical resection and adjuvant radiation and chemotherapy for improved
  survival

RECENT ADVANCES IN THE DIAGNOSIS AND TREATMENT OF BRAIN TUMORS

Proton MR spectroscopy

MR spectroscopy is a recent advance in the diagnosis of different subtypes of brain tumors. Brain tumors have characteristic decreases in *N*-acetyl aspartate compared with normal areas of the brain. Higher-grade tumors have areas of increased cellularity, and this may be demonstrated by increased levels of choline (an element found in the cell membrane) as measured by an increased ratio of choline to creatinine.

In addition, it is also possible to narrow the differential diagnosis for a tumor in a particular location by virtue of the specific characteristics of that type of tumor. For instance, MR spectroscopy of choroid plexus tumors is characterized by a prominent choline peak and absence of *N*-acetyl aspartate [47,48]. Furthermore, the metabolites of the different types of posterior fossa tumors (pilocytic astrocytoma, medulloblastoma, and ependymoma) can also be differentiated by MR spectroscopy [49]. As MR spectroscopy is further studied, it may lead to reliable tumor diagnosis based on imaging alone.

Intraoperative MRI

The use of intraoperative MRI is becoming more widely available at several pediatric hospitals. This useful technology allows patients to undergo repeat imaging during their surgical procedure. Repeat imaging gives additional information to surgeons, allowing them to see whether any residual tumor remains. This additional information has the distinct advantage of being able to confirm complete tumor resection during the initial operation, thereby eliminating the need for early re-operations. This technology is often coupled with navigation software, allowing for more accurate localization of the tumor. The past decade has also seen the use of robotics in surgery. This technology has been used to develop an MR-compatible robot that is able to incorporate neuronavigation information and constantly updated MR images to assist with the resection of tumor [50].

Use of biomarkers for brain tumors

One of the most difficult issues in treating brain tumors is a lack of effective methods to detect novel or recurrent disease. Currently, there are no generally accepted screening protocols for the discovery of asymptomatic brain tumors, particularly primary brain tumors. Early detection of tumors in other organ systems, novel and recurrent, has frequently resulted in markedly improved patient outcomes. It would therefore be desirable to recapitulate the successes achieved in other organ systems through the development of noninvasive biomarkers capable of identifying brain tumors.

Despite recent advances in the imaging and treatment of brain tumors, the ability to prospectively diagnose new tumors or to detect tumor recurrence remains poor. Remodeling of the extracellular matrix (ECM) and dysregulation of angiogenesis (the process of new blood vessel formation) are processes essential to the development and maintenance of many tumors. Matrix metalloproteinases (MMPs) (a multigene family of degradative enzymes) have been implicated in the establishment and maintenance of the vasculature required for tumor progression and metastasis and in the initial angiogenic phase of tumor growth in experimental models and human tumors [51–53]. In the CNS, MMPs have been associated with brain tumor development. Studies of primary brain tumors reveal that MMP-2, MMP-9, and several other MMPs are overexpressed in experimental models and tissue samples from human patients [54–64]. MMPs are detectable in the urine of cancer patients [53] and correlate with the presence and stage of disease in several tumors [7,65–68]. Recent work has explored the use of urinary MMPs as biomarkers for brain tumors [29].

Use of urinary biomarkers as a means to screen for and follow known brain tumors has several appealing features. Collection of urine is risk-free and easy for the patient, in contrast to many radiographic studies. In particular, urine sampling avoids the need for sedation and its attendant risks, which are often required to accomplish radiographic studies in the pediatric population. Urinary sample collection and MMP analysis is considerably less expensive than MRIs. Sampling of urine can easily be done at shorter intervals than are currently practical for imaging studies; enabling earlier detection of recurrent disease. Significantly, the detection of MMPs is an assay of biologic activity and is intrinsically different from standard imaging studies, most of which evaluate anatomic findings. At a minimum, measurement of MMP levels could provide an alternative means of evaluating the presence or recurrence of a brain tumor, complementing existing techniques. At best, it could provide a more sensitive and responsive tool for identifying and monitoring brain tumors.

SUMMARY

Despite many advances in medicine, pediatric brain tumors remain a formidable diagnostic and therapeutic challenge. Recent advances in imaging, noninvasive diagnostic tests, and improved surgical, chemotherapeutic, and radiation techniques offer promise to afflicted patients. However, good outcomes for children affected with these lesions ultimately depend on a combination of the ability of primary care providers to recognize the presence of a tumor, and the capacity for specialists to develop and provide effective treatments.

References

[1] Smith ER, Butler WE, Barker FG 2nd. Craniotomy for resection of pediatric brain tumors in the United States, 1988–2000: effects of provider caseloads and progressive centralization and specialization of care. Neurosurgery 2004;54:553–63 [discussion: 563–65].

[2] Surawicz TS, Davis F, Freels S, et al. Brain tumor survival: results from the National Cancer Data Base. J Neurooncol 1998;40:151–60.

[3] Surawicz TS, McCarthy BJ, Kupelian V, et al. Descriptive epidemiology of primary brain and CNS tumors: results from the Central Brain Tumor Registry of the United States, 1990–1994. Neuro Oncol 1999;1:14–25.

[4] Barker FG 2nd, Curry WT Jr, Carter BS. Surgery for primary supratentorial brain tumors in the United States, 1988 to 2000: the effect of provider caseload and centralization of care. Neuro Oncol 2005;7:49–63.

[5] Farwell JR, Dohrmann GJ, Flannery JT. Intracranial neoplasms in infants. Arch Neurol 1978;35:533–7.

[6] Fernandez CA, Yan L, Louis G, et al. The matrix metalloproteinase-9/neutrophil gelatinase-associated lipocalin complex plays a role in breast tumor growth and is present in the urine of breast cancer patients. Clin Cancer Res 2005;11:5390–5.

[7] Medina LS, Pinter JD, Zurakowski D, et al. Children with headache: clinical predictors of surgical space-occupying lesions and the role of neuroimaging. Radiology 1997;202: 819–24.

[8] Keles GE, Banerjee A, Puri D, et al. Supratentorial gliomas. In: Gupta N, Banerjee A, Haas-Kogan D, editors. Pediatric CNS tumors. Berlin: Springer; 2004.

[9] Kim IY, Niranjan A, Kondziolka D, et al. Gamma knife radiosurgery for treatment resistant choroid plexus papillomas. J Neurooncol 2008;90:105–10.

[10] Ries LAG, Eisner EP, Kosary CL, et al. editors. SEER Cancer Statistics Review, 1975–2000. Bethesda (MD): National Cancer Institutue; 2003.

[11] Dohrmann GJ, Farwell JR, Flannery JT. Astrocytomas in childhood: a population-based study. Surg Neurol 1985;23:64–8.

[12] Taylor T, Jaspan T, Milano G, et al. PLAN Study group. Radiological classification of optic pathway gliomas: experience of a modified functional classification system. Br J Radiol 2008;81:761–6.

[13] Binning MJ, Liu JK, Kestle JR, et al. Optic pathway gliomas: a review. Neurosurg Focus 2007;23:E2.

[14] Mehta V, Chapman A, McNeely PD, et al. Latency between symptom onset and diagnosis of pediatric brain tumors: an Eastern Canadian geographic study. Neurosurgery 2002;51: 365–72.

[15] Pollack IF, Gerszten PC, Martinez AJ, et al. Intracranial ependymomas of childhood: long-term outcome and prognostic factors. Neurosurgery 1995;37:655–66 [discussion: 666–67].

[16] Packer RJ, Sutton LN, Bilaniuk LT, et al. Treatment of chiasmatic/hypothalamic gliomas of childhood with chemotherapy: an update. Ann Neurol 1988;23:79–85.

[17] Bloom HJ, Glees J, Bell J, et al. The treatment and long-term prognosis of children with intracranial tumors: a study of 610 cases, 1950–1981. Int J Radiat Oncol Biol Phys 1990;18:723–45.

[18] Packer RJ, Ater J, Allen J, et al. Carboplatin and vincristine chemotherapy for children with newly diagnosed progressive low-grade gliomas. J Neurosurg 1997;86:747–54.

[19] Gururangan S, Cavazos CM, Ashley D, et al. Phase II study of carboplatin in children with progressive low-grade gliomas. J Clin Oncol 2002;20:2951–8.

[20] Sposto R, Ertel IJ, Jenkin RD, et al. The effectiveness of chemotherapy for treatment of high grade astrocytoma in children: results of a randomized trial. A report from the Childrens Cancer Study Group. J Neurooncol 1989;7:165–77.

[21] Finlay JL, Boyett JM, Yates AJ, et al. Randomized phase III trial in childhood high-grade astrocytoma comparing vincristine, lomustine, and prednisone with the eight-drugs-in-1-day regimen. Childrens Cancer Group. J Clin Oncol 1995;13:112–23.

[22] von Koch CS, Schmidt MH, Perry V. Neuronal tumors. In: Gupta N, Barnerjee A, Haas-Kogan D, editors. Pediatric CNS tumors. Berlin: Springer; 2004. p. 143–55.

[23] Johannssen JH, Rekate HL, Roessmann U. Gangliogliomas: pathological and clinical correlation. J Neurosurg 1981;54:58–63.

[24] Johnson JH Jr, Hariharan S, Berman J, et al. Clinical outcome of pediatric gangliogliomas: ninety-nine cases over 20 years. Pediatr Neurosurg 1997;203–7.

[25] Morris HH, Estes ML, Gilmore R, et al. Chronic intractable epilepsy as the only symptom of primary brain tumor. Epilepsia 1993;34:1038–43.

[26] Wolf HK, Weister OD. Surgical pathology of chronic epileptic seizure disorder. Brain Pathol 1993;3:371–80.

[27] Hassoun J, Soylemezoglu F, Gambarelli D, et al. Central neurocytoma: a synopsis of clinical and histological features. Brain Pathol 1993;3:297–306.

[28] Osborn AG, Blazer S, Saltzman K. Diagnostic imaging: brain. Salt Lake City (UT): AMIRSYS; 2004.

[29] Benifla M, Otsubo H, Ochi A, et al. Temporal lobe surgery for intractable epilepsy in children: an analysis of outcomes in 126 children. Neurosurgery 2006;59:1203–13 [discussion: 1213–14].

[30] Lieuw KH, Haas-Kogan D, Ablin A. Intracranial germ cell tumors. In: Gupta N, Banerjee A, Haas-Kogan D, editors. Pediatric CNS tumors. Berlin: Springer; 2004. p. 107–21.

[31] Wisoff JH, Donahue BR. Craniopharyngiomas. In: Albright AL, Pollack I, Adelson PD, editors. Principles and practice of pediatric neurosurgery. New York: Thieme; 2008.

[32] Du R, Lustig RH, Fisch B, et al. Craniopharyngioma. In: Gupta N, Barnerjee A, Haas-Kogan D, editors. Pediatric CNS tumors. Berlin: Springer; 2004. p. 132–42.

[33] Ellenbogen RG, Winston KR, Kupsky WJ. Tumors of the choroid plexus in children. Neurosurgery 1989;25:327–35.

[34] Moore K, Couldwell WT. Craniopharyngioma. In: Bernstein M, Berger MS, editors. Neuro-oncology: the essentials. New York: Thieme; 2000. p. 409–18.

[35] Taylor MD, Sanford RA, Boop FA. Cerebellar pilocytic astrocytomas. In: Albright AL, Pollack I, Adelson PD, editors. Principles and practice of pediatric neurosurgery. 2nd edition. New York: Thieme; 2008. p. 655–67.

[36] Burkhard C, Di Patre PL, Schüler D, et al. A population-based study of the incidence and survival rates in patients with pilocytic astrocytoma. J Neurosurg 2003;98: 1170–4.

[37] Chi JH, Gupta N. Cerebellar astrocytomas. In: Gupta N, Banerjee A, Haas-Koogan D, editors. Pediatric CNS tumors. Berlin: Springer; 2004. p. 27–47.

[38] Fisher PG, Tihan T, Goldthwaite PT, et al. Outcome analysis of childhood low-grade astrocytomas. Pediatr Blood Cancer 2008;51:245–50.

[39] Pan E, Prados M. Brainstem gliomas. In: Gupta N, Barnerjee A, Haas-Kogan D, editors. Pediatric CNS tumors. Berlin: Springer; 2004. p. 29–43.

[40] Jallo GI, Biser-Rohrbaugh A, Freed D. Brainstem gliomas. Childs Nerv Syst 2004;20: 143–53.

[41] Farmer JP, Montes JL, Freeman CR, et al. Brainstem gliomas. A 10-year institutional review. Pediatr Neurosurg 2001;34:206–14.

[42] Farmer JP, McNeely PD, Freeman CR. Brainstem Gliomas. In: Albright AL, Pollack I, Adelson PD, editors. Principles and practice of pediatric neurosurgery. 2nd edition. New York: Thieme; 2008. p. 640–54.

[43] Horn BN, Smyth M. Ependymoma. In: Gupta N, Barnerjee A, Haas-Kogan D, editors. Pediatric CNS tumors. Berlin: Springer; 2004. p. 65–81.

[44] Grill J, Renaux VK, Bulteau C, et al. Long-term intellectual outcome in children with posterior fossa tumors according to radiation doses and volumes. Int J Radiat Oncol Biol Phys 1999;45:137–45.

[45] Fisher PG. Embryonal tumors. In: Gupta N, Banerjee A, Haas-Kogan D, editors. Pediatric CNS tumors. Berlin: Springer; 2004. p. 83–105.

[46] Packer RJ, Rood BR, MacDonald TJ. Medulloblastoma: present concepts of stratification into risk groups. Pediatr Neurosurg 2003;39:60–7.

[47] Horska A, Ulug AM, Melhem ER, et al. Proton magnetic resonance spectroscopy of choroid plexus tumors in children. J Magn Reson Imaging 2001;14:78–82.

[48] Humphreys RP, Nemoto S, Hendrick EB, et al. Childhood choroid plexus tumors. Concepts Pediatr Neurosurg 1987;7:1–18.

[49] Davies NP, Wilson M, Harris LM, et al. Identification and characterisation of childhood cerebellar tumours by in vivo proton MRS. NMR Biomed 2008;21:908–18.

[50] Sutherland GR, Latour I, Greer AD, et al. An image-guided magnetic resonance-compatible surgical robot. Neurosurgery 2008;62:286–92 [discussion: 292–93].

[51] Bergers G, Brekken R, McMahon G, et al. Matrix metalloproteinase-9 triggers the angiogenic switch during carcinogenesis. Nat Cell Biol 2000;2:737–44.

[52] Fang J, Shing Y, Wiederschain D, et al. Matrix metalloproteinase-2 is required for the switch to the angiogenic phenotype in a tumor model. Proc Natl Acad Sci U S A 2000;97:3884–9.

[53] Moses MA, Sudhalter J, Langer R. Identification of an inhibitor of neovascularization from cartilage. Science 1990;248:1408–10.

[54] Beliveau R, Delbecchi L, Beaulieu E, et al. Expression of matrix metalloproteinases and their inhibitors in human brain tumors. Ann NY Acad Sci 1999;236–9.

[55] Kunishio K, Okada M, Matsumoto Y, et al. Matrix metalloproteinase-2 and -9 expression in astrocytic tumors. Brain Tumor Pathol 2003;20:39–45.

[56] Lampert K, Machein U, Machein MR, et al. Expression of matrix metalloproteinases and their tissue inhibitors in human brain tumors. Am J Pathol 1998;153:429–37.

[57] Laurence KM. The biology of choroid plexus papilloma in infancy and childhood. Acta Neurochir (Wien) 1979;50:79–90.

[58] Lena G, Genitori L, Molina J, et al. Choroid plexus tumours in children. Review of 24 cases. Acta Neurochir (Wien) 1990;106:68–72.

[59] Noha M, Yoshida D, Watanabe K, et al. Suppression of cell invasion on human malignant glioma cell lines by a novel matrix-metalloproteinase inhibitor SI–27: in vitro study. J Neurooncol 2000;48:217–23.

[60] Paek SH, Kim DG, Park CK, et al. The role of matrix metalloproteinases and tissue inhibitors of matrix metalloproteinase in microcystic meningiomas. Oncol Rep 2006;16:49–56.

[61] Park CM, Park MJ, Kwak HJ, et al. Ionizing radiation enhances matrix metalloproteinase-2 secretion and invasion of glioma cells through Src/epidermal growth factor receptor-mediated p38/Akt and phosphatidylinositol 3-Kinase/Akt signaling pathways. Cancer Res 2006;66:8511–9.

[62] Pollack I. Supratentorial hemispheric gliomas. In: Albright AL, Pollack I, Adelson PD, editors. Principles and practice of pediatric neurosurgery. 2nd edition. New York: Thieme; 2008. p. 511–30.

[63] Thier M, Roeb E, Breuer B, et al. Expression of matrix metalloproteinase-2 in glial and neuronal tumor cell lines: inverse correlation with proliferation rate. Cancer Lett 2000;149:163–70.

[64] Zhao JX, Yang LP, Wang YF, et al. Gelatinolytic activity of matrix metalloproteinase-2 and matrix metalloproteinase-9 in rat brain after implantation of 9L rat glioma cells. Eur J Neurol 2007;14:510–6.

[65] Chan LW, Moses MA, Goley E, et al. Urinary VEGF and MMP levels as predictive markers of 1-year progression-free survival in cancer patients treated with radiation therapy: a longitudinal study of protein kinetics throughout tumor progression and therapy. J Clin Oncol 2004;22:499–506.

[66] Moses MA, Wiederschain D, Loughlin KR, et al. Increased incidence of matrix metalloproteinases in urine of cancer patients. Cancer Res 1998;58:1395–9.

[67] Roy R, Wewer UM, Zurakowski D, et al. ADAM 12 cleaves extracellular matrix proteins and correlates with cancer status and stage. J Biol Chem 2004;279:51323–30.

[68] Yan L, Borregaard N, Kjeldsen L, et al. The high molecular weight urinary matrix metalloproteinase (MMP) activity is a complex of gelatinase B/MMP-9 and neutrophil gelatinase-associated lipocalin (NGAL). Modulation of MMP-9 activity by NGAL. J Biol Chem 2001;276:37258–65.

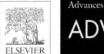

Advances in Pediatrics 56 (2009) 271–299

ADVANCES IN PEDIATRICS

Pediatric Stroke: Past, Present and Future

Neil Friedman, MBChB

Center for Pediatric Neurology/Desk S71, Neurological Institute, Cleveland Clinic, 9500 Euclid Avenue, Cleveland, OH 44195, USA

The past two decades have seen a renewed interest and focus in pediatric stroke. Although pediatric stroke in its various guises (acute infantile hemiplegia, hemiplegic cerebral palsy, and apoplexy) was described as early as the 15th century, it is only more recently that a systematic effort has been made to better define the epidemiology and etiology of pediatric stroke, classify pediatric stroke types, and move toward randomized controlled therapeutic and prevention trials. Although relatively uncommon compared with many other childhood diseases, pediatric stroke carries with it a disproportionately high morbidity and long-term personal and societal cost. Improved and safer noninvasive imaging modalities, and an increasing awareness of pediatric stroke amongst physicians, have allowed for better ascertainment data, which is reflected in the increased incidence in recent years. With more children surviving once-fatal and incurable disease (eg, congenital heart disease [CHD] and malignancies), the incidence of pediatric stroke is likely to increase as neurologic morbidity, in particular stroke, is a well-known sequela of many of these disorders.

This review focuses on arterial ischemic stroke (AIS) in childhood and the perinatal period and does not address other stroke mechanisms such as primary hemorrhagic stroke or sinus venous thrombosis. A brief historical review describes the basis of current knowledge on the incidence, epidemiology, etiology, outcome, and recurrence risk in pediatric stroke, and recent developments in treatment and research are highlighted.

HISTORICAL CONTEXT

The concept of pediatric AIS is defined as any clinical neurologic presentation, including seizure, associated with radiographic evidence of ischemia, infarction, or encephalomalacia in an arterial vascular distribution corresponding to the neurologic deficit or presentation. Acute infarction in confirmed by a hypodensity on computerized tomography (CT) scan in a vascular distribution, or by a diffusion-weighted image abnormality on magnetic resonance imaging

E-mail address: friedmn@ccf.org

0065-3101/09/$ – see front matter
doi:10.1016/j.yapd.2009.08.003

(MRI) study. One exception to this definition is the nonvascular distribution of stroke seen in metabolic disorders such as mitochondrial encephalopathy, lactic acidosis, and stroke (MELAS).

Pediatric stroke was reported in the earliest medical literature as part of case descriptions or clinical series under synonyms such as "cerebral apoplexy," "acute infantile hemiplegia," "acute hemiplegia of childhood," "congenital hemiplegia," and "hemiplegic cerebral palsy." In the absence of imaging studies, and little in the way of pathology, the common denominator was simply the appearance of a hemiplegia in a child. Developmental malformations, tumors, postseizure edema or paralysis, and infectious processes such as cerebral abscesses were all undoubtedly included in this group. With the use of cerebral angiography in children in the late 1950s and early 1960s, radiographic documentation of intracranial vasculopathies was confirmed as the mechanical or etiologic cause of acute hemiplegia in selective children, although the pathophysiology remained elusive [1,2]. CT scans and subsequent MRI and magnetic resonance angiography (MRA) allowed a noninvasive means to image the brain and clarify the nature of the cause of the hemiplegia, although not necessarily the etiology and pathophysiology.

Although the description of stroke has its origins in antiquity in the discussions of Hippocrates and Galen, one of the first documented cases of pediatric stroke in the medical literature may be that of Thomas Willis (1621–1675) in the 17th century [3]. He described a case of neonatal seizures resulting in death within the first month of life of a newborn who was the fourth child of a mother who had already lost 3 previous children in the neonatal period under similar circumstances. At autopsy, Willis described hemorrhage in the brain, but different translations of his original work have raised uncertainty as to the exact site. Although some authors have suggested this was a case of childhood stroke [4], others have argued this case was one of infanticide secondary to a whiplash or shaking injury [3]. Irrespective, a decade or so later, in 1672, Willis did describe a case of suspected venous infarction in a child secondary to presumed septic thrombosis of a cerebral sinus [3].

The 17th century was dominated by the neuroanatomists; however, clinical neurology remained limited by a lack of understanding of the functional anatomy of the brain. Although Willis was the first to realize the clinical importance of the circle or arteries at the base of the brain, subsequently named for him, Gabriel Fallopius (1523–1562) was the first to describe its existence in 1561, and illustrations appeared in the anatomic works of Guilio Casserio (1545–1605) in 1632 and Johann Vesling (1595–1598) in 1647. The presence of the motor cortex was first suggested around this time by Robert Boyle (1627–1691), who described a case of reversible monoplegia ("dead palsy of the arm") following the elevation of a depressed skull fracture in a patient. Advances in understanding of stroke during the 18th century included Giovanni Battista Morgagni's (1682–1771) assertion that lesions occur in the brain opposite the site of hemiplegia (confirmed by anatomically accurate postmortem findings), which was correlated by the works of Emanuel Swedenborg (1688–1772), who described the correct location and regional representation of the motor cortex in the brain. Experimental neurophysiology was introduced by François Pourfour de Petit (1664–1741), whose work in dogs confirmed that the removal of part of the brain resulted in a paralysis on the opposite side of the body. He is also credited with describing the decussation of the pyramidal tracts. The neuropathological basis for apoplexy was also first documented during this era by Giovanni Battista Morgagni, who provided pathologic evidence that the lesion in apoplexy was on the opposite side of the hemiplegia, and Matthew Baillie (1761–1823), who first described cerebral hemorrhage as the consequence of disease of the blood vessels of the brain (but did not recognize the contribution of vascular disease to ischemia of the brain) [5].

It was only during the 19th century that neuropathology started providing some understanding of disease process and with it functional neuroanatomy. The etiologic basis of stroke, which up until that time mostly consisted of hemiplegia on the basis of apoplexy from intracerebral hemorrhage, began to be better delineated by Moritz Heinrich Romberg (1795–1873), who brought structure to the field of neurology by classifying diseases into "neuroses of sensibility" and "neuroses of motility," Jean-Martin Charcot (1825–1893), who clinically demonstrated cerebral localization, and whose work in "cerebral hemiplegia" included defining the blood supply of the brain (especially the internal capsule and basal ganglia), and John Hughlings Jackson (1835–1911), who introduced the concept of paralysis generally resulting from vascular disturbances in the territory of the middle cerebral artery and who studied cerebrovascular disease [5].

That ischemia rather than "vascular congestion" was the cause of "anemia" of the brain and apoplexy was first suggested by John Cheyne (1777–1836) in 1812 after postmortem studies in apoplexy survivors showed cystic cavities or encephalomalacia. Almost 50 years before, Gerard van Swieten (1700–1772) had suggested emboli as a cause of apoplexy in a case of "polyps" in the heart travelling to the arteries in the brain. Rudolf Virchow (1821–1902) demonstrated the role of vascular occlusion producing cerebral infarction in 1856 [5].

Pediatric stroke, in particular, owes much of its origins to the seminal works of Osler [6], Sachs [7], Freud [8], Gowers [9], and Taylor [10], who wrote early monographs on cerebral palsy, which included hemiplegic forms of cerebral palsy. In 1884, Strümpell postulated primary encephalitis (polioencephalitis acuta) as the infectious basis for acquired hemiplegic cerebral palsy, believing this was akin to anterior poliomyelitis of the spinal cord, although there was not much anatomic or pathologic evidence to support this. Gowers was one of the first to emphasize cerebral thrombosis as a cause of hemiplegia in children, but believed it was usually caused by small vessel disease (venous occlusion). Osler and Freud also considered thrombosis as a cause of infantile hemiplegia, but stressed the importance of emboli as a cause. Osler, Sachs, and others believed that a few cases of infantile hemiplegia were secondary to convulsions resulting in cerebral hemorrhage. Taylor further emphasized the vascular nature of acquired infantile hemiplegia. In another influential early work, Ford and Schaffer [11] suggested the possibility that embolus and thrombosis of major arteries result from acute infectious and postinfectious causes in a substantial number of cases of infantile hemiplegia, and that coagulation abnormalities associated with the infectious process may also contribute to the vascular lesions. They also emphasized noninfectious causes apart from cardiac emboli, which they had excluded from their series of nearly 70 cases. They provided a more comprehensive classification as to the etiologic basis of pediatric AIS than had existed, and refuted the position of Strümpell (as did Sachs, Freud, and others) that all cases of acquired infantile hemiplegia were caused by a primary infection of the brain based on a detailed review of the literature. In 1948, Wyllie [12] provided a synopsis of the theories of the pathogenesis of acute infantile hemiplegia based on a review of the literature at that time. Although the first reported cases of surgical intervention for epilepsy in infantile hemiplegia occurred around the turn of the 20th century [7], Krynauw in 1950 presented the first detailed series of hemispherectomy in children for intractable epilepsy [13]. The pathology of the resected specimens in several of his cases detailed infarcts caused by vascular ischemia. Although there have been numerous other contributions to the field of pediatric AIS, the monumental and comprehensive work by Gold and colleagues for the Strokes in Children Study Group in the 1970s needs to be acknowledged [14–17].

EPIDEMIOLOGY

Incidence

The published incidence of pediatric AIS (Table 1) has varied from as low as 0.2/100,000 children/y [18] to as high as 7.9/100,000 children/y [19]. The first North American population-based study of pediatric stroke from 1965 to 1974 found an incidence rate of 0.63/100,000 children/y. Many of the earlier incidence studies were hampered by selection bias and poor imaging modalities in determining stroke. Perhaps the best data, and largest cohort of patients, comes from the prospective Canadian Ischemic Stroke Registry, which showed an incidence of AIS in childhood to be 3.3/100,000 children/y. The highest incidence occurs in the neonatal period with estimates as high as 20–30/100,000 newborns/y. This is equivalent to approximately 1/4000–5000 live births/y [20–23], although a population-based epidemiologic study from Switzerland using MRI confirmation of neonatal AIS showed a higher incidence of 1:2300 live births [24]. Perinatal ischemic stroke (occurring between 20 weeks' gestation and 28 days' postnatal life) comprises approximately 25% to 30% of all AISs in children [25,26] and occurs primarily in term infants [21].

Demographics

AIS occurs more commonly amongst males than females in neonatal and childhood forms [26–30], and has a higher incidence amongst blacks [27]. The reason for the latter remains unclear and cannot be attributed to sickle cell disease (SCD) or trauma alone [27]. Ischemic stroke is more common than hemorrhagic stroke. The mean age of childhood presentation is 4 to 6 years

Table 1
Incidence of arterial ischemic stroke in children

Study	Year	AIS (/100 000/y)	Total (ischemic plus hemorrhagic stroke) (/100,000/y)
United States (Rochester) [4]	1965–1974	0.63	2.52
Sweden (Linköping) [171]	1970–1979		2.1
Japan (Tohoku) [18]	1974–1989	0.2	–
France (Dijon) [19]	1985–1993	7.9	13
Unites States (Cincinnati) [172]	1988–1989	1.2	2.7
Unites States (California) [27]	1991–2000	1.2	2.3
Canada [87]	1992–1998	3.3	6
Australia (Victoria) [29]	1993–2001	1.8	–
China (Hong Kong) [32]	1998–2001		2.1
Switzerland [30]	2000–2002	2.1	–

of age [25,28–32] although detailed analysis of 1187 cases from the International Pediatric Stroke Study (IPSS) group showed a slightly older age of 6.8 years for boys and 7.4 years for girls [26].

Mortality
Pediatric stroke remains one of the top 10 causes of death in childhood, with a mortality rate of 0.6/100,000 pediatric strokes/y [33]. This rate is significantly higher during the first year of life with a mortality of 5.3/100,000/y [34]. A review of pooled data on 18 AIS studies in the past 30 years showed that approximately 9% of children who suffered from AIS died [35]. Earlier studies suggested mortality was higher in males [27], although the more recent IPSS cohort did not find any gender differences in case fatality [26]. Mortality is also higher in black children [36].

Morbidity
More than half of the survivors of pediatric stroke develop some neurologic or cognitive deficit or impairment, and epilepsy is a sequela in just more than a quarter of these survivors. Data regarding outcome have been impaired by the lack of standardization of deficits and because they are descriptive. Nonetheless, studies have been consistent in showing some form of motor deficit in about two-thirds of childhood stroke survivors (Table 2). Motor outcome appears slightly better following neonatal stroke, with just under half having a residual motor deficit (Table 2). This finding is of significance as the deficit results in a lifetime of disability and impairment, with associated economic costs (such as physical and occupational therapy, orthotics, and orthopedic surgery) [37]. Two-thirds of all neonatal strokes are left hemispheric and most often involve middle cerebral artery (MCA) territory [38,39]. Neuroimaging findings may help to predict motor developmental outcome following neonatal stroke. Studies from the Hammersmith group in London suggest the need for concomitant involvement of cerebral hemisphere, internal capsule

Table 2
Motor outcome for AIS in selective pediatric stroke studies

Study	Years	N	Motor abnormality (%)
Neonatal			
Sran and Baumann [68]	1975–1986	17	24
Fujimoto et al [69]	1980–1989	18	28
Sreenan et al [60]	1983–1997	46	48
Golomb et al [173]	1989–2006	111	68
Mercuri et al [40]	1991–1996	22	27
DeVeber et al [25]	1995–1999	33	64
Lee et al [43]	1997–2002	36	58
Mean			45
Childhood			
Schoenberg et al [4]	1965–1974	38	94
Lanska et al [174]	1976–1988	42	76
De Schryver et al [31]	1976–1995	37	59
Steinlin et al [79]	1985–1999	16	63
Giroud et al [19]	1985–1993	17	65
Salih et al [81]	1992–2003	90	81
Barnes et al [29]	1993–2001	95	42
DeVeber et al [25]	1995–1999	90	67
Brower et al [72]	1996	36	61
Mean			67

and basal ganglia for resultant hemiplegia in neonatal stroke [40]. Others, however, have suggested that stroke size/volume is more strongly predictive of motor outcome [41–43]. More recently, diffusion-weighted (DWI) MRI signal abnormalities of the ipsilateral cerebral peduncle and posterior limb of the internal capsule were strongly correlated with subsequent Wallerian degeneration and resultant hemiplegia [44]. This finding was refined by a study from Canada [45], showing a correlation between increased motor impairment and length (>20 mm) and volume ($\geq 0.09\%$) of descending corticospinal tracts DWI signal abnormality, and percentage of peduncle involvement ($\geq 25\%$) [45].

Cognitive, behavioral, and emotional deficits also commonly occur in children following stroke. A leftward shift in the mean intelligence quotient (IQ) has been described in some [46] but not all studies [47]. There appears to be a difference between performance and verbal IQ, with children performing better in the latter following stroke [46,48]. This difference appears to be unrelated to the side of the infarct [49–52] and appears independent of the motor disability itself [50]. However, cognitive outcome was better following left-sided stroke than right-sided stroke [48,53]. Expressive language is more severely affected than receptive language [25,46]. Less-favorable cognitive outcome was associated with stroke onset in children younger than 5 years [46,53–55] and older than 10 years [53]. There was no gender difference [51]. Despite the relevant preservation of global IQ, specific learning disabilities are not uncommon [54]. In a study of 39 pre- or perinatal focal infarcts (hemorrhagic and ischemic), no behavioral or emotional difficulties relative to matched control patients were found. This finding was true irrespective of hemisphere involved, involvement of frontal lobes, or the presence or absence of seizures [56], in contradistinction to earlier studies that suggested that behavioral, emotional, and social skills are impaired following neonatal stroke [46,50]. Social and attention difficulties were seen as a consequence of ischemic stroke, independent of early family adversity [55,57]. The presence of epilepsy as a consequence of stroke negatively affects the degree of cognitive impairment, although specific hemispheric involvement appears unrelated [31,49,58].

There are limited data concerning the incidence of visual field deficits and sensory impairment following pediatric stroke [42,47,59–61]. The first report of hemianopsia with infantile hemiplegia was that of Freud [7].

> "The association of epilepsy with infantile cerebral palsies is perhaps the gravest feature of these diseases."
>
> —B. Sachs 1890 [7]

Data regarding the incidence and risk for the development of epilepsy as a sequela of pediatric stroke have been impaired by there being few prospective studies, small sample size, selection bias, differing definitions and terminology in the classification of epilepsy, and short-term follow-up. Between 12% and 18% of all neonatal seizures are associated with cerebral infarction [21,62–64], with 80% to 90% presenting within 48 to 72 hours of stroke onset. Conversely, more than 80% of all perinatal strokes presenting in the newborn period present with seizures (Table 3). The remainder present with encephalopathy [60,65], hypotonia [39], or focal neurologic features. In an autopsy series of 592 infants, 5.4% were found to have AISs and none showed focal neurologic features during the newborn period; however, 17% had neonatal seizures. The majority of seizures (74%) tend to be focal (Table 4), but generalized and subtle seizures, including apnea, may occur. Electrographic seizures may occur in the absence of clinical findings [66,67]. The seizures are usually easy to control [47,68,69] and typically last 3 to 5 days [69,70]. Prognostically, the presence of an abnormal background on electroencephalogram (EEG) has been associated with subsequent development of hemiplegia, although EEG seizures or epileptic discharges with normal background were not [71]. This study was limited by the use of only 2-channel recording EEGs in most cases. The reported risk for subsequent epilepsy has varied from 0% to 50% depending on the nature of the study, with a "mean" of 22% (Table 3) for all studies. Studies in which hemorrhagic and ischemic stroke could not be differentiated or studies in which ischemic stroke included AIS and sinus venous thrombosis have been excluded from analysis in Tables 3 and 5.

Acute/symptomatic seizures occur in ~30% of childhood stroke (Table 5). Seizures may also occur despite deeper (basal ganglia/thalamic) infarcts [72]. Epilepsy occurs as a neurologic sequela in ~28% of childhood strokes (Table 5). Seizures or altered level of consciousness at presentation are associated with increased mortality at 6 months or unfavorable outcome [42]. Cortical involvement is a risk for subsequent epilepsy [73].

Table 3
Seizures and epilepsy in neonatal arterial ischemic stroke

Study	Year	N	Seizures and epilepsy (%)
Clancy et al [66]	1985	11	Acute 91
Levy et al [62]	1985	7	Acute 100
			Epilepsy 14
Filipek et al [175]	1987	7	Acute 100
			Epilepsy 29
Sran and Baumann [68]	1988	17	Acute 82
			Epilepsy 21
Fujimoto et al [69]	1992	18	Acute 78
			Epilepsy 0
Koelfen et al [176]	1993	8	Epilepsy 50
Trauner et al [47]	1993	29	Acute 31
			Late: 34
			Epilepsy 21
Estan and Hope [21]	1997	12	Acute 100
			Epilepsy 0
Jan and Camfield [70]	1998	7	Acute 100
			Epilepsy 0
Mercuri et al [71]	1999	24	Acute 100
			Epilepsy 0
Sreenan et al [60]	2000	46	Acute 91
			Epilepsy 46
Golomb et al [177]	2001	22	Acute 0
			Late 14
			Epilepsy 23
Kurnik et al [39]	2003	215	Acute 77
Ramaswamy et al [65]	2004	5	Acute 100
Steinlin et al [30]	2005 (prospective)	23	Acute 83
Lee et al [43]	2005	34	Acute 80
			Late 14
			Epilepsy 39
Golomb et al [173]	2007	111	Epilepsy 42
Mean			Acute 81
			Epilepsy 22

Recurrence

The mechanism and etiology of childhood stroke strongly influence recurrence risk. Recurrence rate for childhood AIS has varied between 6% and 37% [25,31,32,42,74–84]. Many studies are limited by short-term follow-up, and others include clinical recurrence (transient ischemic attacks [TIAs]) and radiographic confirmation of stroke recurrence [25,77,80]. The best of these studies would suggest a stroke recurrence risk of ~15% to 20%. Risk factors for recurrence include vascular abnormalities as the cause for the initial stroke [78–80,84], and prothrombotic risk factors, either individually (elevated lipoprotein (a) and protein C deficiency) [78] or as part of multiple risk factors [39,76,80,85]. AIS recurrence risk appears highest in the first 6 months after

Table 4
Seizure semiology at presentation in acute neonatal seizures secondary to arterial ischemic stroke

Study	N	Focal seizures (%)	Generalized seizures (%)	Subtle/Apnea (%)
Levy et al [62]	7/7	43	57	0
Clancy et al [66]	10/11	100	0	10 (also with focal seizures)
Filipek et al [175]	7/7	86	14	0
Sran & Baumann [68]	14/17	86	14	0
Fujimoto et al [69]	14/18	86	14	0
Estan & Hope [21]	12/12	67	25	8
Jan & Camfield [70]	7/7	86	0	14
Sreenan et al [60]	42/46	40	24	36
Kurnik et al [39]	193/215	73	4	13
Total[a]	306/340	74	17	9

[a]Totals more than 100% as one patient had focal seizures and subtle seizures.

initial stroke presentation [78,84]. Clinically, silent infarcts were detected in more than 10% of patients on repeat neuroimaging studies in one series [80]. The issue of silent infracts is being assessed as part of a multicentered study on SCD (Silent Cerebral Infarct Multicenter Transfusion [SIT] Trial), and children with SCD are also known to be at increased risk for stroke recurrence, despite blood transfusions [86].

Recurrence risk data for a repeat AIS in perinatal AIS are poor, with only 2 studies specifically addressing this issue. Both showed a low recurrence risk of 1.8% [39] and 1.2% [84], respectively, although the risk for any thromoembolic event (systemic or cerebral venous sinus thrombosis) was slightly higher at 3.3%.

ETIOLOGY

The trigger that fires the explosion, the convulsion and hemiplegia, is not pulled however, until some time after birth [12].

The basic mechanism of AIS in childhood, like that in adults, includes embolus (cardiac or artery-artery) and in situ thrombosis or occlusion. Perhaps the biggest difference, however, between adult and pediatric stroke, lies in the risk factors and causes of AIS. Unlike adult stroke, degenerative vascular disease (atherosclerosis) and chronic degenerative risk factor diseases such as hypertension, hypercholestolemia/hyperlipidemia, diabetes, and smoking have very little role in pediatric AIS. Although multiple risk factors have

Table 5				
Seizures and epilepsy in childhood arterial ischemic stroke				
Study	Year	N	Age (months/ years)	Seizures and epilepsy (%)
Isler [74]	1984	87	<1 y to >10 y	Epilepsy 50
Lanska et al [174]	1991	42	Birth to 13 y	Epilepsy 19
Yang et al [73]	1995	56	1 mo to 7 y	Acute 54 Epilepsy 30
Giroud et al [99]	1997	31	Mean 10.25 y	Acute 35 Epilepsy 36
De Schryver et al [31]	2000	37	3 mo to 4 y	Acute 22 Epilepsy 26
Ganesan et al [46]	2000	90	3 mo to 15 y	Acute 33 Epilepsy 15
Lanthier et al [76]	2000	46	1 mo to 18 y	Epilepsy 12
Delsing et al [42]	2001	31	2 mo to 14.3 y	Acute 19
Barnes et al [29]	2004	95	Birth to 19 y	Epilepsy 7
Steinlin et al [30]	2005 (prospective)	40	1 mo. to 16 y	Acute 20
Salih et al [81]	2006	104	1 mo. to 12 y	Epilepsy 58
Mean				Acute 31 Epilepsy 28

been identified in pediatric stroke, the understanding of pathogenesis remains limited in many instances, especially in focal cerebral arteriopathy, one of the larger etiologic groups for pediatric AIS. Despite recent advances in pediatric AIS, approximately one-quarter to one-third of all childhood strokes remain "idiopathic" [35,46,75,84,87], and this number is even greater for perinatal AIS. This may, in part, be accounted for by a nonstandardized approach and limitations in the evaluation and assessment of etiologic causes of AIS in the various studies. In 2 larger studies, for example, in which detailed cerebrovascular imaging was performed, abnormalities were present in 79% [28] and 78% [75] of patients, respectively. A population-based cohort study in California showed 5-year cumulative recurrence stroke risk rate in children of 66% in those with abnormal vascular imaging studies, versus no recurrences among children with normal vascular imaging studies [84]. Attempts to accurately classify the etiology for AIS are therefore important to allow correct treatment and establish potential recurrence risk. This is especially true for cardioembolic sources of stroke and progressive arteriopathies such as moyamoya disease and primary progressive central nervous system (CNS) vasculitis.

The commonest etiologic categories for pediatric AIS include arteriopathies, cardiac disease (congenital and acquired), hematological disease, and infection. Multiple risk factors are often present at the time of stroke, including acute or chronic disease and prothrombotic states (primary or secondary). Table 6 lists some of the more common causes of childhood AIS.

Table 6
Risk factors and causes of childhood AIS

CARDIAC
Congenital
  CHD
  Cardiomyopathy
  Cardiac tumors
  Arrhythmias
Acquired
  Cardiomyopathy
  Carditis
  Arrhythmias
  Artifical valves
  Endocarditis
Iatrogenic
  Cardiac catheterization
  Cardiac surgery/cardiopulmonary
    bypass
  Carotid ligation

HEMATOLOGIC
Hemagloniopathies
  SCD
  Thalassemia
Thrombophilia
  – Primary
  – Secondary
Iron deficiency anemia
Thrombocytopenia

INFECTIOUS
Meningitis
  Viral, bacterial, fungal
Encephalitis

ARTERIOPATHIES
Vasculitis
Primary
  Primary angiiitis of the CNS
Secondary
  Postinfectious
    Varicella
    Other
  Infectious
    Encephalitis
    Meningitis
  Associated with collagen vascular
    disease or systemic vasculitides

VASCULOPATHIES
Transient/focal cerebral arteriopathy[a]
Down syndrome
Fabry disease
NF1
PHACE syndrome
SCD
Moyamoya disease (primary)
Moyamoya syndrome (secondary)
  Down syndrome
  NF1
  SCD
  William syndrome
  Postcranial irradiation
Fibromusuclar dysplasia
Vasospams
  Migraine
Dissection

OTHER
Trauma
  Dissection
  Fat/air embolus
Toxins/Drugs
  Cocaine
  L-aspariginase
  Oral contraceptive pill
Metabolic
  Shock/dehydration
  Carbohydrate deficient glycoprotein
    syndrome
  Fabry disease
  Homocysteinuria
  MELAS

[a]Cause is uncertain.

Cardiac disorders

CHD is one of the most common birth defects in the United States, and the annual number of infants born with complex CHD is just more than 6500 [88]. Hypoplastic left heart syndrome and tetralogy of Fallot account for nearly 2500 (almost 40%) of these cases; neurologic dysfunction, including stroke, is the major extracardiac complication in the survivors. In a prospective study in infants undergoing cardiopulmonary bypass surgery, 8% had evidence of stroke before surgery, with a further 19% developing new infarcts after surgery [89]. Stroke relating to CHD is usually embolic and may result from mural thrombus in a dyskinetic atrium or ventricle, clot, or vegetation from an abnormal heart valve, or as a consequence of cardiopulmonary bypass. The latter may result from air embolus from open intracardiac procedures, prosthetic patches, or from particulate microemboli from the bypass circuit itself (artificial surfaces, tubing, filters, and aerators). Moyamoya disease has rarely been described in association with CHD [90,91]. Embolic infarcts from cardiomyopathy are usually the result of hypokinetic cardiac wall motion with subsequent clot formation or of cardiac arrhythmias. In an autopsy series of 84 brains in children who died following heart transplantation, cerebral infarct was the most common finding of the CNS, occurring in 34% of the autopsy cases [92]. Stroke following Fontan repair was reported in 2.6% of a large retrospective series from Boston [93], with higher incidences (5.5%–20%) reported in other smaller series [94–98]. Risk factors for the development of embolic stroke following the Fontan procedure include pulmonary artery banding and residual pulmonary artery stump following ligation of the pulmonary artery [93,97]. Other mechanisms for stroke in cardiac disease include septic emboli from infective endocarditis, paradoxic emboli through a persistent patent foramen ovale or atrial septal defect, emboli secondary to cardiac arrhythmias, iatrogenic emboli following cardiac catherization (atrial balloon septostomy or traumatic dissection), and thrombosis from polycythemia in chronic cyanotic CHD.

Stroke from cardiac disease accounts for approximately 20% to 30% of childhood stroke [27,29,30,32,42,76,87,99,100], although some series have shown a lower frequency of less than 20% [46,83]; this percentage is lower in perinatal stroke. Additional prothrombotic risk factors were identified in a cohort of children with cardiac disease suffering stroke compared with age-matched controls [100]. These risk factors included elevated lipoprotein(a) levels, protein C deficiency, anticardiolipin antibodies, and combined prothrombotic disorders.

Hematologic disorders

SCD, an autosomal recessive disorder, is the most common hemaglobinopathy associated with childhood AIS. Historically, the association between SCD and cerebrovascular disease was first made by Sydenstricked in 1923 [101]. Subsequently, Greer and Schotland [102] and Portnoy and Herion [103] emphasized the high prevalence of cerebrovascular disease among SCD patients. The incidence of stroke in children with SCD is estimated at

7% to 11% [104–107]. Arterial ischemic infarction accounts for the majority of stroke subtypes in childhood. The incidence of ischemic stroke was highest in patients younger than 20 years (0.44/100 patient-years); conversely, the rate of hemorrhage was highest in patients 20 to 29 years of age (0.44/100 patient-years) and was low in children [107]. Silent infarction has been found in up to 22% of children with SCD and was associated with an increased risk of new stroke [108]. The majority of strokes are seen in the setting of homozygous SCD, as opposed to sickle trait or the sickle thalassemias. The precise mechanism by which SCD produces infarction is unknown, although several theories have been proposed. Initial thoughts placed emphasis on small vessel disease [109,110]; however, current views have shifted in favor of large arterial disease [111,112] being the cause of most clinically evident cerebrovascular syndromes. In all likelihood, several factors are implicated in the production of stroke in these patients [113–117]. On angiography, the most commonly affected sites are the supraclinoid internal carotid arteries (ICAs), and the proximal MCAs and anterior cerebral arteries (ACAs). Progressive narrowing of vessels may lead to moyamoya syndrome [118].

The Stroke Prevention Trial in Sickle Cell Anemia (STOP) [119] was a landmark study and showed the first successful preventive strategy in reducing stroke risk in a susceptible population. It showed a 92% reduction of first stroke in children with SCD in the treatment arm (blood transfusion to reduce hemoglobin S values to less than 30%) compared with standard therapy arm if their transcranial Doppler (TCD) ultrasound velocity was more than 200 cm/s in the ICA or MCA. The STOP II trial was designed to see whether children on a regular exchange transfusion protocol for 30 months or more following initial abnormal TCD studies (velocities $\geq$ 200 cm/s) could safely stop their transfusion therapy (because of the risks of long-term transfusion and iron overload). This trial was also halted prematurely because 2 children who had discontinued transfusion therapy suffered strokes, and because there was an unacceptably high rate of TCD reversion back to high risk ($\geq$ 200 cm/s) [120]. The SIT Trial in SCD is enrolling patients with silent cerebral infarcts who are to be randomized to receive blood transfusion therapy or observation (standard care) for 36 months to assess if this will improve progressive neurologic complications [121]. Pilot safety and feasibility trials of low-dose aspirin and overnight respiratory support in SCD have also begun [122].

Thrombophilias

The incidence of prothrombotic disorders in pediatric AIS is estimated at between 20% and 50% [123–126]; however, the strength of its association in the etiology of pediatric AIS remains uncertain. The prothrombotic risk factors most strongly associated with pediatric AIS include protein C deficiency, elevated lipoprotein(a) levels, factor V Leiden mutation (G1691A), prothrombin gene mutation (G20210A), methylenetetrahydrofolate reductase mutation (TT677), and antiphospholipid antibodies [124–129]. Most increase the odds ratio for stroke by 2- to 10-fold [125,126]. Multiple prothrombotic risk factors were found in 10% of patients in one study [125]. Elevated lipoprotein(a) and protein C deficiency are risk factors for recurrent AIS in childhood [78].

Arteriopathies

The arteriopathies, as a group, comprise an important part of pediatric AIS (Table 6). Improved vascular imaging has shown abnormalities of the vessel wall in approximately 80% in some series [28,130], although the incidence has not been so high in other studies, varying from 17% to 53% [75,78,84,131]. Vascular abnormalities are a significant risk for recurrent AIS [78]. The presence of an arterial abnormality does not, however, imply an understanding of the mechanism/pathophysiology or etiology. MRA is a readily available and sensitive tool for assessing the intracranial and extracranial vessels, but requires sedation in younger children unable to lie still for a prolonged period of time. This problem can be overcome by using CT angiography (CTA), however, CTA requires large-bore intravenous access for rapid administration of contrast and exposes the child to high levels of irradiation and potential adverse reaction to the iodide contrast. The sensitivity of MRA in detecting extracranial dissection can be increased by obtaining fat-saturated views. MRA is not sensitive for small vessel disease and may overestimate the degree of stenosis [132]. Formal 4-vessel cerebral angiography (CA) remains the "gold standard" for imaging vessels, especially if the diagnosis remains uncertain, the MRA is "equivocal", or small vessel disease such as vasculitis is a concern. Studies have shown that MRA in pediatric AIS may be as sensitive as CA for large vessel disease [132].

Vasculopathies

The noninflammatory vasculopathies are a heterogeneous group of disorders. The more common vasculopathies seen in pediatric AIS include moyamoya disease and syndrome, dissection, SCD (see discussion earlier in this article), neurofibromatosis, and transient cerebral arteriopathy (TCA).

Moyamoya disease is a disorder of multiple progressive intracranial occlusions of the large cerebral arteries (ICA, MCA, ACA) with compensatory development of lenticulostriate collaterals. Less commonly, the posterior circulation (basilar artery, posterior communicating arteries) may be involved. "Moyamoya" was first used to describe this appearance of collateral networks at the base of the brain in 1969 [133] and comes from the Japanese expression for something "hazy, just like a puff of cigarette smoke drifting in the air." Although the etiology is unknown, familial cases have suggested autosomal dominance inheritance with incomplete penetrance. Genomic imprinting may be associated with the disease as affected mothers are more likely to produce late-onset or asymptomatic female offspring [134]. To date, 3 gene loci have been identified through linkage studies and mapped to chromosome 3p [135], chromosome 17q25 [136], and chromosome 8q23 [137]. A high incidence of moyamoya disease is found in people of

Asian descent, especially Japanese, although it has now been recognized world-wide. It accounts for only about 6% of childhood strokes in Western counties [138] and occurs more frequently in females.

Moyamoya syndrome is differentiated from primary or idiopathic moya-moya disease as it develops secondary to an underlying disorder (acquired or genetic). It is sometimes referred to as "secondary" moyamoya syndrome and has been described in persons with Down syndrome, SCD, William syndrome, neurofibromatosis, and less commonly in other phakomatoses (hy-pomelanosis of Ito and tuberous sclerosis) [139].

Children with moyamoya disease and/or syndrome typically present with symptoms secondary to an acute ischemic infarct or with seizures; hemorrhagic stroke is more common in adults. There is a high risk of recurrence, and progressive cognitive decline secondary to chronic cerebral hypoperfusion may occur [140]. Treatment to restore the cerebral circulation and avoid recurrent stroke has focused on surgical revascularization options. This typically includes "direct" procedures, ie, the direct anastomosis of an extracranial to intracranial vessel, versus "indirect" procedures in which the superficial temporal artery typically is placed directly on the surface of the brain. The procedure appears to be safe, although perioperative stroke may occur in about 4.5%, and effective, with most treated patients deriving symptomatic benefit [141].

Dissection

Arterial dissection results from a tear in the intimal wall of the blood vessel. This may affect the anterior or posterior circulation, and may be intracranial or extracranial. Symptoms typically result from an artery-artery embolism arising from the site of the intimal tear, but may also occur secondary to thrombosis and complete occlusion of the dissected vessel. Dissection accounts for 7.5% to 20% of AIS in children [28,75,142]. Mean age of presentation is 8 to 11 years [142,143]. Intracranial dissection occurs more commonly in pediatric AIS than in adult stroke, and usually affects the anterior circulation, whereas posterior circulation dissection more commonly involves the extracranial vessels (especially at the C1-C2 vertebral body level) [143]. Arterial dissection differs from adult dissection in several other ways, including an increased frequency in boys (even when trauma is excluded), lack of preceding warning symptoms (such as headache or neck pain), and frequent lack of significant head or neck trauma [143]. Trauma, when present, usually results in an extra-cranial dissection. Predisposing factors for dissections such as fibromuscular dysplasia or connective tissue disease are rare. There is often a delay in onset of symptoms following dissection, and children almost universally present with signs and symptoms of ischemia, specifically hemiplegia or hemisensory deficits, although seizures at onset, cranial neuropathies, ataxia, visual disturbances, or headache may occur. Angiographic features include a string sign, luminal flap, aneurysmal dilatation, double lumen sign, or short, smooth tapering stenosis or occlusion of the affected vessel. Although conventional CA remains the gold standard, MRA, complemented by fat-saturated T1 views and CTA can often confirm the diagnosis [138]. Recurrence risk is variable and occurs in about 10% to 12.5% [142,143] but this may be an underestimate since most children are treated with antiplatelet or anticoagulation therapy (for 3–6 months). There are no studies showing superiority of one treatment compared with the other, or superiority of treatment versus nontreatment, in arterial dissection in childhood. In a systematic review of the literature involving 118 reported cases of pediatric AIS from 79 studies, the majority of fatalities occurred in patients not receiving anticoagulation, and complications (specifically hemorrhage) occurred in only 2 patients (1 with a fatal intracranial hemorrhage, and 1 with a large gastrointestinal hemorrhage) [143]. The recent American Heart Association (AHA) guidelines for the treatment of stroke in infants and children [138] give a class III recommendation, (ie, not recommended) to the use of anticoagulation for intracranial dissection (because of concern about possible subarachnoid hemorrhage).

Neurofibromatosis

Neurofibromatosis type 1 (NF1) is an autosomal dominant disorder involving mutations of the NF gene on chromosome 17q11. It affects 1 in 3000 individuals and is a progressive, multisystem disease with complications that can affect any part of the body. NF1 vasculopathy is well recognized and manifests as stenosis, occlusion, arteriovenous fistula, or aneurysm of the large and medium-sized arteries. A 2.5% incidence of NF1 vasculopathy was found in a cohort of 316 pediatric patients with NF1 who underwent brain MRI studies [144]. A recent study from Canada found a minimum prevalence rate of NF1 vasculopathy, amongst a cohort of 419 children with confirmed NF1, of 6% [145]. The incidence of stroke in NF1 vasculopathy is unknown. The most frequently documented vascular abnormality is renal artery stenosis with resultant hypertension [146]. Intracranial occlusive arterial disease is the most common neurovascular manifestation of neurofibromatosis and occurs predominantly in younger patients [146,147]. This disease usually involves the anterior circulation and may be bilateral in about half the cases, resulting in moyamoya syndrome. It may follow intracranial irradiation for optic glioma [148]. The pathogenesis of the vasculopathy in NF1 patients remains to be fully elucidated. Familial occurrence of cerebral vasculopathy in NF1 is rare [149].

Recently, a case of a brainstem stroke in a child with NF2 was reported concurrent with a gastrointestinal illness [150]. No obvious cause for the stroke was found, and what relationship, if any, the NF2 had on the stroke is uncertain. Unlike NF1, vasculopathy is not a known manifestation of NF2.

TCA

TCA describes an idiopathic, nonprogressive focal or segmental, unilateral stenosis of the distal (supraclinoid) ICA or proximal MCA/ACA [151–153], resulting in a lenticulostriate infarction. It appears to be a monophasic event, although angiographic data have shown that the stenosis may worsen in a 3- to 6-month period, with persistent focal narrowing of the vessel in a significant number of patients [151,153]. A recurrence rate of TIA or stroke has been reported in up to 18% in some series [153]. This term has been used interchangeably with focal arterial stenosis in childhood. TCA is one of the most common causes of vasculopathy in pediatric AIS, accounting for about 20% to 30% of cases [131,153,154]. The pathophysiology is still not fully understood but a postinfectious inflammatory mechanism has been proposed given the strong association between TCA and a preceding varicella infection (postvaricella angiopathy), and the natural history, which initially involves a progressive course with subsequent stabilization on angiogram [28,130, 151,153,155,156]. An angiographic TCA appearance has also been associated with other infectious agents [138,153]. Whether the introduction of the varicella vaccine into childhood immunizations will show a significant reduction in the incidence of stroke from TCA remains to be seen. Further studies are needed to determine the optimal treatment for this condition given the frequency, recurrence risk, and outcome. Whether immunosuppressive agents, with or without antivital medication, affect outcome and recurrence is not known. Similarly, it is unclear whether adjunctive antiplatelet or anticoagulation therapy during the acute phase or the long term is necessary.

Vasculitis

Inflammatory vasculitis may occur as an isolated phenomenon affecting the cerebral arteries (primary angiitis of the CNS) or may be part of a collagen vascular disease, systemic vasculitides, or an infectious or postinfectious process (Table 6).

Primary Angiitis of the CNS

Childhood primary angiitis of the CNS (cPACNS) is a rare, noninfectious, progressive arteriopathy isolated to the cerebral vessels without systemic involvement. It is associated with high recurrence rate, morbidity, and mortality. In a recent review [153] it accounted for 6% of all arteriopathies in childhood AIS. It often presents with a more indolent course of headaches, academic or cognitive decline, and encephalopathy compared with the transient cerebral arteriopathies (discussed earlier in this article), which present acutely with ischemic symptoms, typically hemiplegia. It may involve large-to medium-sized blood vessels, or small distal blood vessels [157]. The small vessel involvement can readily be missed on MRA or CTA although MRI shows evidence of ischemic infarct. The hallmark on CA is beading (segmental vessel narrowing with poststenotic dilatation). In contradistinction to adult PACNS, in which angiographic findings are typically bilateral and asymmetrical, angiographic findings in cPACNS are usually unilateral, proximal, and multifocal [158]. Angiogram may be normal [159]. Cerebrospinal fluid analysis may show an elevated opening pressure, mild lymphocytosis, or elevated protein, but may also be normal. Brain biopsy, including dura, may be necessary for diagnosis but given the patchy nature of involvement of the brain can give a false-negative result. A nongranulomatous vasculitis may be found rather than the typical necrotizing granulomatous vasculitis seen in adult

PACNS [157,160]. Systemic inflammatory markers may be present but are nonspecific and not necessary for diagnosis.

Differentiating progressive cPACNS from a TCA or moyamoya syndrome can be difficult but is important for determining treatment. The presence of multifocal parenchymal lesions, neurocognitive dysfunction, and distal stenosis were important predictive markers in one series [161]. Treatment of cPACNS involves immunosuppressive agents, including steroids and pulse cyclophosphamide, in the acute phase [138], with maintenance immunosuppressive therapy such as azothioprine or mycophenolate mofetil for a prolonged period [157]. The concomitant use of anticoagulation or antiplatelet therapy during the acute phase and for a few months thereafter to prevent in situ thrombosis from vessel inflammation is controversial. Given the rarity of this condition, no formal studies of optimal therapy have been conducted.

Treatment

Evidence-based prevention strategies and treatments for pediatric stroke are lacking, with only 1 randomized control trial [119] in SCD and AIS. In recent years 3 guidelines have been published that address for the first time management and treatment issues in pediatric stroke [138,162,163]. However, many of the recommendations are based on small nonrandomized trials, case series, extrapolation from adult data, or expert consensus opinion. For specific treatment recommendations, readers are referred to these guidelines and other reviews that have been published recently [35,164,165]. The most recent and comprehensive guideline from the AHA also provides protocols for the use of unfractionated heparin (UH), low molecular weight heparins (LMWH) and warfarin in childhood AIS [138].

Initial acute supportive measures for childhood AIS are much the same as in adult stroke and include maintenance of normal oxygenation, control of systemic hypertension (although the specific targeted range and level of "permissible" hypertension is unclear given concerns for lowering perfusion pressure), and normalization of serum glucose [138]. Fever should be controlled. Hyperthermia has been associated with increased secondary injury in multiple animal models of stroke [164]. Seizures should be aggressively treated. There is no evidence to support the use of supplemental oxygen in the absence of hypoxemia or antiepileptic medication prophylactically in the absence of clinical or electrical seizures. None of the 3 guidelines recommend the use of acute thrombolysis with intraarterial or intravenous tissue plasminogen activator (t-PA) in childhood AIS. The recent AHA guidelines [138] give a class III recommendation, that is, it is not recommended or should not be used outside a clinical trial. The use of anticoagulation in acute AIS is also controversial, with differing opinions between the guidelines. There appears to be consensus for its use acutely and indefinitely in children with a cardioembolic source of their stroke if the underlying cardiac reason for their stroke cannot be surgically corrected. The use of anticoagulation in extracranial dissection acutely and for 3 to 6 months is also generally accepted, although the AHA guidelines include the alternative use of antiplatelet agents instead of anticoagulation. Anticoagulation is not recommended for intracranial dissection (see section on dissection earlier in this article). The *Chest* guidelines [163] recommend UH or LMWH for up to a week while the cause of the stroke is determined, whereas the UK guidelines [162] recommend aspirin. Anticoagulation is not recommended for neonatal AIS in the absence of a cardioembolic source. Exchange transfusions and hydration to keep sickle hemoglobin less than 30% is recommended for acute AIS in SCD.

For secondary prevention in AIS of unknown etiology or in vasculopathy not caused by vasculitis, moyamoya, or dissection, all 3 guidelines recommend the use of aspirin, given the risk of recurrence. Doses vary from 1 to 3 mg/kg in the UK guidelines to 2 to 5 mg/kg in the *Chest* guidelines. The length of treatment is uncertain. There are no specific recommendations on the use of aspirin for secondary stroke prevention in thrombophilias.

FUTURE

> The physician is no longer content, or at least should not be, to make the diagnosis of apoplexy; of hemiplegia, or of paraplegia, in the adult. It is his aim to determine whether the special form of paralysis be due to hemorrhage, thrombosis, embolism, tumor, abscess, or what not. In short, he studies the symptoms of each case with special reference to pathology of the disease. And so with infantile palsies: it is not enough to recognize spastic hemiplegia, diplegia or paraplegia, but the attempt should be made to determine the special morbid condition underlying each form.
>
> —B. Sachs 1898 [7]

Much remains to be learned about pediatric AIS. Despite more than a century of descriptive studies in pediatric AIS, approximately one-third to one-quarter of strokes remain idiopathic. Etiology and risk factors in pediatric AIS are diverse, with no one risk factor predominating, hence each requires a different research approach [87]. The rarity of pediatric AIS, diverse causes, and mimics of stroke have affected the development of rational and effective treatment strategies. The application of adult data to pediatric stroke is not always appropriate because of intrinsic differences in the pathophysiology, etiology, and risk aversion in pediatric stroke. Vasculopathy in pediatric stroke is common, but does not involve the degenerative risk factors or processes of adult stroke, namely atherosclerosis and hypertension, but rather, healthy vessels and robust collateral circulation. Developmental differences in the coagulation system and issues related to birth also affect pediatric AIS. Since the 1990s, research work has provided improved epidemiologic and population-based data regarding pediatric stroke. Efforts have been made to standardize pediatric stroke classification [152], and advances in imaging have allowed for improved diagnostic yield and better classification of etiology, although not necessarily pathophysiology, of pediatric AIS. A monumental, ongoing unfunded international collaboration for data collection and cooperation in pediatric stroke has been established: the IPSS consortium [26] (http://app3.ccb.sickkids.ca/cstro-kestudy). These are necessary first steps toward the development of standardized diagnostic and evaluation protocols and toward randomized controlled trials for therapeutics and intervention in the treatment and prevention of pediatric AIS. The IPSS has also led to the development and establishment of pediatric stroke centers throughout the world that will promote increasing awareness of pediatric stroke (which remains an ongoing problem), more rapid and comprehensive evaluation of AIS, improved outcomes, and age-appropriate clinical research. The first such trial in pediatric stroke funded by the US National Institutes of Health (NIH) is under way; it is investigating the application of a modified pediatric NIH stroke scale in acute AIS and is based at the Children's Hospital of Philadelphia with the participation of several centers throughout the United States and Canada.

Several obstacles still exist with respect to potential treatment studies for pediatric AIS. Despite the increased awareness of pediatric stroke, delays in presentation and evaluation persist. A study from Stony Brook, New York [166] showed a mean delay in symptom onset to medical contact in AIS of 43 hours (median of 20 hours) and a further 7-hour delay (mean) in the diagnosis of AIS. These findings were confirmed in a more recent study from Toronto in which only 20% of childhood AIS cases were diagnosed within 6 hours [167]. Further confounding the time to diagnosis are the stroke mimics that frequently occur in pediatrics, including migraine (hemiplegic, ophthalmic, and confusional forms), seizures (with resultant Todd paralysis), demyelinating disorders (especially acute disseminating encephalomyelitis), and functional disorders [168,169]. The insensitivity of CT scan and the need for MRI/MRA in pediatric stroke is therefore essential, and brings with it its own set of difficulties, as sedation is often required in children. These problems are magnified in perinatal AIS, in which there is often a paucity of symptoms in the newborn period apart from seizures, and diagnosis is often made only at 4 to 6 months of age when asymmetry in reaching or use of the hands is first noted. New therapies for acute intervention in AIS have become available in adult stroke, but their application and suitability for pediatric stroke still needs to be assessed. Three treatment guidelines for pediatric AIS have recently been published, but these are limited because they are based on small nonrandomized trials, case series, extrapolation from adult data, or expert consensus opinion [138,162,163]. Nonetheless, these publications serve as a foundation for future studies and provide some guidelines in an otherwise difficult area. Among the problems associated with primary stroke prevention strategies in pediatrics are the multitude of causes that may give rise to stroke, many of which are uncommon or rare. However, primary stroke prevention measures are well established for the two largest categories of childhood AIS (SCD and cardiac disease). It remains to be seen whether the implementation of varicella vaccination into the immunization schedule of children reduces the incidence of postvaricella angiopathy, one of the more common causes of TCA in childhood AIS. Evidence for the efficacy of treatment for secondary prevention of recurrence of childhood AIS is lacking, apart from some specific disease entities such as moyamoya. Given the recurrence risk of childhood AIS is ~15% to 20%, depending on the cause, this is an important area for future research.

Although the way forward is difficult for pediatric stroke given the multiple challenges outlined in this article, the lack of funding, and the small number of physicians working in this area, the future is bright given the dedication of purpose of collaboration, such as the IPSS and European collaborative groups, and the advances in the field in the last 1or 2 decades. Ongoing population-based prospective studies are needed with respect to etiology, incidence, recurrence risk, and outcome. Standardized diagnostic and therapeutic algorithms need to be developed so that evaluation and treatment of pediatric AIS is more readily available to all physicians caring for pediatric stroke. This may lead to reduced lifetime morbidity and a reduction in the associated costs for survivors of pediatric stroke. Standardized definitions, classification of stroke subtype, and outcomes are crucial for treatment studies. In this regard, outcome instruments such as the pediatric stroke outcome measure [25] have been helpful, but validated measures of cognitive and behavioral outcomes relating to pediatric stroke are needed. As Kirkham [170] has pointed out, case-controlled studies are preferable to minimize selection bias, but given the difficulty (often for ethical reasons) in obtaining a control group, another option is for studies to use data pooling. Although some early work has been performed to assess the direct cost of pediatric AIS, more information is needed to address the indirect costs of pediatric AIS in the hope of improving funding for research into childhood stroke by showing the burden of pediatric AIS not just to the individual, but to society as a whole. Most children with stroke have vascular abnormalities on imaging and a better understanding is needed of the mechanisms behind this. t-PA is being used in childhood AIS despite a lack of evidence showing safety or even efficacy and this needs to be urgently evaluated in a study. Other future studies will need to focus on small cohorts of homogenous at-risk stroke populations to address possibilities of primary stroke prevention, such as the vasculopathy associated with NF1, and silent strokes seen in CHD. The potential role and application, if any, of newer technologies such as vascular stenting or angioplasty remain to be elucidated in pediatric AIS.

References

[1] Wisoff HS, Rothballer AB. Cerebral arterial thrombosis in children. Review of literature and addition of two cases in apparently healthy children. Arch Neurol 1961;4:258–67.

[2] Bickerstaff ER. Aetiology of acute hemiplegia in childhood. Br Med J 1964;2:82–7.

[3] Williams AN. Winner of the young physician's section of the Gowers' prize 2000. Too good to be true? Thomas Willis–neonatal convulsions, childhood stroke and infanticide in seventeenth century England. Seizure 2001;10:471–83.

[4] Schoenberg BS, Mellinger JF, Schoenberg DG. Cerebrovascular disease in infants and children: a study of incidence, clinical features, and survival. Neurology 1978;28:763–8.

[5] Garrison FH. Garrison's history of neurology. Revised and enlarged with a bibliography of classical, original and standard works in neurology. Springfield (IL): Charles C. Thomas; 1969.

[6] Osler W. Infirmary for nervous diseases (Philadelphia, PA.). The cerebral palsies of children: a clinical study from the infirmary for nervous diseases, Philadelphia. London: H.K. Lewis; 1889.

[7] Sachs B, Peterson F. A study of cerebral palsies of early life, based upon an analysis of one hundred and forty cases. J Nerv Ment Dis 1890;17:295–332.

[8] Freud S. Infantile cerebral paralysis. Translated by Lester A. Russin. Coral Gables (FL): University of Miami Press; 1968.

[9] Gowers W. In: Gowers Sir WR, Taylor James, editors. A manual of diseases of the nervous system. 3rd edition. London: J. & A. Churchill; 1899.

[10] Gowers WR. A manual of diseases of the nervous system. Volume II: Diseases of the brain and cranial nerves, general and functional diseases of the nervous system. 2nd edition. Philadelphia: P. Blakiston's Son and Co; 1907.

[11] Ford FR, Schaffer AJ. The etiology of infantile acquired hemiplegia. Arch Neurol Psychiatr 1927;18:323–47.

[12] Wyllie WG. Acute infantile hemiplegia. Proc R Soc Med 1948;41:459–66.

[13] Krynauw RA. Infantile hemiplegia treated by removing one cerebral hemisphere. J Neurol Neurosurg Psychiatr 1950;13:243–67.

[14] Report of the Joint Committee for Stroke Facilities. IX. Strokes in children. 1. Epidemiology of strokes in children. Stroke 1973;4:835–58.

[15] Report of the Joint Committee for Stroke Facilities. IX. Strokes in children. 1. Neuropathology of strokes in children. Stroke 1973;4:859–70.

[16] Report of the Joint Committee for Stroke Facilities. IX. Strokes in children. 1. Diagnosis and medical treatment of strokes in children. Stroke 1973;4:871–94.

[17] Report of the Joint Committee for Stroke Facilities. IX. Strokes in children. 2. Stroke 1973;4: 1007–52.

[18] Satoh S, Shirane R, Yoshimoto T. Clinical survey of ischemic cerebrovascular disease in children in a district of Japan. Stroke 1991;22:586–9.

[19] Giroud M, Lemesle M, Gouyon JB, et al. Cerebrovascular disease in children under 16 years of age in the city of Dijon, France: a study of incidence and clinical features from 1985 to 1993. J Clin Epidemiol 1995;48:1343–8.

[20] Perlman JM, Rollins NK, Evans D. Neonatal stroke: clinical characteristics and cerebral blood flow velocity measurements. Pediatr Neurol 1994;11:281–4.

[21] Estan J, Hope P. Unilateral neonatal cerebral infarction in full term infants. Arch Dis Child Fetal Neonatal Ed 1997;76:F88–93.

[22] Lynch JK, Hirtz DG, DeVeber G, et al. Report of the National Institute of Neurological Disorders and Stroke workshop on perinatal and childhood stroke. Pediatrics 2002;109: 116–23.

[23] Lee J, Croen LA, Backstrand KH, et al. Maternal and infant characteristics associated with perinatal arterial stroke in the infant. JAMA 2005;293:723–9.

[24] Schulzke S, Weber P, Luetschg J, et al. Incidence and diagnosis of unilateral arterial cerebral infarction in newborn infants. J Perinat Med 2005;33:170–5.

[25] deVeber GA, MacGregor D, Curtis R, et al. Neurologic outcome in survivors of childhood arterial ischemic stroke and sinovenous thrombosis. J Child Neurol 2000;15: 316–24.

[26] Golomb MR, Fullerton HJ, Nowak-Gottl U, et al, International Pediatric Stroke Study Group. Male predominance in childhood ischemic stroke findings from the International Pediatric Stroke Study. Stroke 2009;40:52–7.

[27] Fullerton HJ, Wu YW, Zhao S, et al. Risk of stroke in children: Ethnic and gender disparities. Neurology 2003;61:189–94.

[28] Ganesan V, Prengler M, McShane MA, et al. Investigation of risk factors in children with arterial ischemic stroke. Ann Neurol 2003;53:167–73.

[29] Barnes C, Newall F, Furmedge J, et al. Arterial ischaemic stroke in children. J Paediatr Child Health 2004;40:384–7.

[30] Steinlin M, Pfister I, Pavlovic J, et al. The first three years of the Swiss neuropaediatric stroke registry (SNPSR): a population-based study of incidence, symptoms and risk factors. Neuropediatrics 2005;36:90–7.

[31] De Schryver EL, Kappelle LJ, Jennekens-Schinkel A, et al. Prognosis of ischemic stroke in childhood: a long-term follow-up study. Dev Med Child Neurol 2000;42:313–8.

[32] Chung B, Wong V. Pediatric stroke among Hong Kong Chinese subjects. Pediatrics 2004;114:e206–12.

[33] Arias E, Anderson RN, Kung HC, et al. Deaths: final data for 2001. Natl Vital Stat Rep 2003;52:1–115.

[34] Lynch JK, Nelson KB. Epidemiology of perinatal stroke. Curr Opin Pediatr 2001;13: 499–505.

[35] Lynch JK, Han CJ. Pediatric stroke: what do we know and what do we need to know? Semin Neurol 2005;25:410–23.

[36] Fullerton HJ, Chetkovich DM, Wu YW, et al. Deaths from stroke in US children, 1979 to 1998. Neurology 2002;59:34–9.

[37] Lo W, Zamel K, Ponnappa K, et al. The cost of pediatric stroke care and rehabilitation. Stroke 2008;39:161–5.

[38] Miller V. Neonatal cerebral infarction. Semin Pediatr Neurol 2000;7:278–88.

[39] Kurnik K, Kosch A, Strater R, et al. Recurrent thromboembolism in infants and children suffering from symptomatic neonatal arterial stroke: a prospective follow-up study. Stroke 2003;34:2887–92.

[40] Mercuri E, Barnett A, Rutherford M, et al. Neonatal cerebral infarction and neuromotor outcome at school age. Pediatrics 2004;113:95–100.

[41] Ganesan V, Ng V, Chong WK, et al. Lesion volume, lesion location, and outcome after middle cerebral artery territory stroke. Arch Dis Child 1999;81:295–300.

[42] Delsing BJ, Catsman-Berrevoets CE, Appel IM. Early prognostic indicators of outcome in ischemic childhood stroke. Pediatr Neurol 2001;24:283–9.

[43] Lee J, Croen LA, Lindan C, et al. Predictors of outcome in perinatal arterial stroke: a population-based study. Ann Neurol 2005;58:303–8.

[44] De Vries LS, Van der Grond J, Van Haastert IC, et al. Prediction of outcome in new-born infants with arterial ischaemic stroke using diffusion-weighted magnetic resonance imaging. Neuropediatrics 2005;36:12–20.

[45] Kirton A, Shroff M, Visvanathan T, et al. Quantified corticospinal tract diffusion restriction predicts neonatal stroke outcome. Stroke 2007;38:974–80.

[46] Ganesan V, Hogan A, Shack N, et al. Outcome after ischaemic stroke in childhood. Dev Med Child Neurol 2000;42:455–61.

[47] Trauner DA, Chase C, Walker P, et al. Neurologic profiles of infants and children after perinatal stroke. Pediatr Neurol 1993;9:383–6.

[48] Pavlovic J, Kaufmann F, Boltshauser E, et al. Neuropsychological problems after paediatric stroke: two year follow-up of Swiss children. Neuropediatrics 2006;37:13–9.

[49] Vargha-Khadem F, Isaacs E, van der Werf S, et al. Development of intelligence and memory in children with hemiplegic cerebral palsy. The deleterious consequences of early seizures. Brain 1992;115(Pt 1):315–29.

[50] Goodman R, Yude C. IQ and its predictors in childhood hemiplegia. Dev Med Child Neurol 1996;38:881–90.

[51] Hogan AM, Kirkham FJ, Isaacs EB. Intelligence after stroke in childhood: review of the literature and suggestions for future research. J Child Neurol 2000;15:325–32.

[52] Max JE. Effect of side of lesion on neuropsychological performance in childhood stroke. J Int Neuropsychol Soc 2004;10:698–708.

[53] Aram DM, Eisele JA. Intellectual stability in children with unilateral brain lesions. Neuropsychologia 1994;32:85–95.

[54] Lansing AE, Max JE, Delis DC, et al. Verbal learning and memory after childhood stroke. J Int Neuropsychol Soc 2004;10:742–52.

[55] Max JE, Robin DA, Taylor HG, et al. Attention function after childhood stroke. J Int Neuropsychol Soc 2004;10:976–86.

[56] Trauner DA, Nass R, Ballantyne A. Behavioural profiles of children and adolescents after pre- or perinatal unilateral brain damage. Brain 2001;124:995–1002.

[57] Laucht M, Esser G, Baving L, et al. Behavioral sequelae of perinatal insults and early family adversity at 8 years of age. J Am Acad Child Adolesc Psychiatry 2000;39:1229–37.

[58] Fitzgerald KC, Williams LS, Garg BP, et al. Epilepsy in children with delayed presentation of perinatal stroke. J Child Neurol 2007;22:1274–80.

[59] Tizard JP, Paine RS, Crothers B. Disturbances of sensation in children with hemiplegia. J Am Med Assoc 1954;155:628–32.

[60] Sreenan C, Bhargava R, Robertson CM. Cerebral infarction in the term newborn: Clinical presentation and long-term outcome. J Pediatr 2000;137:351–5.

[61] Kirton A, Deveber G, Pontigon AM, et al. Presumed perinatal ischemic stroke: vascular classification predicts outcomes. Ann Neurol 2008;63:436–43.

[62] Levy SR, Abroms IF, Marshall PC, et al. Seizures and cerebral infarction in the full-term newborn. Ann Neurol 1985;17:366–70.

[63] Aso K, Scher MS, Barmada MA. Cerebral infarcts and seizures in the neonate. J Child Neurol 1990;5:224–8.

[64] Tekgul H, Gauvreau K, Soul J, et al. The current etiologic profile and neurodevelopmental outcome of seizures in term newborn infants. Pediatrics 2006;117:1270–80.

[65] Ramaswamy V, Miller SP, Barkovich AJ, et al. Perinatal stroke in term infants with neonatal encephalopathy. Neurology 2004;62:2088–91.

[66] Clancy R, Malin S, Laraque D, et al. Focal motor seizures heralding stroke in full-term neonates. Am J Dis Child 1985;139:601–6.

[67] Scher MS, Wiznitzer M, Bangert BA. Cerebral infarctions in the fetus and neonate: maternal-placental-fetal considerations. Clin Perinatol 2002;29:693–724, vi–vii.

[68] Sran SK, Baumann RJ. Outcome of neonatal strokes. Am J Dis Child 1988;142:1086–8.

[69] Fujimoto S, Yokochi K, Togari H, et al. Neonatal cerebral infarction: symptoms, CT findings and prognosis. Brain Dev 1992;14:48–52.

[70] Jan MM, Camfield PR. Outcome of neonatal stroke in full-term infants without significant birth asphyxia. Eur J Pediatr 1998;157:846–8.

[71] Mercuri E, Rutherford M, Cowan F, et al. Early prognostic indicators of outcome in infants with neonatal cerebral infarction: a clinical, electroencephalogram, and magnetic resonance imaging study. Pediatrics 1999;103:39–46.

[72] Brower MC, Rollins N, Roach ES. Basal ganglia and thalamic infarction in children. Cause and clinical features. Arch Neurol 1996;53:1252–6.

[73] Yang JS, Park YD, Hartlage PL. Seizures associated with stroke in childhood. Pediatr Neurol 1995;12:136–8.

[74] Isler W. Stroke in childhood and adolescence. Eur Neurol 1984;23:421–4.

[75] Chabrier S, Husson B, Lasjaunias P, et al. Stroke in childhood: outcome and recurrence risk by mechanism in 59 patients. J Child Neurol 2000;15:290–4.

[76] Lanthier S, Carmant L, David M, et al. Stroke in children: the coexistence of multiple risk factors predicts poor outcome. Neurology 2000;54:371–8.

[77] Ganesan V, Chong WK, Cox TC, et al. Posterior circulation stroke in childhood: risk factors and recurrence. Neurology 2002;59:1552–6.

[78] Strater R, Becker S, von Eckardstein A, et al. Prospective assessment of risk factors for recurrent stroke during childhood—a 5-year follow-up study. Lancet 2002;360:1540–5.

[79] Steinlin M, Roellin K, Schroth G. Long-term follow-up after stroke in childhood. Eur J Pediatr 2004;163:245–50.

[80] Ganesan V, Prengler M, Wade A, et al. Clinical and radiological recurrence after childhood arterial ischemic stroke. Circulation 2006;114:2170–7.

[81] Salih MA, Abdel-Gader AG, Al-Jarallah AA, et al. Outcome of stroke in Saudi children. Saudi Med J 2006;27(Suppl 1):S91–6.

[82] Sofronas M, Ichord RN, Fullerton HJ, et al. Pediatric stroke initiatives and preliminary studies: what is known and what is needed? Pediatr Neurol 2006;34:439–45.

[83] Gokben S, Tosun A, Bayram N, et al. Arterial ischemic stroke in childhood: risk factors and outcome in old versus new era. J Child Neurol 2007;22:1204–8.

[84] Fullerton HJ, Wu YW, Sidney S, et al. Risk of recurrent childhood arterial ischemic stroke in a population-based cohort: the importance of cerebrovascular imaging. Pediatrics 2007;119:495–501.

[85] Barreirinho S, Ferro A, Santos M, et al. Inherited and acquired risk factors and their combined effects in pediatric stroke. Pediatr Neurol 2003;28:134–8.

[86] Scothorn DJ, Price C, Schwartz D, et al. Risk of recurrent stroke in children with sickle cell disease receiving blood transfusion therapy for at least five years after initial stroke. J Pediatr 2002;140:348–54.

[87] deVeber G, Roach ES, Riela AR, et al. Stroke in children: recognition, treatment, and future directions. Semin Pediatr Neurol 2000;7:309–17.

[88] Centers for Disease Control and Prevention (CDC). Improved national prevalence estimates for 18 selected major birth defects–United States, 1999–2001. MMWR Morb Mortal Wkly Rep 2006;54:1301–5.

[89] Mahle WT. Neurologic and cognitive outcomes in children with congenital heart disease. Curr Opin Pediatr 2001;13:482–6.

[90] Lutterman J, Scott M, Nass R, et al. Moyamoya syndrome associated with congenital heart disease. Pediatrics 1998;101:57–60.

[91] Ganesan V, Kirkham FJ. Noonan syndrome and moyamoya. Pediatr Neurol 1997;16:256–8.

[92] McClure CD, Johnston JK, Fitts JA, et al. Postmortem intracranial neuropathology in children following cardiac transplantation. Pediatr Neurol 2006;35:107–13.

[93] du Plessis AJ Chang AC, Wessel DL, et al. Cerebrovascular accidents following the Fontan operation. Pediatr Neurol 1995;12:230–6.

[94] Mathews K, Bale JF Jr, Clark EB, et al. Cerebral infarction complicating Fontan surgery for cyanotic congenital heart disease. Pediatr Cardiol 1986;7:161–6.

[95] Day RW, Boyer RS, Tait VF, et al. Factors associated with stroke following the Fontan procedure. Pediatr Cardiol 1995;16:270–5.

[96] Rosenthal DN, Friedman AH, Kleinman CS, et al. Thromboembolic complications after Fontan operations. Circulation 1995;92:II287–93.

[97] Chun DS, Schamberger MS, Flaspohler T, et al. Incidence, outcome, and risk factors for stroke after the Fontan procedure. Am J Cardiol 2004;93:117–9.

[98] Barker PC, Nowak C, King K, et al. Risk factors for cerebrovascular events following Fontan palliation in patients with a functional single ventricle. Am J Cardiol 2005;96:587–91.

[99] Giroud M, Lemesle M, Madinier G, et al. Stroke in children under 16 years of age. Clinical and etiological difference with adults. Acta Neurol Scand 1997;96:401–6.

[100] Strater R, Vielhaber H, Kassenbohmer R, et al. Genetic risk factors of thrombophilia in ischaemic childhood stroke of cardiac origin. A prospective ESPED survey. Eur J Pediatr 1999;158(Suppl 3):S122–5.

[101] Sydenstricked VP, Mulherin WA, Houseal RW. The AJDC archives. August 1923. Sickle cell anemia. Report of two cases in children, with necropsy in one case. by V.P. Sydenstricked [sic], W.A. Mulherin and R.W. Houseal. Am J Dis Child 1987;141:612–5.

[102] Greer M, Schotland D. Abnormal hemoglobin as a cause of neurologic disease. Neurology 1962;12:114–23.

[103] Portnoy BA, Herion JC. Neurological manifestations in sickle-cell disease, with a review of the literature and emphasis on the prevalence of hemiplegia. Ann Intern Med 1972;76:643–52.

[104] Powars D, Wilson B, Imbus C, et al. The natural history of stroke in sickle cell disease. Am J Med 1978;65:461–71.

[105] Adams RJ, McKie VC, Brambilla D, et al. Stroke prevention trial in sickle cell anemia. Control Clin Trials 1998;19:110–29.

[106] Balkaran B, Char G, Morris JS, et al. Stroke in a cohort of patients with homozygous sickle cell disease. J Pediatr 1992;120:360–6.

[107] Ohene-Frempong K, Weiner SJ, Sleeper LA, et al. Cerebrovascular accidents in sickle cell disease: rates and risk factors. Blood 1998;91:288–94.

[108] Pegelow CH, Macklin EA, Moser FG, et al. Longitudinal changes in brain magnetic resonance imaging findings in children with sickle cell disease. Blood 2002;99:3014–8.

[109] Baird RL, Weiss DL, Ferguson AD, et al. Studies in sickle cell anemia. xxi. Clinico-pathological aspects of neurological manifestations. Pediatrics 1964;34:92–100.

[110] Hess DC, Adams RJ, Nichols FT 3rd. Sickle cell anemia and other hemoglobinopathies. Semin Neurol 1991;11:314–28.

[111] Stockman JA, Nigro MA, Mishkin MM, et al. Occlusion of large cerebral vessels in sickle-cell anemia. N Engl J Med 1972;287:846–9.

[112] Gerald B, Sebes JI, Langston JW. Cerebral infarction secondary to sickle cell disease: arteriographic findings. AJR Am J Roentgenol 1980;134:1209–12.

[113] Francis RB Jr. Platelets, coagulation, and fibrinolysis in sickle cell disease: their possible role in vascular occlusion. Blood Coagul Fibrinolysis 1991;2:341–53.

[114] Tam DA. Protein C and protein S activity in sickle cell disease and stroke. J Child Neurol 1997;12:19–21.

[115] Tuohy AM, McKie V, Manci EA, et al. Internal carotid artery occlusion in a child with sickle cell disease: case report and immunohistochemical study. J Pediatr Hematol Oncol 1997;19:455–8.

[116] French JA 2nd, Kenny D, Scott JP, et al. Mechanisms of stroke in sickle cell disease: sickle erythrocytes decrease cerebral blood flow in rats after nitric oxide synthase inhibition. Blood 1997;89:4591–9.

[117] Solovey A, Lin Y, Browne P, et al. Circulating activated endothelial cells in sickle cell anemia. N Engl J Med 1997;337:1584–90.

[118] Adams RJ. Stroke prevention and treatment in sickle cell disease. Arch Neurol 2001;58: 565–8.

[119] Adams RJ, McKie VC, Hsu L, et al. Prevention of a first stroke by transfusions in children with sickle cell anemia and abnormal results on transcranial Doppler ultrasonography. N Engl J Med 1998;339:5–11.

[120] Adams RJ, Brambilla D, Optimizing Primary Stroke Prevention in Sickle Cell Anemia (STOP 2) Trial Investigators. Discontinuing prophylactic transfusions used to prevent stroke in sickle cell disease. N Engl J Med 2005;353:2769–78.

[121] Vendt BA, McKinstry RC, Ball WS, et al. Silent cerebral infarct transfusion (SIT) trial imaging core: application of novel imaging information technology for rapid and central review of MRI of the brain. J Digit Imaging 2009;22(3):326–43.

[122] Kirkham FJ, Lerner NB, Noetzel M, et al. Trials in sickle cell disease. Pediatr Neurol 2006;34:450–8.

[123] deVeber G, Monagle P, Chan A, et al. Prothrombotic disorders in infants and children with cerebral thromboembolism. Arch Neurol 1998;55:1539–43.

[124] Heller C, Becker S, Scharrer I, et al. Prothrombotic risk factors in childhood stroke and venous thrombosis. Eur J Pediatr 1999;158(Suppl 3):S117–21.

[125] Nowak-Gottl U, Strater R, Heinecke A, et al. Lipoprotein (a) and genetic polymorphisms of clotting factor V, prothrombin, and methylenetetrahydrofolate reductase are risk factors of spontaneous ischemic stroke in childhood. Blood 1999;94:3678–82.

[126] Kenet G, Sadetzki S, Murad H, et al. Factor V Leiden and antiphospholipid antibodies are significant risk factors for ischemic stroke in children. Stroke 2000;31:1283–8.

[127] Zenz W, Bodo Z, Plotho J, et al. Factor V Leiden and prothrombin gene G 20210 A variant in children with ischemic stroke. Thromb Haemost 1998;80:763–6.

[128] Chan AK, deVeber G. Prothrombotic disorders and ischemic stroke in children. Semin Pediatr Neurol 2000;7:301–8.

[129] Lynch JK, Han CJ, Nee LE, et al. Prothrombotic factors in children with stroke or porencephaly. Pediatrics 2005;116:447–53.

[130] Danchaivijitr N, Cox TC, Saunders DE, et al. Evolution of cerebral arteriopathies in childhood arterial ischemic stroke. Ann Neurol 2006;59:620–6.

[131] Amlie-Lefond C, Bernard TJ, Sebire G, et al. Predictors of cerebral arteriopathy in children with arterial ischemic stroke: results of the International Pediatric Stroke Study. Circulation 2009;119:1417–23.

[132] Husson B, Rodesch G, Lasjaunias P, et al. Magnetic resonance angiography in childhood arterial brain infarcts: a comparative study with contrast angiography. Stroke 2002;33: 1280–5.

[133] Suzuki J, Takaku A. Cerebrovascular "moyamoya" disease. Disease showing abnormal net-like vessels in base of brain. Arch Neurol 1969;20:288–99.

[134] Mineharu Y, Takenaka K, Yamakawa H, et al. Inheritance pattern of familial moyamoya disease: autosomal dominant mode and genomic imprinting. J Neurol Neurosurg Psychiatr 2006;77:1025–9.

[135] Ikeda H, Sasaki T, Yoshimoto T, et al. Mapping of a familial moyamoya disease gene to chromosome 3p24.2-p26. Am J Hum Genet 1999;64:533–7.

[136] Mineharu Y, Liu W, Inoue K, et al. Autosomal dominant moyamoya disease maps to chromosome 17q25.3. Neurology 2008;70:2357–63.

[137] Sakurai K, Horiuchi Y, Ikeda H, et al. A novel susceptibility locus for moyamoya disease on chromosome 8q23. J Hum Genet 2004;49:278–81.

[138] Roach ES, Golomb MR, Adams R, et al. Management of Stroke in Infants and Children: A Scientific Statement from a Special Writing Group of the American Heart Association Stroke Council and the Council on Cardiovascular Disease in the Young. Stroke 2008;39:2644–91.

[139] Kirkham FJ, Hogan AM. Risk factors for arterial ischemic stroke in childhood. CNS Spectr 2004;9:451–64.

[140] Imaizumi C, Imaizumi T, Osawa M, et al. Serial intelligence test scores in pediatric moyamoya disease. Neuropediatrics 1999;30:294–9.

[141] Fung LW, Thompson D, Ganesan V. Revascularisation surgery for paediatric moyamoya: a review of the literature. Childs Nerv Syst 2005;21:358–64.

[142] Rafay MF, Armstrong D, Deveber G, et al. Craniocervical arterial dissection in children: clinical and radiographic presentation and outcome. J Child Neurol 2006;21:8–16.

[143] Fullerton HJ, Johnston SC, Smith WS. Arterial dissection and stroke in children. Neurology 2001;57:1155–60.

[144] Rosser TL, Vezina G, Packer RJ. Cerebrovascular abnormalities in a population of children with neurofibromatosis type 1. Neurology 2005;64:553–5.

[145] Rea D, Brandsema JF, Armstrong D, et al. Cerebral arteriopathy in children with neurofibromatosis type 1. Pediatrics 2009; [epub ahead of print].

[146] Schievink WI, Michels VV, Piepgras DG. Neurovascular manifestations of heritable connective tissue disorders. A review. Stroke 1994;25:889–903.

[147] Sobata E, Ohkuma H, Suzuki S. Cerebrovascular disorders associated with von Recklinghausen's neurofibromatosis: a case report. Neurosurgery 1988;22:544–9.

[148] Hilal SK, Solomon GE, Gold AP, et al. Primary cerebral arterial occlusive disease in children. II. Neurocutaneous syndromes. Radiology 1971;99:87–94.

[149] Erickson RP, Woolliscroft J, Allen RJ. Familial occurrence of intracranial arterial occlusive disease (moyamoya) in neurofibromatosis. Clin Genet 1980;18:191–6.

[150] Ng J, Mordekar SR, Connolly DJ, et al. Stroke in a child with neurofibromatosis type 2. Eur J Paediatr Neurol 2009;13(1):77–9.

[151] Chabrier S, Rodesch G, Lasjaunias P, et al. Transient cerebral arteriopathy: a disorder recognized by serial angiograms in children with stroke. J Child Neurol 1998;13:27–32.

[152] Sebire G, Fullerton H, Riou E, et al. Toward the definition of cerebral arteriopathies of childhood. Curr Opin Pediatr 2004;16:617–22.

[153] Braun KP, Bulder MM, Chabrier S, et al. The course and outcome of unilateral intracranial arteriopathy in 79 children with ischaemic stroke. Brain 2009;132(Pt2):544–57.

[154] Braun KP, Rafay MF, Uiterwaal CS, et al. Mode of onset predicts etiological diagnosis of arterial ischemic stroke in children. Stroke 2007;38:298–302.

[155] Sebire G, Meyer L, Chabrier S. Varicella as a risk factor for cerebral infarction in childhood: a case-control study. Ann Neurol 1999;45:679–80.

[156] Askalan R, Laughlin S, Mayank S, et al. Chickenpox and stroke in childhood: a study of frequency and causation. Stroke 2001;32:1257–62.

[157] Elbers J, Benseler SM. Central nervous system vasculitis in children. Curr Opin Rheumatol 2008;20:47–54.

[158] Aviv RI, Benseler SM, DeVeber G, et al. Angiography of primary central nervous system angiitis of childhood: conventional angiography versus magnetic resonance angiography at presentation. AJNR Am J Neuroradiol 2007;28:9–15.

[159] Benseler SM, deVeber G, Hawkins C, et al. Angiography-negative primary central nervous system vasculitis in children: a newly recognized inflammatory central nervous system disease. Arthritis Rheum 2005;52:2159–67.

[160] Lanthier S, Lortie A, Michaud J, et al. Isolated angiitis of the CNS in children. Neurology 2001;56:837–42.

[161] Benseler SM, Silverman E, Aviv RI, et al. Primary central nervous system vasculitis in children. Arthritis Rheum 2006;54:1291–7.

[162] Paediatric Stroke Working Group, Royal College of Physicians of London, Clinical Effectiveness and Evaluation Unit. Stroke in childhood: clinical guidelines for diagnosis, management and rehabilitation. London: Royal College of Physicians, Clinical Effectiveness and Evaluation Unit; 2004.

[163] Monagle P, Chalmers E, Chan A, et al. Antithrombotic therapy in neonates and children: American College of Chest Physicians evidence-based clinical practice guidelines (8th edition). Chest 2008;133:887S–968S.

[164] Carpenter J, Tsuchida T, Lynch JK. Treatment of arterial ischemic stroke in children. Expert Rev Neurother 2007;7:383–92.

[165] Bernard TJ, Goldenberg NA, Armstrong-Wells J, et al. Treatment of childhood arterial ischemic stroke. Ann Neurol 2008;63:679–96.

[166] Gabis LV, Yangala R, Lenn NJ. Time lag to diagnosis of stroke in children. Pediatrics 2002;110:924–8.

[167] Rafay MF, Pontigon AM, Chiang J, et al. Delay to diagnosis in acute pediatric arterial ischemic stroke. Stroke 2008.

[168] Shellhaas RA, Smith SE, O'Tool E, et al. Mimics of childhood stroke: characteristics of a prospective cohort. Pediatrics 2006;118:704–9.

[169] Braun KP, Kappelle LJ, Kirkham FJ, et al. Diagnostic pitfalls in paediatric ischaemic stroke. Dev Med Child Neurol 2006;48:985–90.

[170] Kirkham F, Sebire G, Steinlin M, et al. Arterial ischaemic stroke in children. Review of the literature and strategies for future stroke studies. Thromb Haemost 2004;92:697–706.

[171] Eeg-Olofsson O, Ringheim Y. Stroke in children. Clinical characteristics and prognosis. Acta Paediatr Scand 1983;72:391–5.

[172] Broderick J, Talbot GT, Prenger E, et al. Stroke in children within a major metropolitan area: the surprising importance of intracerebral hemorrhage. J Child Neurol 1993;8: 250–5.

[173] Golomb MR, Saha C, Garg BP, et al. Association of cerebral palsy with other disabilities in children with perinatal arterial ischemic stroke. Pediatr Neurol 2007;37:245–9.

[174] Lanska MJ, Lanska DJ, Horwitz SJ, et al. Presentation, clinical course, and outcome of childhood stroke. Pediatr Neurol 1991;7:333–41.

[175] Filipek PA, Krishnamoorthy KS, Davis KR, et al. Focal cerebral infarction in the newborn: a distinct entity. Pediatr Neurol 1987;3:141–7.
[176] Koelfen W, Freund M, Konig S, et al. Results of parenchymal and angiographic magnetic resonance imaging and neuropsychological testing of children after stroke as neonates. Eur J Pediatr 1993;152:1030–5.
[177] Golomb MR, MacGregor DL, Domi T, et al. Presumed pre- or perinatal arterial ischemic stroke: risk factors and outcomes. Ann Neurol 2001;50:163–8.

Advances in Pediatrics 56 (2009) 301–339

ADVANCES IN PEDIATRICS

ELSEVIER
MOSBY

Global Child Health: Promises Made to Children—Not Yet Kept

Burris Duncan, MD

Department of Pediatrics and Public Health, Arizona Health Sciences Center, Mel and Enid Zuckerman, College of Public Health, 1295 N. Martin Ave., Tucson, AZ 85724, USA

T his article represents an overview of the state of the world's children from the late 1970s, starting with the high hopes issued from the International Conference in Alma Ata declaring "Health for all by the year 2000." It progresses through the Revolution for Children including the World Summit for Children in 1990 followed by the Millennium Development Goals of 2000. We are halfway to 2015, the year when the Millennium Development Goals should be realized, but most of these goals are appearing illusive. For millions, many of the promises will not be kept. However, progress toward improving the health and well-being of children has been substantial, and is documented in the last half of the article that ends with a call to get involved.

THE ALMA ATA 1978 DECLARATION: HEALTH FOR ALL BY THE YEAR 2000

The 1978 Declaration at the International Conference held in Alma Ata, then Kazakhstan, stated that: "Governments have a responsibility for the health of their people which can be fulfilled only by the provision of adequate health and social measures. A main social target of governments, international organizations and the whole world community in the coming decades should be the attainment by all peoples of the world by the year 2000 of a level of health that will permit them to lead a socially and economically productive life. Primary health care is the key to attaining this target as part of development in the spirit of social justice"[1]. The attendees representing almost all of the member nations of World Health Organization (WHO) and the United Nations Children's Fund (UNICEF) affirmed that health care is a fundamental human right requiring a change from the generally accepted narrow concept of health to embrace an interdisciplinary, intersectorial approach involving broad community support and collaboration. The International Conference on Primary Health Care extended an urgent call to all nations to join in a collaborative effort "to develop and implement primary health care throughout the world."

E-mail address: bduncan@peds.arizona.edu

0065-3101/09/$ – see front matter
doi:10.1016/j.yapd.2009.08.013

THE REVOLUTION FOR CHILDREN: UNICEF AND JAMES P. GRANT

Motivated by the Declaration of Alma Ata and the visionary leadership of its Executive Director, James Grant, UNICEF launched an ambitious, bold program to bring low-cost, low-level technologies to the developing world. The program was based on the belief that scientific discoveries had advanced at a faster rate than had the application of that knowledge. The plan was to decrease child morbidity and child mortality by training community health workers in 4 basic programs: Growth monitoring, Oral rehydration, Breast feeding, and Immunization: GOBI.

Growth monitoring

Several important facts make this a cornerstone to the Revolution for Children. (1) The development of malnutrition is insidious. The day-to-day slow loss of body mass often goes unrecognized by the child's family until it is brought to the mother's attention by a family member or friend who has not seen the child for some time. (2) The vicious cycle of infection, malnutrition, and immunoincompetence is unrelenting. The cycle can begin at any one of the interlacing points of the triangle. Infection in a child is invariably associated with anorexia. If the illness is prolonged or if the child is on the edge of malnutrition, the tumble into acute malnutrition is precipitous and predictable. (3) Diets in poor countries are often deficient in essential micronutrients such as iron and vitamin A; a lack of either encourages a swift decline into severe malnutrition and infections. Meats are too expensive. Iron-containing foods are seldom a part of the child's meal. Staples are either rice or corn. Other vegetables and fruits are lacking. Any intake of β-carotene or vitamin A is low. (4) Malnutrition is an integral component of a least 50% of the deaths of the children younger than 5 years. (5) Early detection of a declining nutritional status followed by appropriate intervention could break the vicious cycle.

James Grant expanded the ideas of Dr. David Morley, an English pediatrician who had worked in West Africa where he instituted the Under-Five Clinics. These centers were basically well child clinics that emphasized good nutrition and growth. An important component of these clinics was the "Road to Health Chart" (Fig. 1) [2,3].

The chart has some very unique features. The horizontal axis represents the child's age, but not as the age in months; the columns are identified by the calendar months starting with the month the child was born. This chart eliminates the need for the health care worker to estimate the age of the child, minimizing mistakes. Only weights are recorded and only 2 reference lines (rather than 7) are shown on the graph. On this chart; the upper line is the 50th percentile for boys and the lower line is the third percentile for girls. The chart uses the National Centre for Health Statistics (NCHS) as a reference; not as a standard [4]. The child's individual line is plotted to show the mother the trajectory of her child's weight. The smaller box in the left upper corner shows 3 possible trajectories: an upward line is the best trajectory, a flat line indicates

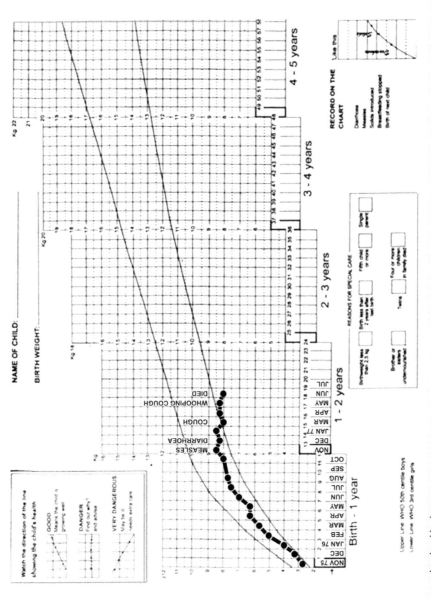

Fig. 1. The road to health chart.

danger, and a downward trajectory shouts an alarm. The chart also contains space to record any perinatal problems or complications at birth as well as birth weight, length, and head circumference, the clinic the child usually attends, and all immunizations the child receives. The health worker is advised to note when the child was weaned from the breast and when the next child was born. Significant illnesses are recorded on the chart in the month they occurred. Any change in weight trajectory with these sentinel events are points for discussion with the mother. There is also information extolling the benefits of breast feeding and when important developmental milestones should be met. The time when immunizations are due is also given on the chart.

The Road to Health Chart is given to the mother in a plastic, watertight bag at the birth of her child. She is instructed to keep it safe and to bring it to the clinic each month. Scenes like the one represented in Fig. 2 are a part of the life of the mother and her new child. Each month the child is weighed, and the weight plotted on the graph along with any significant illnesses the child had had since the last visit. With counsel, the mother can easily see the slope of the child's weight and compare the trajectory with the 3 lines in the smaller box. Intervention can be instituted with the first sign of "danger" before any serious consequences develop.

Oral rehydration
In much of the developing world, clean uncontaminated water is a rarity. Women and young children must often travel many miles to a river or well each day for portable but, all too frequently, not potable water. Piping water

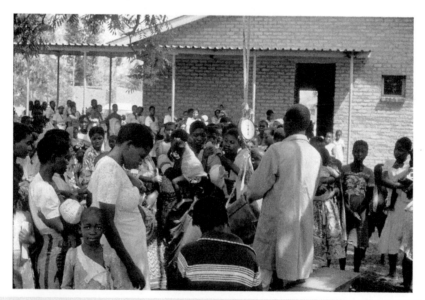

Fig. 2. A typical weight-in scene in East Africa.

to villages and rural homes is very expensive, and "at-source" purification is not frequently practiced. In this environment, every child younger than 5 years will have a minimum of 3 episodes of diarrhea each year [5]. Diarrheal deaths account for 21% of all deaths in children younger than 5 living in developing countries [6]. Although 37% fewer people died of diarrhea in 2002 compared with 1990, 1.8 million continue to die each year, most of which are preventable deaths [7–9].

In the mid 1970s, children with diarrhea and severe dehydration were admitted to "rehydration centers" scattered throughout the cities in developing countries. These centers administered intravenous fluids through butterfly needles. These needles were in short supply, hence the same needles were used repeatedly and interchanged between children. "Sterilization" of the needles was done by soaking them in a dilute "antiseptic" solution. In the 1980s, with the introduction of oral rehydration therapy (ORT), all of that changed. The oral rehydration solution (ORS) was developed in the treatment of cholera, with the discovery that the greatest absorption of water occurred when the ratio of sodium and glucose was close to 1:1. ORS contained 90 mmol/L of sodium and 111 mmol/L of glucose along with potassium and bicarbonate. One packet of the powdered mixture (Fig. 3) was dissolved in one quart (0.95 L) of water. At a cost of less than 10 US cents, many countries manufactured their own packets. This solution was effective in 90% of the cases of diarrhea, even in the presence of hyper- and hyponatremic dehydration. In children who were in shock or who had greater than 10% dehydration, a push of intravenous fluids was initiated, followed by the oral solution. Once hydration

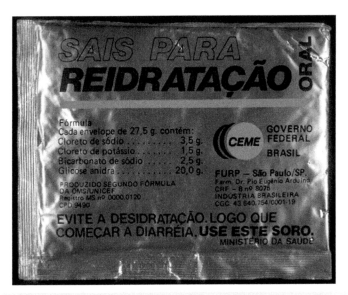

Fig. 3. A 10-cent package of rehydration salt to be mixed with 1 quart of clean water.

was reestablished, the ORS was given in quantities equal to the fluid lost in the stool, but this did not immediately stop the watery diarrhea. The mother was told the solution would help her child but when she continued to see diarrhea she was confused, and acceptance was slow. Other formulations were tried in an attempt to thicken the stools, but success was mixed. However, the effect of ORT was dramatic. Each year, 1 million fewer children were dying a diarrheal death. Eight years after the introduction of this treatment (1980–1988), 36% of the cases of diarrhea were being treated with ORT [10]. If this therapy could be extended to all diarrhea episodes, another 2.5 million deaths would be averted. By 2005, 43% of the children with diarrhea in 31 countries in the developing world were receiving ORS; further along, but not there yet (Fig. 4) [11].

Breast feeding

Spurred by the unscrupulous behavior of some infant formula companies that were promoting their product as superior to breast milk, the WHO published The International Code of Marketing of Breast Milk Substitutes [12]. The Code was designed to promote the safety, adequacy, and benefits of breast milk. Its guidelines state that the promotion of artificial milk substitutes by manufacturers and their representatives must be limited to discussing scientific and factual matters with health professionals, and were not to imply that bottle feeding is equal to or superior to breastfeeding. Advertisements to the general public and particularly to pregnant women that either explicitly or implicitly indicated that breast milk was inferior to a milk substitute would not be permitted. Representatives of these companies would not be allowed in the nurseries to promote their products to the unsuspecting new mothers. Samples would not be distributed. Health providers would extol the advantages of breast milk and discuss the disadvantages of substitutes.

Shortly after the International Code in 1991, the WHO and UNICEF launched the Baby-friendly Hospital Initiative [13]. Just 15 years later, more than 20,000 hospitals in 152 countries had been designated Baby-friendly. Exclusive breast feeding for at least the first 6 months of life in countless infants had expanded.

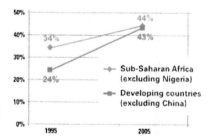

COVERAGE OF RECOMMENDED TREATMENT SIGNIFICANTLY INCREASED FROM 1995 TO 2005

Yet, data are limited

Percentage of children under five with diarrhoea receiving oral rehydration or increased fluids with continued feeding, based on an analysis of findings from 31 developing countries (1995–2005)

Fig. 4. (*From* UNICEF. Progress for children—a world fit for children: statistical review. Number 6, December 2007. http://www.unicef.org/progressforchildren/2007n6/index_41401.htm; with permission.)

The ten steps to successful breastfeeding inherent in a Baby-friendly Hospital [14]:

1. Have a written breastfeeding policy that is routinely communicated to all health care staff.
2. Train all health care staff in the skills necessary to implement this policy.
3. Inform all pregnant women about the benefits and management of breastfeeding.
4. Help mothers initiate breastfeeding within a half-hour after birth.
5. Show mothers how to breastfeed, and how to maintain lactation even if they should be separated from their infants.
6. Give newborn infants no food or drink other than breast milk, unless medically indicated.
7. Practice rooming-in: allow mothers and infants to remain together 24 hours a day.
8. Encourage breastfeeding on demand.
9. Give no artificial teats or pacifiers (dummies or soothers) to breastfeeding infants.
10. Foster the establishment of breastfeeding support groups and refer mothers to them on discharge from the hospital or clinic.

Of all the arguments extolling the virtues of breast milk or "breast is best," perhaps the most convincing is the "enteromammary system" [15]. Any antigen that inhabits the intestinal tract of the lactating mother stimulates the production of IgA antibodies in the Peyer patches in her intestinal tract. Those specific antibodies enter the adjacent lymphatic nodes; travel to the thoracic duct, and into the blood stream. The antibodies then *hone* to the mother's breast. The specific IgA levels in her breast milk are higher than the levels in her blood stream. Two molecules of IgA fuse forming secretory IgA, the predominant immunoglobin in human milk. The infant ingests these antibodies, which enter the infant's intestinal tract where they attach to the epithelial cells. Invasion by the antigen is prevented. This system is so effective that pathogenic viruses, bacteria, and even some parasites have been cultured or found in the infant's stool yet the infant is not diseased!

Immunizations

When the Revolution for Children began in the early 1980s, immunization rates for children younger than 2 years living in the developing world were from 5% to 10%. Fourteen years later, rates for 5 of the 6 targeted diseases, diphtheria, pertussis, tetanus, polio, and measles, were close to 80% and the sixth, the BCG vaccine against tuberculosis given at birth, was greater than 80%. However, only 40% of pregnant women had received the second dose of tetanus (Fig. 5). This low rate kept the incidence of neonatal tetanus high [16]. Mortality and morbidity from these diseases decreased proportionately. By 2006, global coverage of infants with 3 doses of diphtheria/polio/tetanus vaccine was still close to 80% but 114 countries (59% of all countries) had achieved 90% coverage. However, there is a sharp disparity. In many African

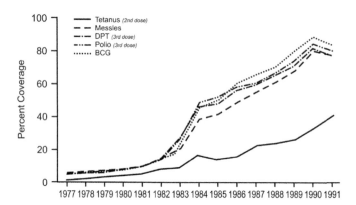

Fig. 5. Global immunization coverage 1977 to 1991. (*Data from* Expanded Programme on Immunizations Programme report for the year 1992. Incorporating the recommendations of the global advisory group, October 1992. World Health Organization. January 1993. http://whqlibdoc.who.int/hq/1993/WHO_EPI_GEN_93.1.pdf.)

countries, coverage is 82%, whereas in the Americas it is 94% and in Europe, 95% [17,18].

The efficacy of both the polio and measles vaccines decreases when the "cold chain" is broken. This finding prompted the use of thermal indicators packed with these vaccines to alert health care workers if the "cold chain" has been violated and the efficacy of the vaccine has been reduced. Appropriate authorities are notified to prevent recurrence of the problem.

In the fall of 1991, the last case of polio was seen in the Americas and by 2003 polio had been eradicated from all but 3 countries in the world. Then a few cases were imported from Nigeria and soon 21 countries were reporting polio cases. The involved countries rapidly instituted "Supplementary Immunization Activity" to quickly abort any new cases. It is expected that very soon polio will meet the same fate as smallpox: elimination [19].

Eradicating measles has been a more difficult job. Whereas coverage has improved, it has been slow. Dr. Margaret Chan, WHO Director-General, reported that measles deaths decreased by 60% (873,000 to 345,000) from 1999 to 2005 [20] (Fig. 6), a remarkable achievement, but unfortunately coverage is insufficient. Too many children are still dying from this preventable illness.

One hundred and twenty-three countries have added the Rubella vaccine to the list of immunizations [17]. By 2006, many countries had expanded coverage of children to include hepatitis B and *Haemophilus* influenza type B (Fig. 7) [11].

FFF: THREE OTHER LOW-COST, LOW-LEVEL TECHNOLOGIES WERE ADDED

Female education

It is generally accepted that the more education a women has, the healthier she and her family are, the fewer children she has, and the greater is her potential

MEASLES IMMUNIZATION COVERAGE HAS INCREASED STEADILY SINCE 1990
IN 47 PRIORITY COUNTRIES AND WORLDWIDE

Trends in first-dose coverage of measles-containing vaccine (MCV; 1990–2006)

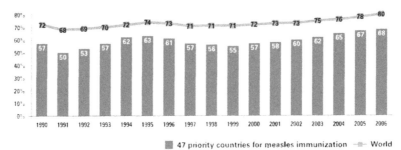

47 priority countries for measles immunization   World

Fig. 6. (*From* UNICEF. Progress for children—a world fit for children: statistical review. Number 6, December 2007. http://www.unicef.org/progressforchildren/2007n6/index_41401. htm.; with permission.)

SINCE 1990, MOST COUNTRIES HAVE BEGUN IMMUNIZING AGAINST
HEPATITIS B (HepB) AND *HAEMOPHILUS INFLUENZAE* TYPE B (Hib)

Number of countries that have introduced HepB and Hib into infant immunization schedules,
with global percentage of target population reached with three doses of HepB vaccine (1990–2006)

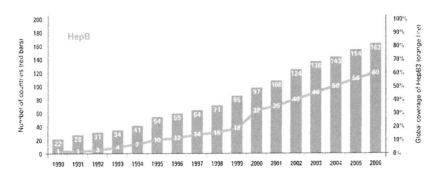

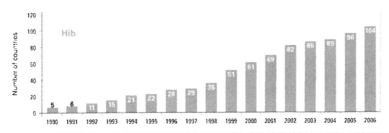

Fig. 7. Immunization against hepatitis B and *Haemophilus influenzae.* (*From* UNICEF. Progress for children—a world fit for children: statistical review. Number 6, December 2007. http://www.unicef.org/progressforchildren/2007n6/index_41401.htm; with permission.)

for income generation. In the early 1980s, the disparity in primary and secondary education between the genders was large and unacceptable [21]. Perhaps the best example of the impact female education can have on the whole population is in the State of Kerala in India. The per capita income in Kerala is less than throughout most of India, yet in Kerala the commitment to female education is strong. In India, one-half of girls drop out of school before completing 5 grades, and only 34% of women are literate. In Kerala, the dropout percentage is zero before grade 5, and 87% of the women are literate. The average number of births per woman in 1990 in India was 4. In Kerala, it was half that (1.9), and twice as many women in Kerala use birth control. In 1990, infant mortality was 83 per 1000 live births in India. In Kerala it was only 17 per 1000 live births. The life expectancy in Kerala for women was 15 years longer than in the whole of India (74 compared with 59) [22].

Family spacing

The rallying cry of nongovernmental organizations (NGO) as well as many governments was "too young, too many, too soon." In many developing countries, the custom is for young adolescent girls to marry older men and start having babies at a very early age. Fertility is good. Sterility is not. A 1992 survey in Niger found that 47% of women aged 20 to 24 years had married before they were 15 years old and 87% had married before the age of 18. More than half had had a child before they had left the teenage years [23].

Complications from a teen pregnancy are numerous and include a high percentage of school dropouts as well as a high prevalence of anemia, and due to the smaller pelvis of young mothers, obstructed labor is more frequent. The WHO estimates that maternal mortality rates are fivefold greater for girls between 10 and 14 and twice as high for adolescents who are between 15 and 19 compared with women who are 20 to 24 years old. In societies where the infant and childhood mortality rates are high, families have grown to anticipate that several of their children will die prematurely. To ensure a significant work force, women have more children. In country after country, as infant and childhood mortality rates decrease and more children live, fertility rates also decrease, although it may take a generation or two to realize this [24]. From 1960 to1980, infant and childhood mortality rates fell close to 60% and fertility rates decreased by 48%. The "too soon" refers to too short a period between one pregnancy and the next. The "simple" strategy of waiting 2 to 3 years between pregnancies will cut infant mortality almost by half and if the interval is greater than 4 years, infant mortality decreases by 60%. Due to the contraceptive effects of *exclusive* breast feeding, delaying weaning has helped lengthen the time between pregnancies.

Food supplementation

Many studies have reported the benefits of supplementing diets of pregnant women and young children. Perhaps the most well known is the Guatemala study conducted by the Institute of Nutrition of Central America and Panama (INCAP) [25–27]. Two randomly chosen villages received a nutritious supplement (atole, containing 163 kcal of energy and 11.5 g of protein for each 180 mL of fluid). Two other randomly chosen villages received a less nutritious supplement (fresco, which contained approximately one-third as many calories and no protein). The women in the study who supplemented their usual diet with 20,000 kcal or more during pregnancy had half the risk of delivering a low birth weight infant. Infant mortality rates were reduced by 66% in the atole villages compared with 24% in the fresco villages. A follow-up study in 1987 to 1988 reported that half of the women who as children had received the fresco supplement had short stature compared with only one-third of the women who had received the more nutritious atole supplement [28]. Short stature is associated with a small pelvis. Thus, the infants fared better and the girls were less likely to have obstructed labor when they became pregnant themselves.

The Guatemala food supplementation programs has also had very significant long-term economic effects [29,30]. A follow-up study involved 60% of the 2392 children, aged 0 to 7 years, from the original INCAP study. Linear regression models were adjusted for confounding variables to estimate the annual income, hours worked, and average hourly wages of the adults. The adult men, who as children had received the more nutritious supplement atole from birth to age 2, had a 46% increase in average wages compared with those who received the less nutritious supplement. Boys who had received the atole during their first 3 years of life had an increase of 37% in hourly wages. However, there was no difference in hourly wages in those who received the atole after age 3.

MICRONUTRIENT DEFICIENCIES CAUSED CONCERN AND ACTION

Iodine

In 1993, it was estimated that iodine deficiency was responsible for cretinism in 5.7 million and for mental retardation in another 26 million of the 1.6 billion at-risk populations. In 1990, a goal was set to eliminate all new cases of iodine deficiency by the year 2000. To achieve that goal, every country was to have iodized 95% of the salt supplies by 1995 [22]. The goal has not been met; but by 2003 approximately 70% of the world's salt consumed by humans was iodized. Areas where there is much work yet to be done include some West and East African countries, some Middle Eastern countries, and Russia. China is a story of success. In a span of just 10 years, the population of that huge country had increased its use of iodized salt from 50% to 95% [31].

Vitamin A

In 1994, of the 562 million children younger than 5 years living in the developing world, 500,000 suffered severe eye damage or were blind as a result of vitamin A deficiency; another 3 million had xerophthalmia, and another 13.5 million had "night blindness." Forty-four percent of the entire under-5 population was deficient in vitamin A, inviting a 20% to 30% increased risk of death from common diseases [22]. The risk was even higher for those children who contracted measles. This exanthem is a highly desquamating disease, with loss of epithelium in numerous organs. Vitamin A is essential in the repair of these epithelial cells. With a deficiency of vitamin A, corneal necrosis (keratomalacia) occurs and ulcerates, with the potential expulsion of the lens and blindness. The denuded epithelium-lined tracts are susceptible to bacterial invasion through pneumonia, gastroenteritis, and nephritis. Sepsis is often the result. Without epithelial repair, death can occur as long as 9 months after the measles exanthem. An observant ophthalmologist, Dr. Al Sommer, reported that the survival of children who are deficient in vitamin A can be increased by 35% if they are given a high dose of vitamin A supplementation (200,000 units on 2 successive days) [32]. A meta-analysis by Fawzi and colleagues concluded with the recommendation that "Vitamin A supplements should be given to all measles patients in developing countries whether or not they have symptoms of vitamin A deficiency" [33].

UNICEF and other NGOs, and some countries started programs to orally administer 200,000 units of vitamin A every 5 to 6 months to all children between the ages of 12 months and 5 years. The vitamin A is dispensed in a capsule containing oil to improve absorption, which costs less than 10 cents. The vitamin is stored in the liver, and an adequate supply is maintained unless the child develops repeated illnesses that call on an excessive amount of vitamin A to repair damaged epithelial cells. In southern Nepal, a high percentage of pregnant women are deficient in vitamin A [34]. If the pregnant woman's diet remains inadequate in β-carotene or vitamin A and is without supplementation, her newborn will be deficient and will remain so due to inadequate levels in her breast milk. Until the intake is sufficient, the newborn will be more susceptible to disease and death.

Iron

It is estimated that more than 1 billion people have iron deficiency anemia; 16% of the world's population [35]. In 1990, half of the pregnant women in the developing world suffered from iron deficiency anemia. These women were tired and having difficulty doing all the chores of daily living, and were at an increased risk of death in childbirth. Their infants were more likely to be small, with lower birth weights and with impaired development [36]. In some areas it was even worse; 90% of pregnant women living in an urban area in Pakistan had anemia [37]. The anemia was mild in 75% of these women, with hemoglobin (Hg) level between 9 and 10.9 g/dL, and in 14% it was moderate, with Hg level between 7 and 8.9 g/dL. More than 40% of children younger than 5 years have a Hg level less than 11 g/dL. In the short term this is responsible for considerable morbidity and mortality. Long-term consequences include a diminution in cognitive abilities and less income potential. This major problem has not been adequately addressed.

Zinc

Thirty percent of the world's population is deficient in zinc, largely due to the fact that zinc is mainly found in red meat (expensive) and there are no tissue stores. The areas with the highest deficiencies are in Central and East Africa, Angola, Zambia, Zimbabwe, Afghanistan, India, and South East Asia. Zinc supplementation benefits children with diarrhea and respiratory illnesses, and improves linear growth. Pooled analysis of zinc studies has not shown a reduction in *infant* mortality, but has shown an 18% reduction in mortality in children between 12 months and 5 years old. The lack of effect on mortality in infants has a biological basis, as this age group is not thought to have a deficiency of zinc [38].

A recently published community-based, cluster-randomized, double-masked, placebo-controlled, and zinc supplemental trial involved 41,276 children aged 1 to 35 months living in southern Nepal [39]. The 4 groups received daily doses of: (1) placebo; (2) zinc (10 mg); (3) iron (12.5 mg) and folic acid (50 µg); or (4) zinc plus iron and folic acid. The mortality in children younger than 12 months was not affected by the supplemental zinc. Although mortality was 20% lower in the older children, the difference did not reach statistical significance. Contrary to the 1999 report of the Zinc Investigators Collaborative Group [40], the study in Nepal found no difference in the frequency and duration of diarrhea and respiratory infections between the groups. The discrepancy was explained with the observation that most of the studies cited in the Collaborative review involved high-risk children; those just recovering from acute diarrhea or who had persistent diarrhea, and children who were underweight or stunted. Results from studies on unselected populations published after the Collaborative Group report are mixed. The final chapter on morbidity data has not been written.

THE INTEGRATED MANAGEMENT OF CHILDHOOD ILLNESS (IMCI)

Within the past few years, the WHO and UNICEF have adopted a more comprehensive approach to child care that emphasizes not just the child's acute illness and nutritional deficiencies but the child's total well-being. The child's presenting complaint is dealt with first. The community health care worker makes a careful and systematic assessment of common symptoms and well-selected specific clinical danger signs that provide sufficient information to guide rational and effective actions. The emphasis is on the severity of the acute problem rather than on a specific diagnosis. Algorithms have been developed to assist the health care worker who may have had limited training to make an informed determination as to where and how best to treat the child. The worker follows a chart color-coded by red (danger), yellow (caution), or green (safe). For example, danger signs are depicted on a chart whose center has a big red stop sign surrounded by danger words ("lethargy or unconscious," "inability to drink or breast feed," and "convulsions"). If the child has the danger signs, immediate referral is made to the nearest appropriate facility. If the danger signs are not present and the child can be treated at home, the family is given an explanation of the problem, why it has occurred, and instructions on how to implement the care suggested.

After addressing the acute problem, the focus shifts to addressing what is necessary to promote the child's growth and development. In addition to the assessment and management of the child's acute condition, more chronic issues are identified and addressed, including nutritional status and immunization coverage. The child younger than 5 years receives the greatest scrutiny.

IMCI not only includes both curative and preventative elements, but also strives to engage the family and the entire community in health promotion. IMCI is a full program that also involves improving the training of the health workers, educating the community in preventive measures to decrease morbidity and mortality of the children, upgrading the available care in the local health clinics, strengthening the available care in the hospital for those children too sick to be treated at the local clinic, and helping local governments plan and include the program as part of the national health policy [41].

The Revolution for Children predicted that if the low-cost, low-technology strategies were put in place, half of the children who would have died would now be alive. The goal was within reach. The cost was not great. The success has largely been the result of implementing the vision of James Grant. He pushed the agenda for nations and NGOs to adopt these simple strategies, and knew that the main obstacles would be creating the political will to place children at the level of highest priority (Table 1).

THE CONVENTION ON THE RIGHTS OF THE CHILD

This document was presented at the World's Summit for Children in the fall of 1990. In 1989, the General Assembly of the United Nations had adopted this Convention and by the time of the Summit, it had a sufficient number of signatures to become law [42]. This international Convention enumerates the civil, political, economic, social, and cultural rights of children, and a country's signature binds the country to carry out the Articles through international law. The Convention has now been ratified by every country except two: Somalia and the United States. The United Nation's Committee on the Rights of the Child monitors each country to ensure that its Articles are observed.

Table 1
Significant improvement in major health indicators in the past 40+ years

Revolution for children

Indicator	1960	2006–2007	Change
Child deaths	20,000,000	9,700,000 in 2007	51% less
Infant mortality ratio	126	49 in 2006	61% less
Under-5 mortality	197	72 in 2006	63% less
Fertility rate	5.0	2.5 in 2006	48% less
Life expectancy	56 in 1970	68 in 2006	12 more years

THE WORLD'S SUMMIT FOR CHILDREN

Close to one-half of the world's Presidents and Prime Ministers convened in New York in September of 1990 to ensure that the welfare of children would be placed highest on their political agendas. The challenge of the Summit was: "Enhancement of children's health and nutrition is a first duty, and also a task for which solutions are now within reach. The lives of tens of thousands of boys and girls can be saved every day because the causes of their death are readily preventable. Child and infant mortality is unacceptably high in many parts of the world, but can be lowered dramatically with means that are already known and easily accessible."

From the Summit came the World Declaration on the Survival, Protection and Development of Children and Plans of Action [43]. In September 1990, the following Declaration was signed by 71 heads of state and governments and has subsequently been endorsed by 181 countries.

1. We will work to promote earliest possible ratification and implementation of the Convention on the Rights of the Child. Programs to encourage information about children's rights should be launched worldwide, taking into account the distinct cultural and social values in different countries.
2. We will work for a solid effort of national and international action to enhance children's health, to promote prenatal care, and to lower infant and child mortality in all countries and among all peoples. We will promote the provision of clean water in all communities for all their children, as well as universal access to sanitation.
3. We will work for optimal growth and development in childhood, through measures to eradicate hunger, malnutrition, and famine, and thus to relieve millions of children of tragic sufferings in a world that has the means to feed all its citizens.
4. We will work to strengthen the role and status of women. We will promote responsible planning of family size, child spacing, breastfeeding and safe motherhood.
5. We will work for respect for the role of the family in providing for children and will support the efforts of parents, other caregivers, and communities to nurture and care for children, from the earliest stages of childhood through adolescence. We also recognize the special needs of children who are separated from their families.
6. We will work for programs that reduce illiteracy and provide educational opportunities for all children, irrespective of their background and gender; that prepare children for productive employment and lifelong learning opportunities, ie, through vocational training; and that enable children to grow to adulthood within a supportive and nurturing cultural and social context.
7. We will work to ameliorate the plight of millions of children who live under especially difficult circumstances—as victims of apartheid and foreign occupation; orphans and street children and children of migrant workers; the displaced children and victims of natural and man-made disasters; the disabled and the abused, the socially disadvantaged and the exploited. Refugee children must be helped to find new roots in life. We will work for special protection of the working child and for the abolition of illegal child labor. We will do our best to ensure that children are not drawn into becoming victims of the scourge of illicit drugs.

8. We will work carefully to protect children from the scourge of war and to take measures to prevent further armed conflicts, in order to give children everywhere a peaceful and secure future. We will promote the values of peace, understanding, and dialogue in the education of children. The essential needs of children and families must be protected even in times of war and in violence-ridden areas. We ask that periods of tranquility and special relief corridors be observed for the benefit of children, where war and violence are still taking place.

9. We will work for common measures for the protection of the environment, at all levels, so that all children can enjoy a safer and healthier future.

10. We will work for a global attack on poverty, which would have immediate benefits for children's welfare. The vulnerability and special needs of the children of the developing countries, and in particular the least developed ones, deserve priority. But growth and development need promotion in all States, through national action and international cooperation. That calls for transfers of appropriate additional resources to developing countries as well as improved terms of trade, further trade liberalization, and measures for debt relief. It also implies structural adjustments that promote world economic growth, particularly in developing countries, while ensuring the well-being of the most vulnerable sectors of the populations, in particular the children.

In 2000, The Millennium Development Goals (MDGs) were signed by 189 countries, and were to be accomplished in the next 15 years (2015) [44].

Goal 1 Eradicate extreme poverty and hunger: Decrease by half from 1990 the proportion of people whose income is less than 1 dollar a day and the proportion of people who suffer from hunger. Achieve full and productive employment and decent work for all, including women and young people.

Goal 2 Achieve universal primary education: Ensure that children everywhere, boys and girls alike, will be able to complete a full course of primary schooling.

Goal 3 Promote gender equality and empower women: Eliminate gender disparity in primary and secondary education at all levels.

Goal 4 Reduce child mortality: Reduce the under-5 mortality rate by two-thirds from 1990.

Goal 5 Improve maternal health: Reduce the maternal mortality ratio by three-quarters from 1990. Achieve universal access to reproductive health.

Goal 6 Combat human immunodeficiency virus (HIV)/AIDS, malaria, and other diseases: Have halted and begun to reverse the spread of HIV/AIDS. Achieve universal access to treatment for HIV/AIDS for all those who need it. Have halted and begun to reverse the incidence of malaria and other major diseases.

Goal 7 Ensure environmental sustainability: Integrate the principles of sustainable development into country policies and programs; reverse loss of environmental resources. Reduce biodiversity loss and a significant reduction in the rate of loss. Halve the proportion of people without sustainable access to safe drinking water and basic sanitation. By 2020, achieve a significant improvement in the lives of at least 100 million slum dwellers.

Goal 8   Develop a global partnership for development: Further develop an open trading and financial system that is rule-based, predictable, and nondiscriminatory, and that includes a commitment to good governance, development and poverty reduction; nationally and internationally. Address the special needs of the least developed countries, including tariff and quota free access for their exports; enhanced program of debt relief for heavily indebted poor countries; and cancellation of official bilateral debt; and more generous official development assistance for countries committed to poverty reduction. Address the special needs of landlocked and small-island developing States. Deal comprehensively with the debt problems of developing countries through national and international measures in order to make debt sustainable in the long term. In cooperation with developing countries, develop and implement strategies for decent and productive work for youth. In cooperation with pharmaceutical companies, provide access to affordable essential drugs in developing countries. In cooperation with the private sector, make available the benefits of new technologies, especially information and communications.

WORLD HEALTH ORGANIZATION ALTERING COURSE: VERTICAL TO HORIZONTAL PROGRAMS

Dr. Margaret Chan, the WHO's Director-General, recently stated that international evidence overwhelmingly demonstrates that the primary health care approach is the most efficient and cost-effective way to organize a health system and is the way to achieve "Health Care for All" [45–47]. She observed that whereas it was once thought that attacking single diseases (the vertical approach) would strengthen health care systems, the opposite has occurred. In fact, when some targeted projects implemented by some NGOs or large foundations initiated strategies to ameliorate a specific disease their good intentions often actually disrupted basic health care services. The limited numbers of health care workers were drawn from their government-sponsored jobs of delivering primary health care to these outside higher-paying, more attractive, and more narrowed focused jobs. Dr. Chan argued for a return to primary health care as the only means to meet the 8 Millennium Developmental Goals. This call is emphasized in the World Health Report 2008, Primary Health Care Now More than Ever [48].

Dr. Chan confirmed her strong commitment to social justice and equity in health care, and noted the ever widening gaps between wealthy urban populations and poor rural populations. She recognized the link between health and poverty, and described the vicious circle of how poor health induces poverty and poverty is embedded in poor health. Both must be addressed actively, vigorously, and urgently. She emphasized the necessity of the multisectorial approach outlined at the Alma Ata Conference on Primary Health Care. Dr. Chan extolled governments to strengthen health policies, with particular attention to poor communities. Equity of access was a strong theme of her remarks, and is given further emphasis in the World Health Report 2008 [46,47].

THE PROGRESS FOR CHILDREN: A WORLD FIT FOR CHILDREN 2007

During the 25 years from 1980 to 2005, under-5 mortality fell 34%; from 110 in 1000 to 72 in 1000 live births (Fig. 8). Worldwide, the annual mortality dropped from 13.5 million to 9.7 million. In Latin America, North Africa, the Middle East, Europe, and Southeast Asia, the annual rate of decline was more than 4%. But from 1970 to 2005 in the subregions of West, East, and Central Africa the total number of deaths actually rose 25% [49]! The inequality is explained by a slower decline in under-5 mortality in these regions in Africa, only minimal reductions in the fertility rate with an increase in total population, and the HIV/AIDS epidemic. It is estimated that by 2015, 56% of all under-5 deaths will occur in sub-Saharan Africa; an increase from 19% in 1970. Another 31% will occur in south Asia. In China between 1980 and 1985, the rate of decline was 5%, but since 1985 the decline has slowed to less than 3% [49].

The current rates of decline are not enough to achieve the MDG #4. Diversity of rates within countries and regions presents opportunities to identify the most effective policy changes that should be adopted and implemented.

The Progress for Children: a World Fit for Children [11] presents data proclaiming many important achievements related to the MDGs [11,44,50].

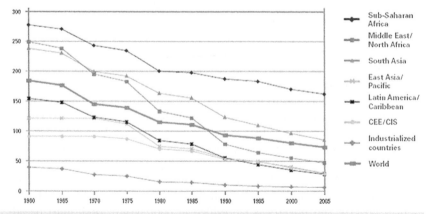

TRENDS IN CHILD MORTALITY

Under-five mortality rate (per 1,000 live births), by region (1960–2005)

Fig. 8. (*From* UNICEF. Progress for children—a world fit for children: statistical review. Number 6, December 2007. http://www.unicef.org/progressforchildren/2007n6/index_41401.htm; with permission.)

Promoting healthy lives
- In 2006, the number of deaths in children younger than 5 years fell below 10 million (9.7 million)—half what it was in 1960 (20 million)
- In 2005, 4 times as many children received 2 doses of vitamin A as in 1999.
- The use of insecticide-treated bed nets tripled in 16 of 20 African countries.
- From 1990 to 2006, in the 47 countries which account for 95% of measles deaths, measles immunization coverage had increased 11% (57% 68%).
- More than 1.2 billion people gained access to improved drinking water sources.
- Sanitation increased but not at a rate to meet the MDG #7.
- Insufficient progress has been made to reduce maternal mortality.

Providing a quality education
- From 2002 to 2006, the number of school-aged children out of school decreased by 18 million or 19% (115 to 93 million).
- But, in sub-Saharan Africa only 1 out of 4 children of secondary school age attend secondary schools.

Combating HIV/AIDS
- Almost two-thirds of all people with HIV live in sub-Saharan Africa.
- Only 11% of over 2 million pregnant women living with HIV/AIDS received antiretroviral therapy to prevent transmission to their unborn child.
- Only 15% of children younger than 15 years in need of antiretroviral therapy received that therapy.

MORTALITY AND MORBIDITY: HOW ACCURATE ARE THE NUMBERS?

Murray and colleagues site 5 problems that raise questions concerning the accuracy of the statistical reports from the WHO and UNICEF [49]: (1) child mortality data are missing in some countries; (2) figures do not distinguish between actual measurements and predictions; (3) Methods used to obtain the numbers are not transparent and are not reproducible; (4) data from different countries are not obtained with the same precision; and (5) there has been a trend to overestimate mortality in several sub-Saharan countries (Fig. 9).

THE 2008 HIV/AIDS PROGRESS REPORT (MDG #6): POSITIVE AND NEGATIVE STATISTICS

From 2006 to 2007, access to antiretroviral therapy in low- and middle-income countries increased 7.5-fold, an increase of almost 1 million; but coverage remains low, with only 31% of those in need receiving therapy and in 2007 an estimated 2.5 million becoming newly infected. Decreases in mortality of those receiving treatment is the same for low- and middle-income countries as for high-income countries. In 2007, 33% of HIV-positive pregnant women in low- and middle-income countries received antiretroviral drugs to prevent transmission to their child; almost a 3-fold increase from 2004 when only 12% received the drugs. Tuberculosis is the leading cause of death among people with HIV. Unfortunately, many people do not know their HIV status

SUB-SAHARAN AFRICA HAS THE MOST PEOPLE LIVING WITH HIV

Estimated number of people living with HIV, by region (1990–2006)

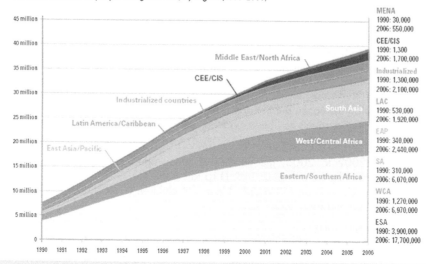

Fig. 9. Human immunodeficiency virus. (*From* UNICEF. Progress for children—a world fit for children: statistical review. Number 6, December 2007. http://www.unicef.org/progress-forchildren/2007n6/index_41401.htm.; with permission.)

and a large number live with undiagnosed HIV. Unless that status is checked and only the tuberculosis is treated, satisfactory results are elusive. Targeting of high-risk groups is effective [51].

New evidence from the Comprehensive International Program for Research in AIDS suggests that diagnosis of infants as young as 6 weeks followed by a combination of 3 antiretroviral drugs (lopinavir-ritonavir, zidovudine, and lamivudine) substantially reduces infant mortality (75%) as well as the progression of HIV (76%). The randomized study involved infants 6 to 12 weeks old; 252 received early treatment and 125 received treatment delayed by a mean of 40 weeks. Four percent of the infants in the early treatment group died compared with 16% in the delayed group [52].

Male circumcision reduces the risk of heterosexually acquired HIV infection in men. A large Randomized Clinical Trial (RCT) of HIV-negative men aged 15 to 49 years were assigned either to an immediate circumcised group (2474) or to a 24-month delayed circumcision group (2522) [53]. The subjects were followed with HIV testing, physical examination, and interviews at baseline, and at 6, 12, and 24 months. The groups were similar at baseline and at each evaluation period. There was 90% to 92% retention in both groups. Over the 24 months, the incidence of HIV conversion in the group who received immediate circumcision was 0.66 cases per 100 person-years compared with an incidence of 1.33 cases per 100 person-years in those who had delayed circumcision.

Breast milk transmitted HIV

The HIV/AIDS epidemic and the strong likelihood of vertical transmission of the virus through breast milk to the suckling infant and milk substitutes introduced considerable controversy. Were deaths more likely from newborns ingesting breast milk contaminated with the AIDS virus or from drinking formula mixed with water contaminated with bacteria or enteroviruses? In areas where water contamination is not a serious problem, mothers who are HIV-infected are advised not to breastfeed their newborn infant. In regions where the water supply is not optimal, breast milk was safer; provided it was the *exclusive and only* nutrient the infant ingested. Maternal characteristics that enhance transmission include recently acquired HIV infection, a high viral load, lower CD4 counts, and breast abnormalities or breast infections. Infant characteristics that promote transmission are oral lesions or sores such as candidiasis [54]. Breast milk contaminated with HIV is responsible for transmitting the virus to 200,000 (40%) of the 500,000 new infections occurring in children each year. Observational cohort studies in Africa indicate that postnatal transmission of HIV through breast feeding increases the risk of infection by a factor of 7.5 [55]. *Exclusive* breast feeding for the first 4 to 6 months will reduce the risk of transmission. A single dose of peripartum prophylaxis with antiretroviral agents reduces intrapartum transmission, but the effect does not extend beyond 4 to 6 weeks. The large RCT study by Kumwenda and colleagues provided evidence that extended antiretroviral prophylaxis reduces breast milk transmission. These investigators screened 46,186 pregnant women for HIV in Malawi and enrolled 3016 infants in the 3-armed study [56]. All infants in the control group (788) received only a single dose of nevirapine plus 1 week zidovudine given twice daily. Infants in another group (800) received what the control group received plus daily prophylaxis with nevirapine for 14 weeks. Infants in the third group (801) received what the control group received, plus daily nevirapine and zidovudine for 14 weeks. The frequency and duration of breast feeding did not differ between the 3 groups. Nearly 90% were breastfeeding at 6 months but only 27% to 32% were still nursing at 9 months. The control group had consistently higher conversion rates from 6 weeks through 18 months than the infants in either the second or third group, with no statistical difference between the latter 2 groups. At 9 months, conversion rates were 10.6%, 5.2%, and 6.4%, respectively. Regardless of HIV infection, 9.5% or 285 of the 3016 infants in the study died. At 9 months, mortality in the control group was 8.9% and 6.8% in group 2 and 6.3% in group 3 (no statistical difference). The primary causes of death were gastroenteritis and pneumonia. Survival in the HIV-negative infants was significantly better in both extended prophylaxis groups at 9 months and in the extended nevirapine group at 15 months [57]. (For reference: in 2006, the infant mortality rate in Malawi was 76/1000 or 7.6%.)

THE WHO CONSENSUS STATEMENT ON HIV AND INFANT FEEDING (NEW FINDINGS)

"The most appropriate infant feeding option for an HIV-infected mother should continue to depend on her individual circumstances, including her health status and the local situation, but should take greater consideration in the health services available and the counseling and support she is likely to receive. *Exclusive* breastfeeding is recommended for HIV-infected women for the first 6 months of life unless replacement feeding is acceptable, feasible, affordable, sustainable and safe for them and their infants before that time. When replacement feeding is acceptable, feasible, affordable, sustainable and safe, avoidance of all breastfeeding by HIV-infected women is recommended. At 6 months, if replacement feeding is still not acceptable, feasible, affordable, sustainable and safe, continuation of breastfeeding with additional complementary foods is recommended, while the mother and baby continue to be regularly assessed. All breastfeeding should stop once a nutritionally adequate and safe diet without breast milk can be provided" [58].

The new findings that prompted the statement included: *exclusive* breastfeeding (BF) for up to 6 months is associated with a 3- to 4-fold decrease in the risk of HIV transmission compared with nonexclusive BF; where free infant formula was provided the combined risk of HIV transmission and death was similar whether infants were formula fed or breast fed from birth; early cessation of breast feeding was associated with reduced HIV transmission but with an increase risk of morbidity and child mortality.

In places where water contamination was inevitable, if formula was supplied and hygienic preparation was insured, would it make a difference [59]? Based on the following observations, the answer is no. Promotion of *exclusive* BF in HIV-endemic countries would prevent 13% of current deaths whereas use of nevirapine and formula feeding would prevent only 2% of current childhood deaths. In a comprehensive "formula plus" program in Haiti, including weekly visits for formula milk and education of proper preparation and growth monitoring, HIV transmission was greatly reduced but infant mortality was very high (217/1000 live births). In 1999, a program in Botswana provided free formula to HIV-infected mothers. In the first quarter of 2006, an area in that country experienced a diarrhea epidemic, and reported 35,000 cases of diarrhea and 532 deaths compared with 100 cases and 21 deaths during the same period a year earlier. Powdered formulas are not sterile products and may contain pathogenic bacteria. Health care professionals need to go beyond the "molecular-level" of disease and address larger issues such as "social, economic, and political determinants of health and sickness." This issue will be addressed more extensively later, but note that lack of clean water kills 5 times more children than HIV/AIDS, and hampers economic growth. Of the 6 billion people in the world, 1.1 billion lack proper access to clean water and 2.6 billion lack access to sanitation. Sub-Saharan Africa loses 5% of its Gross Domestic Product (GDP) every year due to a lack of proper access to clean water and sanitation. That is more money than it obtains from aid.

The "water crisis" is "deeply rooted in poverty, inequality, and unequal power relationships."

THREE ROOT CAUSES OF CHILD MORBIDITY AND MORTALITY

Health professionals working in the international child health arena need to look beyond the long lines of patients that gather at the health facilities. The numbers defy the resources. The diseases they present are but the consequences of fundamental underlying problems. The diseases are merely symptoms of more basic issues. Until the root causes are ameliorated, the lines will not go away. As populations increase, so will the hordes of patients. The lines will grow longer and longer. The needs will continue to increase and even further outstrip the limited resources.

There are at least 3 basic "wrongs" or disparities that are responsible for the still unacceptably high rate of infant and childhood mortality and of maternal mortality, as well as the enormous levels of morbidity seen in many parts of the developing world. In the leading author's (B.D.) view, the big 3 priorities are: (1) the elimination of severe poverty, (2) improving the levels of education particularly for females, and (3) the provision of accessible potable water and adequate sanitation.

Raising the level of income gives families the ability to purchase nutritious food and to send their children to school. Thus, improving economic levels will increase the likelihood that the children will receive higher education, resulting in a spiral of better jobs and improved income. An informed, educated mother will see that her child gets immunized and is taken to the health facility early in the course of an illness. The treatment of diarrhea is ORS, but the solution is clean water.

1. Elimination of severe poverty (MDG #1, #4, and #8)

Growth and development are more dependent on socioeconomic status than genetics

In April 2006, the WHO published a set of new growth charts for children from birth to 5 years of age [60]. The charts were based on a prospective international sample of infants and children selected to represent optimal growth from 6 diverse countries; Brazil, Ghana, India, Norway, Oman, and the United States. Prospective longitudinal data were collected from a favorable socioeconomic population of more than 8000 single, term infants without any significant morbidity, who had been exclusively breastfed for at least 4 months and had been born to mothers who did not smoke before or after delivery. This study found that the growth of children is less influenced by genetics or divergent populations than it is from the environment and feeding practices. Although individual children grow differently, the growth pattern of the children in these 6 countries was very similar. The charts also documented times when key motor milestones should be met.

Most of the world has been using the National Center for Health Statistics charts published over 30 years ago as a growth reference [4]. Those curves were based on a limited sample of children living in the United States, most of whom had been fed formula rather than breast milk.

The new WHO growth charts were compared with the ones developed by the Centers for Disease Control and Prevention (CDC) in 2000, based on United States children; a revised version of the 1977 NCHS charts [61]. The WHO charts show a mean weight for age above that in the CDC charts during the first 6 months, crossing it at 6 months, and remaining below it until 32 months. The CDC charts revealed a heavier and shorter sample, resulting in the body mass index (BMI)-for-age curves (BMI calculated as the weight in kilograms divided by height in meters squared) on the WHO charts depicting a higher rate of over-weight and obesity than seen on the CDC charts [62,63]. Likewise, the WHO curves result in lower estimates of undernutrition (Fig. 10).

The new WHO growth curves represent *how all children should grow* rather than *how children did grow in a specific time and place*.

Poverty and child health

UNICEF estimates that poverty is responsible for the deaths of 25,000 to 30,000 children younger than 5 years who die *each day*. Many of these children are dying in small villages far away from adequate medical care. These deaths are invisible to the industrialized nations. Of the 1.9 billion children living in the developing world, 1 in 3 is without adequate shelter, 1 in 5 has no access

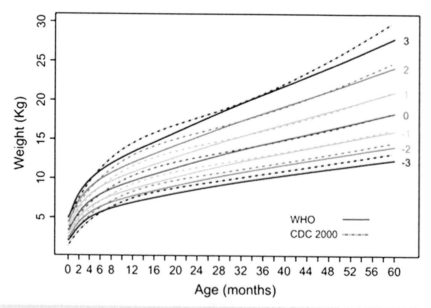

Fig. 10. Comparison of the WHO and CDC weight-for-age Z-score curves for boys. (*From* de Onis M, Garza C, Onyango, et al. Comparison of the WHO child growth standards and the CDC 2000 growth charts. J Nutr 2007;137:144–8; with permission.)

to safe water, 1 in 7 has no access to health services, and 2.2 million children die each year from illnesses that could have been prevented, but were not. These 2.2 million children would be alive if only they had received the recommended immunizations and had been afforded adequate health care. A civilized world cannot/should not accept this appalling situation.

In 2005, 12% of the world's citizens were living on US$1 per day and almost half of all the children on this planet were living below the poverty line. Twenty percent were living on less than $2 per day and over 3 billion were trying to survive on less than $2.50 per day. Eighty percent or 5.1 billion of the 6 billion of all the earth's inhabitants earned less than $10 per day [64].

SOCIAL RISK FACTORS AND CHILD SURVIVAL IN THE UNITED STATES

There is much to do both at home and abroad. Larson and colleagues examined the effects of 8 social risk factors on a child's general health in the United States (ie, dental health, socio-emotional health, and overweight) [65]. Their study emphasized some of the disparities in the United States and the need to address multiple levels of social problems if the health of children here in the United States is to be improved.

These investigators used data from the 2003 National Survey of Children's Health, a telephone survey of 102,353 parents of children between birth and 17 years of age. The 8 risk factors included no education beyond high school of any household member, uninsured children, a family income less than 200% of the federal poverty level, not a 2-parent household, race/ethnicity, family conflicts, low maternal mental health, and living in an unsafe neighborhood. More than half of the children had 2 or more risk factors and one-quarter had 4 or more risk factors. Low maternal mental health, black or Hispanic race/ethnicity, less than 200% below the federal poverty line, low household education, living in an unsafe neighborhood, and lack of health insurance increased the odds for poor health.

What interventions work?

There is a strong association between undernutrition and mortality. In addition, micronutrient deficiencies account for 10% of childhood deaths. Ninety percent of these children live in sub-Saharan Africa and South-Central Asia. It is estimated that worldwide, there are 178 million children who are stunted (height-for-age Z score more than 2 SD below the mean), 55 million who are wasted (weight for height Z score less than 2 SD below the mean), and 19 million who have severe wasting or severe acute malnutrition (weight for height Z score less than 3 SD below the mean). Bhutta and colleagues conducted an extensive review of 209 articles spanning the past 25 years, with the vast majority of the studies published after 2000. These investigators sought to determine whether food supplementation interventions actually improve maternal and childhood nutrition and survival [66]. Food supplementation can reduce the prevalence of stunting by one-third; reduce mortality from birth to 36 months by one-fourth; reduce disability-adjusted life-years (DALYs) associated with stunting, severe wasting, intrauterine growth restriction, and child mortality associated with micronutrient by one-fourth; and with universal supplementation of calcium, iron, and folic acid during pregnancy can prevent almost one-fourth of all maternal deaths. The long-term effects of stunting on cognition and earning potential are other important considerations.

Because it is difficult to affect stunting after 36 months of age, interventions must be directed at pregnant women and at children from birth to 24 months. Supplemental feeding programs that focus on older children will not affect linear growth. Moreover, rapid weight gain from supplemental programs directed at older children may result in an increase in BMI with probable adverse long-term effects. Food supplementation programs like the one in Guatemala have shown beneficial long-term economic benefits [29,30].

Evidence-based intervention programs show beneficial outcomes. What is needed is the technical expertise to determine "which interventions should be given the highest priorities and ensure their effective implementation" and "the political will to combat undernutrition in the very countries that need it most" [66].

Two solutions to combat poverty and improve health

Conditional cash transfer programs: a "magic bullet for health"
Conditional cash transfer (CCT) programs began in Mexico 10 years ago (1998) when Fernald and colleagues randomly assigned 506 low-income communities for either immediate enrollment (320 communities with 6311 households) or after a wait of 18 months, enrollment of 186 communities with 4029 households [67]. The families would receive a monthly fixed stipend, but the money transfer would occur only on the condition that the family would obtain preventive medical care and agree to use the funds to purchase more nutritious foods. A second type of transfer was through educational scholarships that were received by the family, but only if their children attended school a minimum of 85% of the time and did not repeat a grade more than twice. Only 1% of the families were denied cash transfers because of noncompliance. Nine years later,; the total cost of the program was $3.7 billion and had reached more than 5 million families, for an average expenditure of $740 per family. The outcome of 2449 children aged between 24 and 38 months who had been enrolled in the program since birth was assessed. The results were encouraging: 70% of the cash transfer was spent on purchase of "better quality calories," there was a lower prevalence of stunting and a lower prevalence of overweight, as determined by a decrease in BMI for age; language development; and an improvement in mental development in short-term or working memory, which is most sensitive to differences in socioeconomic status and is a measure of executive function.

A literature search by Lagarde and colleagues uncovered 28 articles on CCT, of which only 6 met their criteria for study design. There were 5 programs in

Latin America (Mexico, Honduras, Columbia, Nicaragua, and Brazil) and 1 in Africa (Malawi) [68]. In general, CCT programs resulted in an increased use of health services, improved nutritional and anthropometric outcomes, and preventive behaviors. The nutritional improvement was greatest in the younger children. Immunization rates varied. The "overall effect on health status was less clear." The results were somewhat dependent on the size of the monetary transfers but, most importantly, on the availability and ease of access to primary health care services.

In 2007, New York City launched its own CCT pilot program, the first to be established in the United States. A third component (workforce-participation) was added to the 2 traditional components of health and education.

Microenterprise or Microcredit
Muhammad Yunus received the 2006 Nobel Peace Prize for his innovation of microcredit for the poorest of the poor. Realizing that the poor have no collateral and hence no way to secure loans from commercial banks, he established a different kind of bank: the Grameen Bank. The Bank offered small loans of 30 to 40 US dollars to individuals using the only collateral they had; their word that they would repay the loan. The Bank felt women would use the funds more wisely than men and were more responsible, as their lives and the lives of their children were in the balance. These loans enabled families to start small businesses. A global movement of microcredit was launched. Thousands of institutions have now adopted this strategy, and it is present in 43 different countries. More than 100 million poor people have taken advantage of microloans and many are escaping poverty. The loans are paid back at a rate of greater than 98%. Dr Yunus is extending the program from starting businesses to helping people pay for education and housing. His goal over the next 10 years is to extend the loans to half a billion people who are living in poverty [69,70].

MDG #8: A global partnership for development
Data 2007 is the second annual report on the progress of commitments made by the Group of Eight (G8) in Gleneagles in 2005; "the year of Africa" and the Global Call to Action Against Poverty [71]. The G8 is composed of the 8 richest industrialized countries: France, Germany, Italy, Japan, the United Kingdom, the United States, Canada, and Russia. Some important gains have been achieved. Debt cancellation for some African nations and targeted aid has helped 20 million African children enter school. In 2002, only 50,000 or 1% of Africans in need of antiretroviral treatment had access to it but by 2006, the number had increased to 1.34 million, yet was reaching only 26% of those in need of treatment. More effective aid has improved economic growth and decreased poverty; for example, in Mozambique, from 2002 to 2004 aid increased from $49 to $63 per capita and the country's annual GDP growth rate increased from 2% to 8%, while the under-5 mortality rate dropped from 178 to 152 per 1000 live births. The Lubombo region of South Africa has used this aid to buy insecticide-treated bed nets, resulting

in a 90% reduction of malaria prevalence with a potential of further decreasing the 3000 daily malaria-related deaths in Africa.

Individual G8 nations are keeping their promise in specific areas: Japan and the United Kingdom have increased aid; the United Kingdom and Canada have invested in education; The United States has made good on its promises for aid in the fight against HIV/AIDS and malaria; Germany, France, and Italy have invested in water and sanitation. However, all is not positive. Total G8 assistance increased only $2.3 billion, less than half of the $5.4 billion promised; the United Kingdom and Japan have kept to their deal but the United States, Canada, Germany, and France have not, and Italy has actually cut its aid. Only small increases in aid were scheduled for 2007 and 2008. A lack of global agreement on trade and failure to focus on Africa will prevent even well-governed African countries from succeeding in their efforts to reduce poverty. The way the G8 decided to account for debt relief masks the real picture of development assistance. Piecemeal progress on specific issues will not lead to the overall results promised by the G8 countries.

2. Improving the levels of education and the numbers of educated females (partially addressed earlier under female education, MDG #2, #3, and #5)

Economic discrepancies related to maternal and child health

Health outcomes are directly related to household income, as are educational levels, particularly of women. Houweling and colleagues examined the inequalities among 4 economic groups (the urban rich, the urban poor, the rural rich, and the rural poor) living in 45 developing countries [72]. Assignment to these 4 wealth-related groups was done by using household ownership of durable goods, housing quality, and water and sanitation facilities. Five indicators were used to estimate the level of health care; professional delivery attendance, professional antenatal care, fully immunized children, and childhood treatment of diarrhea and of acute respiratory infections. No discrepancies were seen in respect to these child care indicators. However, wealth and maternity care are linked; the less wealth, the less care with the poor-rich inequalities, looming larger in respect of deliveries by professional trained care providers than provision of antenatal care. Professional delivery attendance is higher in urban than in rural areas, but in most countries the urban poor and the rural rich have very similar levels. The percentage of poor mothers who receive antenatal care is high, but the percentage being delivered by professional trained providers is very low. Relative inequalities tend to be larger in the countries where there are lower overall levels of health care use. Cultural differences may partially explain some of the discrepancies: poor women may favor traditional birth attendants or family members to assist in the deliveries and may favor home deliveries; women in richer families are often better educated and have a more "modern view;" and some families may be less willing to spend money on women's health (perhaps particularly true in South East Asia). Availability of resources are implicated in explaining the difference in health outcome for maternal and child health services: there are serious insufficiencies of well-trained personnel who are trained to recognize danger signs in the pregnant woman; there is a lack of 24-hour easy accessible delivery service facilities equipped with the supplies and personnel to handle emergencies; there is a serious lack of available timely transportation for the woman in labor who is experiencing problems; and then there is the expense, as adequate and appropriate physical infrastructure is more costly for deliveries than for the child care indicators. A few countries have addressed these barriers. Indonesia has concentrated on improving the availability of a narrow range of maternity care services whereas Honduras, Cuba, Sir Lanka, and the Kerala State in India have improved a broader range of health services that include maternity services.

This study provides important insights into why there has been so little progress in decreasing the unacceptably high maternal mortality rates in many counties and with the different populations within countries. We are far from reaching the MDG #5 of reducing maternal mortality by 75% by 2015, with just 7 years left. Pediatricians are very much aware of this issue, as a maternal death is a death toll for her infant. Mortality within the first 28 days of life accounts for 27% of all childhood deaths. Reducing maternal deaths will in turn help reduce childhood mortality.

Maternal mortality and safe motherhood strategies (MDG #5)

Compared with the gains made in infant and under-5 mortality over the past 25 years, there has been little change in maternal mortality. Saving the mother's life not only averts the death of her newborn infant, it also prevents emotional trauma to her other children and the likelihood of their ill health and starvation. Each year, half a million women die a maternal death; a death during pregnancy, at the time of labor, or during the 42 days following delivery. Ninety-nine percent of these deaths occur in the developing world. The lifetime risk of a woman dying a maternal death in industrialized countries is 1 in 8000, but for a woman living in sub-Saharan Africa the risk is 1 in 22 [11]. Hemorrhage is responsible for approximately 25% of the deaths, infections and eclampsia each another 13%, and obstructed labor 8%. All of these complications demand early recognition and prompt referral to a facility equipped to deal with the emergency.

Safe motherhood practices have been instituted in only a relative few areas. One such area is Nepal. Freedman and colleagues stress the importance of strengthening the capacity of the district health system to implement integrated "functioning services that are accessible to and used by all segments of the population" [73]. Isolated changes are not enough. The focus must be a broad-based multisectorial change. Establishing such a system will also have a positive effect on other emergency and referral services. Practical lessons can be learned from the 4 major global safe motherhood initiatives of the past decade. Three key elements are crucial: family planning, skilled care for all deliveries, and access to emergency obstetric care for women who are identified as having life-threatening complications. What to do is known, but how to do it will vary with the local situation. Geographic distribution, skilled personnel, the high cost of keeping adequate obstetric facilities open 24 hours a day, and transportation all present challenging problems. The ultimate goal is for every birth to be attended by a skilled health professional, one who can recognize risks and complications and initiate an appropriate referral to a center where the women can receive appropriate obstetric care. A needs assessment is fundamental to identify how to proceed in implementing the most important positive changes. Such an assessment allows the building blocks of the health care system to be put in place.

Maternal mortality rates over a 30-year period in 2 adjacent areas in Bangladesh with different levels of care have been compared [74]. In 2002, the population in these areas was 220,000 and the 2 areas were similar in socioeconomic criteria. One area was served by the International Center for Diarrhoeal Disease Research (ICDDR). There, maternal and child health services were introduced in the late 1970s and a safe motherhood program was piloted in 1987. The health centers were staffed by trained midwives and transportation was provided to a referral hospital when necessary. The other area received routine government services.

Over the 30-year period, maternal mortality fell substantially. In the ICDDR area the decrease was 68%, from 412 to 131 per 100,000 live births. In the Government service area the decrease was 54%, from 451 to 206. From 1990 onward the decline was 7% and 4% per year, respectively. Introduction of the safe motherhood program did not produce a statistically significant difference. Nor was there a statistically significant difference with the shift from home births to facility-based births or the availability of antibiotics. The proportion of pregnant women with formal education increased 50%. Mortality was 3 times lower in women who had 8 or more years of education compared with women with no formal education, and abortion mortality was 11 times lower in the highly educated women. The number of pregnant women who lived in the lowest asset quintile decreased from one-third to less than 1%. The gap in mortality between the rich and the poor and between the educated and uneducated was striking.

Investment in trained birth attendants and the availability of emergency services are important in reaching the MDG #5, but female education and decrease in poverty are essential to sustain any of the success that was achieved in Bangladesh.

3. The provision of accessible potable water and adequate sanitation (MDG #7)

From 1990 to 2004, there has been considerable improvement in the provision of safe drinking water to developing world countries, from 71% to 80%, with a goal of 86% by 2015. The greatest strides were seen in South Asia (71% to 85%, with a goal of 86%), less in the East Asia/Pacific area (72% to 79%, with a goal of 86%), but far too little progress in sub-Saharan Africa (48% to 55%, with a goal of 74%) (Fig. 11).

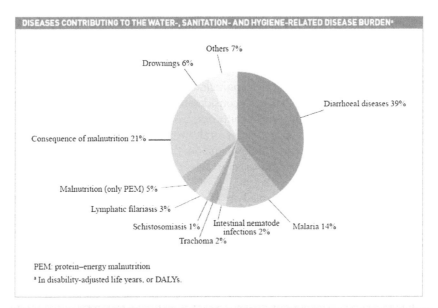

Fig. 11. Diseases related to water and sanitation. (*From* Pruss-Ostun A, Bos R, Gore F, et al. Safe water, better health. Costs, benefits, and sustainability of interventions to protect and promote health. Geneva: World Health Organization; 2008; with permission.)

MDG #7 calls for decreasing the number of people without sustainable access to safe water by 50% from what it was in 2000. This MDG seeks to combat the impact of contaminated water on diarrheal disease that kills 2 million children every year. A critical review of 118 articles that assessed what works in fighting diarrheal diseases in developing countries noted that piped water and sanitation are vital in the fight to reduce childhood mortality, but 30% of those who live in the rural areas of the developing world lack a safe and accessible water supply [75]. Unfortunately, in poor rural areas piping water to every scattered household is expensive and currently not practical. Hence, the focus has been on providing community-level water infrastructure.

Several strategies work in preventing and treating diarrheal diseases: exclusive breast feeding works; the 2 new Rotavirus vaccines work; ORT works; micronutrient supplementation with zinc and vitamin A works; point-of-use water treatment systems work (chemical disinfection of water in the home with household bleach or use of flocculants, adsorption, filtration, boiling, or solar disinfection), reducing diarrheal disease by 20% to 30%; and increased hand washing works. A Cochrane review of 14 RCTs from different counties, across socioeconomic levels, and in both community and institutional settings evaluated the effectiveness of hand washing on the incidence of diarrhea. The target was children and if supplies were availed, the outcome was good. Pooled analysis revealed that the incidence of diarrhea decreased 32% in the community setting and 39% in the institutional setting [76]. Education by itself was the least cost-effective measure, particularly when maternal literacy was low.

2008 is the international year of sanitation

From 1990 to 2004, there has been considerable improvement in the provision of sanitation to developing world countries, from 35% to 50%, but well below the goal of 68% by 2015. The greatest strides were seen in the East Asia/Pacific area (30% to 51%, with a goal of 65%) and South Asia (17% to 37%, with a goal of 59%), but little progress is apparent in sub-Saharan Africa (22% to 27%, with a goal of 66%).

A longitudinal study determined the effect on diarrheal morbidity in children younger than 3 years following an intervention that improved sewage coverage from 26% to 80% in households in Salvador, Brazil. The intervention had a significant effect, with diarrhea days per child-year decreasing by 22% [77].

Data on the economic status, level of childhood underweight, availability of clean water, and type of sanitation and indoor air pollution from household fuels from 52 countries in Latin America, the Caribbean, South Asia, and sub-Saharan Africa was used to estimate what reduction would occur in child mortality if child nutrition was improved and if clean water, sanitation, and clean fuels were provided [78]. The effects of the interventions were related to the economic status of those receiving the interventions. If these strategies reached all the children who needed them, the predicted result would reduce child deaths each year by 49,700 (14%) in Latin America and the Caribbean, by 0.8 million (24%) in South Asia, and by 1.47 million (31%) in sub-Saharan Africa. As expected, the poor were at greatest risk for all the factors assessed. If the strategies targeted the poor first, the reductions would be 30% to 75% larger than if the same 50% coverage reached the wealthier households before the poor households. Targeting the poor first would have the greatest impact and would help close the disparity in child mortality between the poor and the wealthy.

Large-scale investments in water and sanitation infrastructure can have a strong positive impact on child mortality. In the United States, filtration and chlorination technology was responsible for one-half of the decline in child mortality. An increase of 10% of the homes with improved water and sanitation on Native American Reservations in the United States resulted in a 4% decrease of child mortality. Community water sources often do not have a significant health impact, particularly if the source is surface water, as it is often contaminated with pathogens and, unfortunately, wells often fall into disrepair due to poor maintenance. Nearly half of the borehole wells in Kenya are in disrepair. One-quarter of India's water infrastructure is in need of repair. More than one-third of the rural water infrastructure in South Asia is not functional. There is a high degree of recontamination of water in transport or in storage. Sanitation and hygiene is as important or more important than water quality.

The ultimate goal is piped water to all households, but until then emphasis should be on: (1) concentrating efforts on point-of-use water treatment programs; (2) encouraging village councils headed by women as they are more likely to invest in public infrastructure for drinking water; (3) giving communities direct control or ownership over key decisions.

Access to safe water and basic sanitation would result in 200 million fewer episodes of diarrhea each year and prevent 2.1 million deaths each year. Improving water supply, sanitation, hygiene. and management of water resources could reduce the global disease burden by 10% [79].

The rapid growth of slums has slowed reaching the MDG #7 target

The quality of available water and the adequacy of sanitary facilities are even worse in the sprawling slums of the major cities in the developing world. A cross-sectional study assessed the effect of overcrowding and resultant proximity of water supply and pit latrines in an urban slum in Eldoret, Kenya [80]. Forty percent of the pit latrines were less than the recommended 15 m from the water source, and 30% of children did not use latrines but defecated in the field. Most people (91%) used wells for their water supply, but the wells were highly contaminated with fecal matter. Shallow wells were used by 89% of the population and *Escherichia coli* was found in all samples taken from these shallow wells. The shallow wells lacked concrete slabs, often the opening was not covered at all, and none met the WHO requirements for drinking water. Deep wells had a pipe system but were used by only 2% of the population, and 3 of 4 samples taken from these deep wells were contaminated with coliform organisms. Only 42% of those using well water boiled the water used for drinking.

In Kenya, the number of people living in slums nearly doubled in the 18 years from 1980 to 1998. Slums are home to 70% of all urban residents in sub-Saharan Africa. Many governments either do not accept any responsibility for the health of squatting slum dwellers or do not have sufficient funds to provide clean water, drainage, sewerage, and rubbish removal. The percentage of people living in the urban slums who lack these vital services is already high, and the numbers are growing. The prevalence of diarrhea among slum dwellers was double what it was for the city and for the national average. Moreover, the under-5 mortality in slum residents in Nairobi is 35% higher than in the city or among rural populations.

There are many factors that lure rural farmers from the land to the city. The size of family plots has decreased due to governmental acquisition and to division among the children. "Fair trade" practices of foreign governments and the subsidies given to in-country farmers make it difficult for the local farmers to compete in the market place. It is increasingly difficult for farmers to make a living in the rural areas. All of this plus the lure of the city and the dream of getting rich has driven many to urban areas. Municipal governments have not prepared for this influx. The sprawl begins, but the usual vital utilities are not there. Poverty and disease infuse the area and crime rises. The problem is huge and growing. In Ethiopia and Chad, 99.4% of the urban populations live in slums. The next highest percentage of slum dwellers is in Afghanistan (98.5%) and Nepal (92%). Ten to 12 million people live in the slums of Mumbai, and 9 to10 million live in the slums of Mexico City [81].

GLOBAL CLIMATE CHANGE AND CHILDREN'S HEALTH

The American Academy of Pediatrics (AAP) statement on climate change emphasizes the fact that children are a particularly vulnerable group that "is likely to suffer disproportionately from both direct and indirect adverse health effects of climate change." The AAP cites several adverse examples that the anticipated climate change will cause: reduction in the availability of food resulting in an increase in malnutrition; water availability will become less in some regions, potentiating dehydration in children; flooding will occur in other areas; and people living in coastal areas will be displaced. Greater adverse effects will be seen on the less mobile and more dependent citizens, the children. The AAP makes a series of recommendations to pediatricians and to governments to mitigate the effects of climate change [82].

A UNICEF report focused on what affect climate change may have on the MDGs, and concluded that climate change will likely reduce any likelihood that several of the 8 goals will be met [83]. As the world warms and rains fail, crops will wither and livestock will die. A lack of food will result in an increase in malnutrition and childhood mortality. Malnutrition will also have an adverse affect on pregnant women, and their fetuses will suffer. The WHO estimates that in 2000, climate change was responsible for 2.4% of worldwide episodes of diarrhea and 6% of malaria in some middle-income countries. As the world warms, water shortages will increase; by 2020 an estimated 75 million people in Africa alone will experience water stress. Weather-related events like hurricanes and flooding will intensify, coastal areas will be inundated, and millions will be displaced. Children are more affected, and more will die of starvation while many will become orphans. In the first half of the 20th century, 12 natural disasters occurred annually. In 2004, the number was 350.

There is already some response to this impending problem. In Niger, community gardens are encouraged and are nourishing hope. Conservation through tree planting is increasing; the Ethiopian Government has set a goal of planting 20 million trees and the United Nations Environment Program launched the "Plant for the Planet: Billion Tree Campaign" with the goal of planting 1 billion trees by 2007. Community-based advocacy programs are involving youth in planning and decision making. The United Nations Environment Program and UNICEF are developing an Environmental Education Resource Pack for Child-Friendly Schools offering comprehensive solutions to empower children.

INTERNATIONAL HEALTH TRAINING IN PEDIATRIC RESIDENCY PROGRAMS

Ten years ago, the AAP's Section on International Child Health surveyed pediatric residency programs in the United States to document the interest in international electives [84]. Nelson and colleagues recently conducted a similar survey of 201 accredited pediatric residency programs in the United States, Puerto Rico, and the Caribbean. More than half of the responding programs offer a "global health" elective as compared with just 25% from the survey done 10 years earlier [85]. Half of these programs had a global health curriculum including didactic lectures and case reports. Six percent had a formal global health track, and another 7% said they were intending to initiate one within the next 2 years. Only 36% of the programs provided prerequisite clinical training or cultural orientation as recommended by the AAP, but the majority offered pretravel briefing, faculty mentorship, and debriefing sessions. A quarter of the programs reported that "at least half" of their residents had had an international health experience before beginning residency training. The majority of the residents take the elective during their third year, and the programs reported a mean total of 3 participating residents from their program. The programs listed several potential barriers to establishing a global health elective, including call-free time and funding. (The Residency Travel Grants of $500 offered by the AAP's Section on International Child Health were established to assist with the expense.)

The growing interest in international health should encourage programs to incorporate the opportunity for a global health elective for their residents. Barriers are there but are not insurmountable. A short-term international experience has the potential to improve the lives of children and give a broader

What Would You Like to be When You Grow Up?

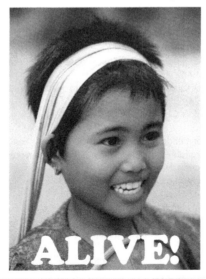

Fig. 12. Yes, you can help. (Copyright UNICEF; reproduced with permission.)

perspective and understanding of the way the majority of the world lives. A word of caution: such a venture has the potential of altering the way a physician views the world and just might influence life-changing decisions.

It is inappropriate for pediatricians from the "developed" world to even try to make or even suggest policy changes without involving the local pediatricians, and they will invariably fail if they try to do so. However, the "guests" are in a unique position to assist their colleagues who live this reality every day, pushing their governments to put children higher on the priority scale and fulfill the contracts they agreed to when they signed the World Declaration on the Survival, Protection and Development of Children, the Plans of Action, and the Convention of the Rights of the Child. Only by realigning governmental priorities will the MDGs stand a chance of being met.

SUMMARY
Perhaps this article can be best summed up by the UNICEF poster (Fig. 12).

References
[1] Declaration of Alma Ata of 1978. Available at: http://www.righttohealthcare.org/Docs/DocumentsC.htm. Accessed October 2008.
[2] Asuzu MC. A comparative study of the commonly used nutritional assessment tools for primary health care. East Afr Med J 1991;68(11):913–22.
[3] Schoeman SE, Hendricks MK, Hattingh SP, et al. The targeting of nutritionally at-risk children attending a primary health care facility in the Western Cape Province of South Africa. Public Health Nutr 2006;9(8):1007–12.
[4] Owen GM. The new National Center for Health Statistics growth charts. South Med J 1978;71(3):296–7.
[5] Kosek M, Bern C, Guerrant RL. The global burden of diarrhoeal disease, as estimated from studies published between 1992 and 2000. Bull World Health Organ 2003;81:197–204.
[6] Parashar UD, Bresee JS, Glass RI. The global burden of diarrhoeal disease in children. Bull World Health Organ 2003;81:236.
[7] Murray CJL, Lopez AD. The Global Burden of Disease. Boston: Harvard University Press; 1996.
[8] Murray CJL, Lopez AD. Global and regional cause of death patterns in 1990. Bull World Health Org 1994;72:447–80.
[9] Murray CJL, Lopez AD. Quantifying disability: data, methods, and results. Bull World Health Org 1994;72:481–94.
[10] The State of the World's Children 1990. Oxford, New York: UNICEF Oxford University Press; 1990. page 23.
[11] UNICEF. Progress for children—a world fit for children: statistical review. Number 6, December. 2007. Available at: http://www.unicef.org/progressforchildren/2007n6/index_41401.htm. Accessed October 2008.
[12] International Code of Marketing of Breast Milk Substitutes. Available at: http://www.ibfan.org/english/resource/who/fullcode.html (reviewed 11/08).
[13] Baby-friendly Hospital Initiative. Available at: http://www.who.int/nutrition/topics/bfhi/en/index.html (reviewed 11/08).
[14] World Health Organization/UNICEF document. published in 1989 by WHO, Geneva, Switzerland.
[15] Kleinman RE, Walker WA. The Enteromammary immune system: an important new concept in breast milk host defense. Dig Dis Sci 1979;24(11):876–82.

[16] Expanded Programme on Immunizations Programme report for the year 1992. Incorporating the recommendations of the global advisory group, October 1992. World Health Organization. January 1993. Available at: http://whqlibdoc.who.int/hq/1993/WHO_EPI_GEN_93.1.pdf.

[17] WHO vaccine preventable disease monitoring system. Available at: www.who.int/vaccines-documents/globalsummary/globalsummary.pdf (reviewed 11/08).

[18] WHO vaccine-preventable diseases: monitoring system—2007 global summary. Expanded Programme on Immunization of the Dept. of Immunization, Vaccines, and Biologicals.

[19] Supplementary Immunization Activities (SIAs) operations and quality. Available at: http://www.comminit.com/en/node/223738/292 (reviewed 11/08).

[20] Coghlan A. Measles deaths tumble by 60% worldwide. New Scientist.com news service. 12:21.January 19, 2007 (quoting Dr. Margaret Chan, WHO Director-General).

[21] The state of the world's children 2004. Oxford, New York: (Focus on girl's education) UNICEF Oxford University Press; 2004.

[22] The state of the world's children 1995. UNICEF. Oxford, New York: Oxford University Press; 1995.

[23] Peterson SA. Marriage structure and contraception in Niger. J Biosoc Sci 1999;31: 93–104.

[24] The state of the world's children 1994. Oxford, New York: UNICEF Oxford University Press; 1994.

[25] Martorell R, Habicht J-P, Rivera JA. History and design of the INCAP longitudinal study (1969–77) and its follow-up (1988–89). J Nutr 1995a;125:1027S–41S.

[26] Habicht JP, Martorell R. Objectives, research design and implementation of the INCAP longitudinal study. Food Nutr Bull 1993;14:176–90.

[27] Rivera J, Martorell R, Castro H. Data collection of the INCAP follow-up study: Organization, coverage, sample sizes. Food Nutr Bull 1993;14:258–69.

[28] Ruel MT, Rivera J, Habicht JP, et al. Differential response to early nutrition supplementation: long-term effects on height at adolescence. Int J Epidemiol 1995;24(2):404–12.

[29] Hoddinott J, Maluccio JA, Behrman JR, et al. Effect of a nutrition intervention during early childhood on economic productivity in Guatemalan adults. Lancet 2008;371: 411–6.

[30] Grosse S, Roy K. Long-term economic effect of early childhood nutrition [Editorial]. Lancet 2008;371:365–6.

[31] Mannar MGV. Iodized salt for the elimination of iodine deficiency. Available at: http://206.191.51.240/documents/Iodized%20Salt%20for%20the%20Elimination%20of%20IDD.pdf (reviewed 11/08).

[32] Sommer A. Xerophthalmia, keratomalacia and nutritional blindness. Int Ophthalmol 1990;14(3):195–9.

[33] Fawzi WW, Chalmers TC, Herrera MG, et al. Vitamin A supplementation and mortality. A meta-analysis. JAMA 1993;269(7):898–903.

[34] Sankaranarayanan S, Suárez M, Taren D, et al. The concentration of free holo-retinol binding protein is higher in vitamin A-sufficient than in deficient Nepalese women in late pregnancy. J Nutr 2005;135(12):2817–22.

[35] Trowbridge F, Martorell R. Forging: effective strategies to combat iron deficiency. Summary and recommendations. J Nutr 2002;132:875S–9S.

[36] World Health Organization. The prevalence of anemia in women: a tabulation of available information. Geneva: WHO; 1992.

[37] Baig-Ansari N, Badruddin SH, Karmaliani R, et al. Anemia prevalence and risk factors in pregnant women in an urban area of Pakistan. Food Nutr Bull 2008;29(2):132–9.

[38] Lazzerini M. Effect of zinc supplement on child mortality (editorial). Lancet 2007;370: 1194–5.

[39] Tielsch JM, Khatry SK, Katz J, et al. Effect of daily zinc supplementation on child mortality in southern Nepal: a community-based, cluster randomized, placebo-controlled trial. Lancet 2007;370:1230–9.

[40] Bhutta ZA, Black RE, Brown KH, et al. Prevention of diarrhea and pneumonia by zinc supplementation in children in developing countries: pooled analysis of randomized controlled trials. Zinc Investigators' Collaborative Group. J Pediatr 1999;135(6):689–97.

[41] Integrated Management of Childhood Illness. Available at: http://www.who.int/child_adolescent_health/topics/prevention_care/child/imci/en/index.html (reviewed 11/08).

[42] Convention on the Rights of the Child. Available at: http://www.unhchr.ch/html/menu3/b/k2crc.htm (reviewed 11/08).

[43] World Declaration on the Survival. Protection and development of children and plans of action. Available at: http://www.unicef.org/wsc/declare.htm (reviewed 11/08).

[44] Millennium Development Goals. Available at: http://un.org/millenniumgoals/bkgd.shtml (reviewed 9/08).

[45] Chan M. Margaret Chan puts primary health care centre stage at WHO [editorial]. Lancet 2008;371:1811.

[46] Chan M. Keynote address at the International Seminar on Primary Health Care in Rural China. Beijing, China: International Seminar on Primary Health Care in Rural China; 2007.

[47] Chan M. Return to Alma-Ata. Lancet 2008;372(9642):865–6.

[48] The World Health Report. Primary health care now more than ever. Geneva 27, Switzerland: World Health Organization; 2008.

[49] Murray CJL, Laakso T, Shi buya K, et al. Can we achieve Millennium Development Goal 4 (reduce under-five mortality by two-thirds)? New analysis of country trends and forecasts of under-5 mortality to 2015. Lancet 2007;370:1040–54.

[50] Countdown Coverage Writing Group. Countdown to 2015 for maternal, newborn, and child survival: the 2008 report on tracking coverage of interventions. Lancet 2008;371:1247–58.

[51] Toward Universal Access: Scaling up priority HIV/AIDS interventions in the health sector – progress report 2008. WHO, UNAIDS, UNICEF.

[52] Violari A, Cotton MF, Gibb DM, et al. CHER Study Team. Early antiretroviral therapy and mortality among HIV-infected infants. N Engl J Med 2008;359(21):2233–44.

[53] Gray RH, Kigazi G, Serwadda D, et al. Male circumcision for HIV prevention in men in Rakai, Uganda: a randomized trial. Lancet 2007;369:657–66.

[54] Read JS, Committee on Pediatrics AIDS. Human milk, breastfeeding, and transmission of human immunodeficiency virus type 1 in the United States. Pediatrics 2003;112(5):1196–205.

[55] Gray GE, Saloojee H. Breast-feeding, antiretroviral prophylaxis, and HIV [Editorial]. N Engl J Med 2008;359(2):189–91.

[56] Kumwenda NI, Hoover DR, Mofenson LM, et al. Extended antiretroviral prophylaxis to reduce breast-milk HIV-1 transmission. N Engl J Med 2008;359:119–29.

[57] The state of the world's children 2008. Oxford, New York: Oxford University Press; 2008.

[58] The WHO consensus statement on HIV and infant feeding (new findings). Available at: http://www.infactcanada.ca/Newsletters/2007-Winter/who_statement.htm (reviewed 11/08).

[59] Coutsoudis A, Coovadia HM, Wilfert CM. HIV, infant feeding and more perils for poor people: new WHO guidelines encourage review of formula milk policies. Bull World Health Organ 2008;86(3):210–4.

[60] WHO Multicentre Growth Reference Study Group. WHO child growth standards based on length/height, weight, and age. Acta Paediatr Suppl 2006;450:76–85.

[61] de Onis M, Garza C, Onyango AW, et al. Comparison of the WHO child growth standards and the CDC 2000 growth charts. J Nutr 2007;137:144–8.

[62] Kuczmarski RJ, Ogden CL, Grummer-Strawn LM, et al. CDC growth charts: United States. Advance data from vital and health statistics no. 314. Hyattsville (MD): National Center for Health Statistics; 2000.

[63] Kuczmarski RJ, Ogden CL, Guo SS, et al. 2000 CDC growth charts for the United States: methods and development. Vital Health Stat 20 2002;11(246):1–190.

[64] Poverty. Available at: http://www.globalissues.org/article/26/poverty-facts-and-stats (reviewed 11/08).

[65] Larson K, Russ SA, Crall JJ, et al. Influence of multiple social risks on children's health. Pediatrics 2008;121(2):337–44.

[66] Bhutta ZA, Ahmed T, Black RE, et al. Maternal and Child Undernutrition Study Group. What works? Interventions for maternal and child under nutrition and survival. Lancet 2008;371:417–40.

[67] Fernald LCH, Gertler PJ, Neufeld LM. Role of cash in conditional cash transfer programs for child health, growth, and development: an analysis of Mexico's Oportunidades. Lancet 2008;371:828–37.

[68] Lagarde M, Haines A, Palmer N. Conditional cash transfers for improving uptake of health interventions in low- and middle-income countries: a systematic review. JAMA 2007;298:1900–10.

[69] Yunus M. Banker to the poor: micro-lending and the battle against world poverty. New York: Public Affairs a member of Perseus Books Group; 1999.

[70] Yunus M. Creating a world without poverty: social business and the future of capitalism. New York: Public Affairs a member of Perseus Books Group; 2008.

[71] The Data Report 2007. Keep the G8 promise to Africa. Available at: http://www.thedatareport.org/pdf/DATAREPORT2007.pdf (reviewed 12/08).

[72] Houweling TAJ, Ronsmans C, Campbell OMR, et al. Huge poor-rich inequalities in maternity care: an international comparative study of maternity and child care in developing countries. Bull World Health Organ 2007;85:745–54.

[73] Freedman LP, Graham WJ, Brazier E, et al. Practical lessons from global safe motherhood initiatives: time for a new focus on implementation. Lancet 2007;370:1383–91.

[74] Chowdhury ME, Botlero R, Koblinsky M, et al. Determinants of reduction in maternal mortality in Matlab, Bangladesh: a 30-year cohort study. Lancet 2007;370:1320–8.

[75] Zwane AP, Kremer M. What works in fighting diarrheal disease in developing countries? A critical review. World Bank Res Obs 2007;22(1):1–24.

[76] Ejemot RI, Ehiri JE, Meremikwu MM, et al. Hand washing for preventing diarrhoea. Cochrane Database Syst Rev 2008;23(1):CD00426.

[77] Barreto M, Genser B, Strina A, et al. Effect of city-wide sanitation programme on reduction in rate of childhood diarrhoea in northeast Brazil: assessment of two cohort studies. Lancet 2007;370:1622–8.

[78] Gakidou G, Oza S, Fuertes CV, et al. Improving child survival through environmental and nutritional interventions: the importance of targeting interventions toward the poor. JAMA 2007;298:1876–87.

[79] Pruss-Ostun A, Bos R, Gore F, et al. Safe water, better health. Costs, benefits, and sustainability of interventions to protect and promote health. Geneva: World Health Organization; 2008.

[80] Kimani-Murage EW, Ngindu AM. Quality of water the slum dwellers use: the case of a Kenyan slum. J Urban Health 2007;84(6):829–38.

[81] Davis M. Planet of slums. New York: Verso; 2006.

[82] Global climate change and children's health. AAP policy statement from the Committee on Environmental Heath. Pediatrics 2007;120(5):1149–52.

[83] Climate change and children UNICEF AM Veneman Executive Director Dec.2007.

[84] Torjesen K, Mandalakas A, Kahn RS, et al. Survey of pediatric residency programs offering international child health electives. Arch Pediatr Adolesc Med 1999;153:1297–302.

[85] Nelson BD, Lee ACC, Newby PK, et al. Global health training in pediatric residency program. Pediatrics 2008;122:28–33.

Printed and bound by CPI Group (UK) Ltd, Croydon, CR0 4YY

03/10/2024

01040362-0005